Peak Performance for Soccer

In this book, over 40 of the world's leading practitioners working in elite soccer—over 6 continents—share advanced knowledge of the environment as well as a scientific understanding of the game and players. This book explores those traits at an intricate level through shared experiences of some of the best performance coaches working in elite soccer. The content in this book is derived from practical and evidence-based concepts that have been applied at the elite level.

Uncovering the coaching strategies as well as contemporary issues in elite soccer, this comprehensive textbook illustrates what it takes to thrive as a performance coach at the top level. Collaborating with the industry leaders in soccer, the chapters address a myriad of topics such as:

- the multiple roles and responsibilities;
- youth development;
- strength and conditioning application;
- nutrition and recovery strategies;
- tracking and monitoring fitness and fatigue;
- powerful communication methods and staff cohesion; and
- return to play and injury prevention strategies

Peak Performance for Soccer is essential reading for all coaches and practitioners, at any level, who work in soccer.

Alex Calder is the head of sports science with Houston Dynamo, competing in the Major League Soccer (MLS). He is an accredited level 3 elite coach with the Australian Strength and Conditioning Association (ASCA), as well as holding accreditations through the National Strength and Conditioning Association (NSCA) and Collegiate Strength and Conditioning Coaches Association (CSCCa). Having worked in a variety of sports, he has coached at different levels of competition worldwide for the past decade. He has published several articles in relation to physical preparation and analysis.

Adam Centofanti is currently the head of fitness for the Seattle Sounders FC, having previously served as the head of academy strength & conditioning for Houston Dynamo FC. Formally with Melbourne City FC, Adam held various roles with the club including conditioning coach/sports scientist in the academy sector as well as overseeing the women's performance program, achieving multiple championships. He currently holds a master's in sports science (Football Performance) and an undergraduate degree in sports science. Adam is accredited as a level 2 coach by the Australian Strength and Conditioning Association (ASCA). Additionally, Adam holds a B-License for coaching with the Football Federation Australia (FFA).

Peak Performance for Soccer
The Elite Coaching and Training Manual

**Edited by Alex Calder
and Adam Centofanti**

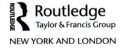

NEW YORK AND LONDON

Cover image: Houston Dynamo FC
Logo design: odd creative

First published 2023
by Routledge
605 Third Avenue, New York, NY 10158

and by Routledge
4 Park Square, Milton Park, Abingdon, Oxon, OX14 4RN

Routledge is an imprint of the Taylor & Francis Group, an informa business

© 2023 selection and editorial matter, Alex Calder and Adam Centofanti; individual chapters, the contributors

The right of Alex Calder and Adam Centofanti to be identified as the authors of the editorial material, and of the authors for their individual chapters, has been asserted in accordance with sections 77 and 78 of the Copyright, Designs and Patents Act 1988.

All rights reserved. No part of this book may be reprinted or reproduced or utilised in any form or by any electronic, mechanical, or other means, now known or hereafter invented, including photocopying and recording, or in any information storage or retrieval system, without permission in writing from the publishers.

Trademark notice: Product or corporate names may be trademarks or registered trademarks, and are used only for identification and explanation without intent to infringe.

ISBN: 978-1-032-06036-1 (hbk)
ISBN: 978-1-032-06031-6 (pbk)
ISBN: 978-1-003-20042-0 (ebk)

DOI: 10.4324/9781003200420

Typeset in Gill Sans
by codeMantra

Contents

List of figures vii
List of tables xii
List of contributors xiv

1 **Role of the practitioner** 1
   GARY WALKER, OLIVER MORGAN, ANTON MATINLAURI,
   ANTHONY NARCISI, ALEX CALDER AND CLAIRE DAVIDSON

2 **From academy to professional** 21
   ALEX BERGER, JACK CHRISTOPHER, NATHAN PLASKETT,
   THOMAS CARPELS AND ADAM CENTOFANTI

3 **Needs analysis and testing** 57
   JARRED MARSH, ALEX CALDER, JORDAN STEWART-MACKIE
   AND MARTIN BUCHHEIT

4 **Strength, power and injury prevention** 83
   MIKE BEERE, CHRISTIAN CLARUP, CODY WILLIAMSON
   AND ADAM CENTOFANTI

5 **Conditioning** 108
   GARY WALKER, MARK READ, DARREN BURGESS, ED LENG
   AND ADAM CENTOFANTI

6 **Player monitoring and practical application** 139
   ANDREA RIBOLI, LEWIS MACMILLAN, ALEX CALDER
   AND LORCAN MASON

7 **Wearable technology** 165
   JOSHUA RICE, DAMIAN KOVACEVIC, ALEX CALDER
   AND JOEL CARTER

8 Recovery and nutrition — 189
FRANCISCO TAVARES, ANTÓNIO PEDRO MENDES,
FRANCISCO PEREIRA, BRETT SINGER, MICHAEL WATTS
AND HANNAH SHERIDAN

9 Return to play — 223
RYAN TIMMINS, JOHN HARTLEY, RISTO-MATTI TOIVONEN,
ALEXANDER MOUHCINE AND ALEX CALDER

10 Periodisation — 259
MARK READ, RICK RIETVELD, DANNY DEIGAN, MATT BIRNIE,
LORCAN MASON AND ADAM CENTOFANTI

11 Coach and staff integration — 289
JARRED MARSH, DAVID COSGRAVE, SCOTT GUYETT, PAUL CAFFREY
AND PHILIPPA MCGREGOR

Index — 323

Figures

1.1	Professional soccer hierarchy	1
1.2	Horizontal hierarchy of sports staff in a professional soccer setting	2
1.3a	A continued professional educational pathway for practitioners in elite soccer (Modified from Springham et al. [1])	3
1.3b	A hypothetical pathway of further study and specialisation options for interested practitioners in elite soccer (Modified from Springham [1])	4
1.3c	A hypothetical continued professional development pathway for practitioners in elite soccer (Modified from Springham [1])	4
1.4	Roles within the industry	13
1.5	Demands of working in elite soccer than potentially cause stress for a practitioner	18
1.6	Potential long-term negative effects associated with constant stress exposure in the workplace	18
2.1	Stages of peak height velocity (PHV) and the physical development windows of opportunity	24
2.2	Weekly activation layout example	29
2.3	Long-term athletic development pyramid	30
2.4	Mobility vs stability of joints in the human body	32
2.5	Movement skill breakdown	33
2.6	An example of progression system for key movements	35
2.7	Plyometric progression system	38
2.8	An example of exercise selection and how it relates to progression system	41
2.9	Y-drill progressions	41
2.10	Energy system development guide	42
2.11	Chronological (o), biological (●), and training age (□) of hypothetical U14s players A, B, and C	47
2.12	Anthropometric measurement and calculation to determine predicted maturity offset and age at peak-height velocity (PHV). S = stature, SH = seated height, LL = leg length (= S-SH), CA = chronological age, BM = body mass (Adjusted equations for predicted maturity offset by Kozieł, S.M. and R.M. Malina [64]	48

viii Figures

3.1	A systematic approach to solving problems and questions within a performance department of an elite soccer organisation	61
3.2	The sensitivity-specificity quadrant	62
3.3	Testing categories with associated influential attributes	66
3.4	Needs analysis based on the groups: cohort, positional, and individual	68
3.5	Types of tests based on the objective. Injury risk tests assess the likelihood of injury risk within a player. Performance-based tests assess output-related qualities of a player	69
3.6	Cohort considerations when selecting tests from the outlined objectives: injury risk and performance-based tests	70
3.7	Examples of tests with cohort-related benchmarks	70
3.8	Positional considerations when selecting tests from the outlined objectives: injury risk and performance-based tests	71
3.9	Examples of tests with positional-related benchmarks	72
3.10	Individual considerations when analysing test results from the outlined objectives: injury risk and performance-based tests	73
4.1	Example of common strength and power tests performed in professional soccer	88
4.2	Force–velocity relationship applied to training methodologies	90
4.3	Common complaints from players, due to misconceptions of strength training in elite soccer	100
4.4	Strategies to increase compliance to strength training prescription	100
5.1	Venn diagram depicting a generalised integrated approach to quantifying and interpreting the physical match performance of soccer players (Adapted from Bradley and Ade [10])	110
5.2	Overview of the relationship between different physiological systems and the development of different fitness components. (Adapted from Morgans et al. [38])	111
5.3	Training approach to conditioning	115
5.4	Extracted GPS data from a 1st half (45-minute period). A 5-minute rolling average applied to speed ($m \cdot min^{-1}$) and acceleration ($m \cdot s^{-2}$). The red dot indicates the peak intensity for a 5-minute period during match-play for the associated variables	117
5.5	Extensive top-up conditioning: fullback position specific	119
5.6	Examples of constraints within technical drills	120
5.7	A 5v5 small-sided game example	121
5.8	Common errors with the drill design process	123
5.9	Identifying the constraints and barriers to performance within a professional soccer environment	124
5.10	Position-specific high-speed-running protocol	131
6.1	A systematic approach to solving problems and questions within a performance department of an elite soccer organization	140

6.2	An investigation of the athlete workload injury cycle, its effects, and modification of risk factors (Adapted from Windt and Gabbett [145])	152
6.3	Injury delay period. Showing weekly loads and the occurrence of a 'spike' (Week 5) causing a 'delayed injury' (Week 9) and return to training protocol (Adapted from Charlton and Drew [169])	154
6.4	The sweet spot. Shows reduction in injury risk when the A:C workload ratio is between 0.8 and 1.3 (Adapted from Blanch and Gabbett [147])	155
7.1	The training outcome is the consequence of the internal training load determined by (1) individual characteristics, such as genetic factors and previous training experience, and (2) the quality, quantity and organisation of the external training load (Extracted from Impellizzeri et al. [3])	166
7.2	Factors that can be quantified by wearable technology in elite soccer	167
7.3	The process for practitioners in elite soccer examining physiology related data	175
7.4	An example of a daily GPS report for a MD-2. HSR = Total distance accumulated above 5.5 $m \cdot s^{-1}$. ACC/DEC = Total exposures above or below 3.0 $m \cdot s^{-2}$. Sprint = Total distance accumulated above 7.0 $m \cdot s^{-1}$	177
7.5	An example of a weekly report. HSR = Total distance accumulated above 5.5 $m \cdot s^{-1}$. ACC/DEC = Total exposures above or below 3.0 $m \cdot s^{-2}$. Sprint = Total distance accumulated above 7.0 $m \cdot s^{-1}$	178
8.1	Schematic representation of hypothetical training capacity/preparedness to train (vertical axis), according to the three different intervals between training stimulus (blue arrow). (a) The interval is too long and no adaptation occurs (undertraining); (b) the interval is appropriate and desired adaptations will occur; and (c) the interval is too short and the training capacity decreases as the accumulated fatigue increases (overreaching) (Adapted from Bishop et al. [6])	192
8.2	Representation of a possible protein distribution throughout the day for a 75 kg player	195
8.3	Example of a carbohydrate loading day for a 75 kg player	196
8.4	Two examples of meeting MD nutrition requirements (three hours before kick-off) for a 75 kg player	198
9.1	Matrix indicating the relationship between incidence and severity when determining injury burden (Extracted from Bahr [5])	224
9.2	Match injuries. Development of injury incidence, injury severity, injury burden and re-injury rate for all injuries, muscle injuries and ligament injuries in matches over the	

x Figures

      study period. Injury incidence is defined as the number of injuries per 1,000 hours of match exposure with 95% CI. Injury severity is defined as the average number of absence days following match injuries with 95% CI. Injury burden is defined as the number of absence days caused per 1,000 hours of match exposure with 95% CI. Re-injury rate is defined as the number of re-injuries per 1,000 hours of training exposure with 95% CI (Extracted from Ekstrand et al. [4])   225

9.3 Training injuries. Time course of injury incidence, injury severity, injury burden and re-injury rate for all injuries, muscle injuries and ligament injuries over the study period. Injury incidence is defined as the number of injuries per 1,000 hours of training exposure with 95% CI. Injury severity is defined as the average number of absence days following training injuries with 95% CI. Injury burden is defined as the number of absence days caused per 1,000 hours of training exposure with 95% CI. Re-injury rate is defined as the number of re-injuries per 1,000 hours of training exposure with 95% CI (Extracted from Ekstrand et al. [4])   226

9.4 Time to return to play and rate of re-injury for injuries without intramuscular tendon involvement and injuries with varying degrees of intramuscular tendon involvement (Adapted from Van der Made et al. [13, 14])   228

9.5 An illustration of the relationship between muscle strain and eccentric force in HSI occurrences. The red line represents the theoretical maximum capacity of the muscle. If we have an eccentric force that exceeds this (e.g. sprinting) then we have injury. If we have strain that exceeds this (e.g. kicking, stretching), an injury often occurs   233

9.6 An example of manipulative variables of rehabilitation   238

9.7 An example of a hamstring RTP exercise progression. Exit-criteria for each stage is listed below the exercise menu   239

9.8 A decision-based RTP model (Extracted from Creighton et al. [74])   241

9.9 Commonly used performance tests throughout RTP procedures. CMJ = Countermovement jumps, MDPP = Most demanding passages of play   242

9.10 A decision-making tree examining progressions based on hamstring strength testing (Extracted from Wollin et al. [75])   243

9.11 An example of field-based progressions using GPS-related metrics from match-play. GL = Game Load, MDPP = Most demanding passage of play, extracted from match-play   245

9.12 Example of weekly increments of volume and intensity markers in an RTP setting (Extracted from Taberner, Allen, and Cohen [84])   247

9.13	The various disciplines involved in an athlete-centred approach in elite soccer	248
9.14	Return-to-play continuum outlining the overlap of involvement of practitioners throughout the process	249
9.15	Elements of RTP process during the acute phase	249
9.16	Elements of RTP process during the subacute phase	250
9.17	Elements of end-stage RTP process during the return-to-play phase	250
10.1	Visual representation of the structure of periodisation (Derived from Matveyev and Zdornyj [7])	259
10.2	Utilizing the warm-up – the 4- and 5-day lead-in	271
11.1	GRPI model (Adapted from Beckhard [1])	289
11.2	Essentialism: The disciplined pursuit of less (Adapted from Greg McKeown [2])	291
11.3	Team of teams: New rules of engagement in a complex world (Adapted from McChrystal [3])	292
11.4	Key points to consider when engaging with conflict	296
11.5	Steps for managing conflict	297
11.6	Skill set of transformational leaders (Adapted from Bass [24])	298
11.7	Mapping the stakeholders within an elite soccer environment	307
11.8	Categorising the power/interest relationships with players in elite soccer	308
11.9	Actions to be taken as a practitioner/leader in relation to the power/interest relationship	308
11.10	Identifying the varieties of hard tactics and soft tactics	309

Tables

2.1	Early specialisation model vs late specialisation models of development	23
2.2	Example of a ten-week training cycle to develop change of direction (COD) qualities in the foundation phase	26
2.3	Implicit vs explicit learning descriptions and example	27
2.4	Movement patterns and examples	36
3.1	Example of testing battery in elite soccer	74
4.1	Example of an on field plyometric prescription	92
4.2	Key exercises frequently utilised in professional soccer	93
4.3	Gym session scheduling example for a seven-day microcycle	95
4.4	Example of a strength-training prescription during fixture congestion	97
5.1	Example of constraints within a 5v5+Goalkeepers drill	122
5.2	A sample template of constraints for a pre-season 'games-based' conditioning programme	129
5.3	Post-match top up – position-specific tempo-run prescription example	132
5.4	A proposed schedule for conditioning and athletic development stimuli during a two-game week separated by four days*	134
6.1	Examples of external and internal measures, separated by subjective and objective categories	142
6.2	Example of a wellness questionnaire (ASRM*)	149
7.1	Examples of absolute and relative speed and acceleration-based thresholds	172
7.2	Heart rate zones, corresponding weight factors and training descriptors	175
8.1	Protocol characteristics and individual and external factors to be considered when designing a water immersion recovery protocol	208
8.2	Example of a cold recovery scheme for elite and amateur team-sport athletes during an in-season week	210
9.1	Stages of a head injury in elite soccer	232
9.2	Mechanisms of hamstring injury strains in elite soccer	233

9.3	Optimal loading approach following a soft tissue injury	236
9.4	Progressions of integrating a player into team training during the return to play phase	240
10.1	Planning considerations for developing a training structure	263
10.2	Four separate microcycles to approach a match day	266
10.3	Advantages and disadvantages to each match 'lead-in' approach	273
10.4	An example of a two games per week microcycle	275
10.5	General speed endurance guidelines	281
10.6	Two microcycles for starters and non-starters (one and two matches per week)	283
11.1	Grouping of soccer players, categorised by their current satisfaction with environment	306

Contributors

Mike Beere has almost a decade of service for Cardiff City FC in the English Football League Championship (EFL), and is one of the most respected practitioners in the game. Mike is currently the senior strength and conditioning coach for the EFL side and is obtaining his PhD from the University of South Wales. Mike has also served the academy, with Cardiff City FC, and previously with Swansea City FC. He is also a registered practitioner with the UK Strength and Conditioning Association (UKSCA).

Alex Berger has extensive coaching experience in the English Football tiers, specifically with Charlton Athletic FC, West Bromwich Albion FC, and Leicester City FC. Alex offers a wealth of knowledge in terms of physical preparation for soccer. Alex holds multiple certifications with The Football Association and the Australian Weightlifting Federation.

Matt Birnie has over 15 years of experience in the field of elite professional football, working across a multitude of age groups. He currently holds the position of first team fitness coach at Chelsea FC, where his priority is the design of daily and weekly training structure. Matt understands the 'pressure cooker' environment to perform at the optimum level and compete in multiple competitions throughout the season. He holds a UEFA B Licence and an MSc in strength and conditioning, and is BASES accredited.

Martin Buchheit is a sport scientist, a strength and conditioning coach, and current head of performance for LOSC Lille in the French top flight, Ligue 1. Buchheit previously served as the head of performance for Paris Saint Germain Football Club (PSG). Additionally, Buchheit worked as an exercise physiologist for ASPIRE Academy in Qatar, and he has served as a lecturer, consultant, and strength and conditioning coach for various organizations. Buchheit received his doctorate in physiology (PhD) from the University of Strasbourg in France. His main research focuses on assessing, improving, and monitoring the physiological determinants of team sport performance, with a greater emphasis on soccer. Based on his field and research experiences, Buchheit developed the 30-15 Intermittent Fitness tests (used to programme high-intensity training) to improve high-intensity training prescription, and the 4'+3' running test to track changes in training status using heart rate (variability) and GPS/accelerometer data. He has also performed some research on the acute and chronic responses to hypoxic and/or heat exposure, and their possible ergogenic effects on team sports physical performance. Buchheit has published more than 160 papers in peer-reviewed journals, with more than 100 as a first author.

Darren Burgess is one of the industry's highest-regarded practitioners and is currently Melbourne Football Club's high performance manager. Burgess has previously had spells with Liverpool FC, Arsenal FC, Parramatta Power, and the Socceroos (Australian National Team). With decades of experience at the elite level, Burgess has worked with some of the best footballers to play the game. Having served multiple prestigious coaches in several countries and competitions, Burgess's wealth of knowledge encompasses all aspects of physical preparation. Burgess obtained a PhD in sports science from the Australian Catholic University in 2011, and continues to publish articles in various international journals.

Paul Caffrey holds experience in Major League Soccer (MLS) and with the United States national team programme. Caffrey has served as Houston Dynamo FC's head of performance since 2015. He spent 2014 at Chivas USA as the first assistant coach under Wilmer Cabrera. He served as an assistant coach and fitness coach with the Colorado Rapids on Oscar Pareja's staff from 2012 to 2013. Caffrey also was the first assistant coach under Cabrera with the United States under-17 national team from 2007 to 2011 and oversaw the physical preparation and fitness training of the team. Caffrey has an extensive playing career, including professional stints with Bohemian FC and University College Dublin AFC (UCD). Caffrey holds a United States Soccer Federation 'A' License as well as certifications as a certified strength and conditioning specialist (National Strength and Conditioning Association) and functional movement specialist (Functional Movement Systems). He also carries master's degrees in business administration, physical education, and football strength and conditioning.

Thomas Carpels has two master's degrees (MSc in training and coaching football and MSc in sport and exercise science and medicine), and is currently working towards his PhD through the University of Glasgow. After working for four seasons as a sports scientist at Rangers Football Club and as head of performance at Orange County SC during the 2021 USL Championship season, Thomas has recently taken up the role of first team physical coach at Royal Antwerp Football Club in the Belgian top division. The Belgian-native also holds the UEFA-A coaching license and is an accredited anthropometrist through the International Society for the Advancement of Kinanthropometry (ISAK).

Joel Carter is serving English Premier League club, Crystal Palace FC, as the academy senior performance coach; his role is to provide sound high-performance knowledge and comprehensive evidence-based performance coaching to service the current and next generation of athletes. The Australian-native has spent the past few years overseas in India and England working with elite players at the top level. Joel holds licences through the Australian Strength and Conditioning Association (ASCA) and Football Federation Australia (FFA).

Jack Christopher has spent the past decade with Chelsea FC in the English Premier League, serving a variety of positions throughout his tenure. Currently serving as the head of academy sport science and physical fitness, Jack has a wealth of knowledge regarding physical development for youth soccer players. Jack completed an MSc in high performance sport and is an accredited sport scientist (BASES) and nutritionist (CISSN), whilst holding credentials with the UK Strength and Conditioning Association. He is also a co-founder and performance coach at MyPerform, helping athletes around the world unleash their true potential.

Christian Clarup is currently serving the Scandinavian giants FC Midtjylland as the head of the sports science and strength and conditioning departments. He is an expert within the field of training elite football players on and off the pitch and gained his expertise from working in elite environments for the past 15 years. His work has contributed to securing international football on a regular basis (UEFA Champions League, UEFA Euro League, and UEFA Conference League) plus several national titles for his current club. He has gained major experience working within a high-performance environment under constant pressure due to vast competitive success.

David Cosgrave is the senior director of Sports Medicine and High Performance at Orlando City Soccer Club in the Major League Soccer (MLS). A graduate of the master of sports directorship in Manchester Metropolitan University, he oversees the programmes that create elite levels of physical capability, low levels of injury, high levels of mental resilience, and development of organizational culture. Cosgrave's experience in the strategic and operational leadership of medical, physical performance, nutrition, and sports science is a result of his experience in top European clubs, including England's Tottenham Hotspur FC, Liverpool FC, Bolton Wanderers FC, Stoke City FC and Fulham FC, and FC Copenhagen of the Danish Superliga.

Claire Davidson is an HCPC registered sport and exercise psychologist who has worked within both senior first team and international football for the past ten years. During this time, she has also supported a number of Olympic athletes. Currently she works as the lead performance psychologist at the English Football Association for the men's pathway teams supporting the coaches, support staff, and athletes involved in the U15-U21 age groups.

Danny Deigan is the current strength and conditioning coach for Mumbai City FC, and has a substantial amount of experience as a strength and conditioning coach in multiple international and club football environments. Danny

Contributors xvii

has previously worked on the international stage with respective roles with New Zealand Football and the Indian National Football teams. Danny holds multiple certifications through the Asian Football Confederation, Australian Strength and Conditioning Association, and Altis.

Scott Guyett is the current assistant coach for the Australian A-League team Brisbane Roar. Prior to this, he spent over a decade with the English Premier League team, Crystal Palace FC, as head of sport science and strength and conditioning and was responsible for overseeing the football performance elements of the first team. Prior to his time at Crystal Palace FC, Scott was a professional soccer player with multiple clubs across England. Scott is currently a UEFA Pro License participant, whilst holding credentials with the National Strength and Conditioning Association (NSCA), and UK Strength and Conditioning Association (UKSCA).

John Hartley has over 20 years of experience as a physiotherapist in professional sport. John is at present the head physiotherapist at Derby County FC. He has previously worked for Aston Villa FC, Blackburn Rovers FC, Warrington Wolves RLFC, and England RLFC. He is registered as a practitioner through the International Federation of Sports Physical Therapists (IFSPT) and the National Strength and Conditioning Association (NSCA). John is currently pursuing a professional doctorate at the University of Birmingham.

Damian Kovacevic is a full-time researcher within the College of Sport and Exercise Science at Victoria University. Prior to working at Victoria University, he was head of sport science and strength and conditioning for 2019 J League champions, Yokohama F. Marinos. Between 2017 and 2019, Damian held key roles within the academy of Melbourne Victory FC, including lead sport scientist and strength and conditioning coordinator. Damian obtained a master's in sport science (majoring in football performance) and a bachelor's in sport development whilst holding accreditation with the Australian Strength and Conditioning Association, and a football conditioning licence with Football Federation Australia.

Ed Leng is currently lead sport scientist for Manchester United's First Team. Ed has spent the past decade working with some of the most prestigious coaches and players in the game. With over six years at Tottenham Hotspur and global experience as head of sports science with Melbourne City FC as part of the City Football Group, Ed has developed knowledge and understanding across many facets of physical performance. He has a particular expertise and passion for data-led strategies to influence injury risk and drive physical performance, demonstrated in his PhD from the University of Bath and his recent international publications.

Lewis MacMillan has spent five years with Fulham FC, and currently serves as the club's first team sport scientist. Lewis is also currently pursuing his PhD in exercise physiology with the University of Glasgow, whilst holding a position as a guest lecturer. Lewis' role with the English Premier League club, Fulham FC, is implementing impactful and meaningful analysis of sporting performance to optimize athletic development.

Jarred Marsh has been involved in professional football for over six years with experience at both club and international level. As head of sport science for one of Africa's largest football clubs, Jarred has been able to create a robust high performance structure and culture that, above all else, remains player-centred. Having completed his master's in exercise science, as well as being a certified strength and conditioning specialist (NSCA), Jarred has merged the use of evidence-based principles and football systems to drive his teams to peak competition level.

Lorcan Mason is a sports scientist and strength and conditioning coach based in Ireland. He is currently working with youth and senior athletes in soccer and Gaelic Games having had previous experience working in professional football. He is a recent graduate from Athlone Institute of Technology with a first class honours BSc in sports science with exercise physiology and has a keen interest in furthering his academic career. Lorcán also has an educational service 'Mind Map Coaching' where he provides research summaries through the creation of mind maps on a variety of sports science topics.

Anton Matinlauri is a first team fitness coach and head of performance at Fortaleza FC/CEIF in Colombia. He was previously in similar role at HJK Helsinki and also possesses first team experience from Sevilla C.F. in Spain and San Jose Earthquakes in the United States along with being part of developing the coaching education for Finnish FA. Anton holds UEFA A licensure from Finnish FA and possesses experience and degrees in both athletic training (BSC from the United States and ATC licensure) and strength and conditioning (MSC from Spain and CSCS licensure).

Philippa McGregor is a performance psychologist working across sport, education, and business sectors. Spending the past ten years working predominately in professional football, Philippa started her career at Fulham Football club 2009–2015. She then moved to Manchester City, where she was head of psychology for the academy until 2017, before moving to work as part of the wider City Football Group, supporting players who were out on loan and City's global network of clubs. In 2019, Philippa set up her own business nThrive2Perform Ltd. and is now working as a self-employed consultant. Her clients have included the English Football Association, Liverpool Women, Aberdeen and West Brom FC, Durham Cricket, and UK Coaching, as well as individual athletes competing in international golf and gymnastics. Alongside her work in sport, Philippa also works across education and business environments applying performance psychology research, theory, and principles to support culture projects, leadership programmes, and mental and wellbeing development. Philippa has a PhD from Loughborough University that looked at talent development environments, emotional regulation, and performance. Philippa also holds her professional accreditation with the British Association of Sport and Exercise Science, and is a chartered scientist and awaiting her HCPC registration.

António Pedro Mendes is the head of Nutrition for Sporting Clube de Portugal, a department that involves four full-time nutritionists. He has previously worked for FC Paços de Ferreira, FC Porto, and Al Nassr FC (Saudi Arabia). He is currently the head of Sports Nutrition at Clínica Espregueira – FIFA Medical Centre of Excellence – and co-Founder of Nutriens Academy, a school focused on teaching nutrition at the highest level. António holds a BSc in nutrition, and he is currently pursuing his PhD.

Oliver Morgan is currently head of performance support at Leicester City FC Academy, having previously worked at Celtic Football Club and Liverpool Football Club, helping to produce professional players to become English and Scottish Premier League champions as well as Champions League winners. With a passion for research, Oliver has completed a master's by Research into talent identification and currently completing a professional doctorate investigating multi-directional movement demands of elite youth soccer players. Oliver's main areas of interest lie within long-term athlete development, maturation, change of direction and agility, return to play strategies, and performance management.

Alexander Mouhcine is a performance and rehabilitation specialist, currently working at Borussia Mönchengladbach in the German Bundesliga. As head of rehabilitation and performance testing, he is responsible for decision making throughout the whole return to play process. While regularly competing internationally (UEFA Champions League/UEFA Europa League), he is well aware of the challenge to work in a high-pressure environment facing time as always being the limiting factor. He contributed to several manuals concerning return to play algorithms, and as a coach, his aim is to translate scientific evidence into practice the best possible way.

Anthony Narcisi is the current strength and conditioning coach with Major League Soccer (MLS) team, Houston Dynamo FC. Previously serving as the head of performance for RGV FC Toros of the USL Championship, he holds a master's in high performance sport and a bachelor of science in kinesiology. Anthony is a certified strength and conditioning specialist through the National Strength and Conditioning Association (NSCA).

Francisco Pereira has been working with professional football teams since 2018, together with his private practice. Currently, he is the head nutritionist of the United Arab Emirates Football Association, where he works with the youth and senior national teams (men and women). In addition, he is a post-graduate student with the Institute of Performance Nutrition (IOPN) and has concluded his diploma in football strength and conditioning with the Football Science Institute.

Nathan Plaskett, an Australian-native, is Derby County FC's current strength, conditioning, and rehab coach. Nathan has international experience working with multiple A-league clubs, Football Federation Australia, and various rugby clubs. With a master's degree in high-performance sport, Nathan also holds accreditations with Exercise and Sports Science Australia (ESSA), the Australian Strength and Conditioning Association (ASCA), and The Football Association (FA).

Mark Read has spent over five years with one of the most successful Swedish teams in soccer, Malmö FF. Currently the club's head of physical performance, Mark has also held roles with their academy. He has previous coaching experience with Swansea City FC and West Bromwich Albion FC. Mark holds a UEFA B Coaching badge, and licences with the National Strength and Conditioning Association (NSCA) and International Society for the Advancement of Kinanthropometry (ISAK).

Andrea Riboli is an accredited physical performance coach, sport scientist, and consultant experienced with both youth and adult elite football players. He holds a PhD in sport sciences and is an adjunct professor in performance analysis at the University of Milan. After experiences as exercise physiologist and performance coach at different levels of competition, he holds the position of head of performance in professional women's basket. He worked as physical performance coach in Como F.C., A.C. Milan, and Atalanta B.C. Academies from 2009 to 2014. In 2014, he moved to Atalanta B.C. first team and led the Sport Science Department of the Club from 2016 to 2020. He published papers in sport-science and medicine peer-reviewed international journals about performance development in elite football players. He is currently leading research projects about training load management and performance development in football.

Joshua Rice is currently a physical development coach at Tottenham Hotspur FC, having previously worked at both Liverpool FC and Everton FC respectively. Josh also completed his PhD last year (2021) at The University of Birmingham with the project entitled 'Examining the importance & effectiveness of physical development strategies in the developing footballer'.

Rick Rietveld is the first team sport scientist at AZ Alkmaar, which is an ambitious club in the top of the Dutch Eredivisie. After his bachelor's and master's in human movement science at VU Amsterdam, Rick started to work at the AZ Alkmaar Academy as an exercise physiologist. During his time with AZ Alkmaar's academy, he was responsible for the periodisation, monitoring, and physical testing of the whole academy. In late 2018, Rick joined the first team of AZ Aklmaar, taking on a similar role. Translating the data and making objective decisions about players and training is one of the key roles of his current position.

Contributors xxi

Hannah Sheridan has worked with a range of elite athletes since 2014. She is currently the lead nutritionist at Tottenham Hotspur Football Club, where she has supported the team throughout the last four seasons, including the Champions League final in 2019. Hannah has developed the Nutrition Department at Spurs, which now involves two full-time nutritionists within the first team and an academy nutritionist. Hannah is also a consultant nutritionist at a private practice and a registered Sport and Exercise Nutritionist (SENr).

Brett Singer is a dietitian with Memorial Hermann IRONMAN Sports Medicine Institute. Brett has had the opportunity to work with individual athletes from elite to junior levels for over ten years. Within his role, Brett serves as the lead dietitian for Houston Dynamo FC, coordinating match day nutrition tactics, supplementation programming, and overall nutrition education for the club. Outside of his role with Memorial Hermann, Brett serves on the Board of Directors for Collegiate Professional Sports Dietitians Association. He has also served as an adjunct professor at the University of Houston for several years.

Jordan Stewart-Mackie is a highly accomplished, ambitious, and current head of sport science with Buriram United FC. Jordan supports and motivates the physical progression of elite professional athletes by delivering tailored training techniques, rehabilitation programmes, and nutritional guidance. Jordan has a strong portfolio of achievements and experience within the sport science and strength and conditioning arena having enjoyed roles with West Bromwich Albion FC, Leicester City FC, and Buriram United FC. Jordan holds a UEFA B licence, and certifications with the National Strength & Conditioning Association (NSCA), the British Association of Sport and Exercise Sciences (BASES), and FIFA.

Francisco Tavares is the performance coordinator for Sporting Clube de Portugal, and has previously worked as a strength and conditioning coach in elite rugby with the Chiefs Super Rugby franchise and the PRO14 team Glasgow Warriors. He holds a PhD in sport sciences from the Waikato University in New Zealand and an MSc also in sport sciences from the University of Lisbon – Faculty of Human Kinetics in Portugal. Francisco is a certified strength and conditioning coach from the National Strength and Conditioning Association (NSCA) and the Australian Strength and Conditioning Association (ASCA-level 2). He is a published author in the areas of neuromuscular responses and adaptations from training, and recovery from training.

Ryan Timmins, PhD, is an ACU researcher in the field of hamstring injury. He completed his PhD in 2015 focusing on hamstring muscle architecture and its role in injury and response to training interventions. He has over 40 publications in the area, as well as being the author of a textbook chapter on hamstring anatomy. Dr Timmins' research focus is on sports injury prevention and rehabilitation practices that are applicable to sporting environments and realistic with their applications. He has been an invited speaker at the ASPETAR Sports Medicine and Orthopaedic Hospital, Oslo Sports Trauma Research Centre, and at the first Copenhagen Hamstring Injury Seminar. For the past decade, Dr Timmins has worked in the A-League, having spent four years at Brisbane Roar and seven years with Melbourne Victory. During this time, his roles have included rehabilitation and injury prevention coordinator, physiotherapist assistant, strength and conditioning coach, and working within the football operations.

Risto-Matti Toivonen is currently serving one of Finland's powerhouse soccer clubs, HIFK Fotboll. Risto-Matti has a considerable amount of European soccer coaching experience. As HIFK Fotboll's sport scientist/strength and conditioning coach/physiotherapist, Risto-Matti has an enormous skillset surrounding the overall football performance for his club. The triple-role practitioner knows how to thrive under adverse conditions, whilst still enhancing overall performance of the team.

Gary Walker is currently the director of sports performance for FC Cincinnati, leading the medical, sports science, strength and conditioning, and nutrition support services to Major League Soccer (MLS) players. Prior to this, he worked for over a decade as the head of strength and conditioning and first team fitness coach at Manchester United FC. Gary holds a PhD from Loughborough University and an MSc in sports directorship from Salford University Business School and is certified with the UK Strength & Conditioning Association (UKSCA), as well as the National Strength and Conditioning Association.

Michael Watts has been researching and applying his knowledge within the health, wellness, longevity, and performance industry for the past 19 years. He spent 12 years working full time in Elite soccer in the English Premier League and at National Team level before a move to the USA to work full time for Under Armour as director of athlete performance. Michael has a very holistic approach to human performance which includes sleep, breathing, recovery, nutrition, and mindset to optimize performance. Holding an MSc in sport science, Michael is currently doing his LMT and a post baccalaureate in sports performance and integrative nutrition at the Maryland University of Integrative Health.

Cody Williamson is the head physiotherapist at Macarthur Football Club in the A-league. Cody completed his physiotherapy studies at La Trobe University and also has a master's degree in strength and conditioning. Cody has previously held roles at Melbourne City Football Club. Specializing in athlete rehabilitation in football, Cody has consulted with clubs across the globe including teams located in the United States, the United Kingdom, and Asia.

1 Role of the practitioner

Gary Walker, Oliver Morgan, Anton Matinlauri, Anthony Narcisi, Alex Calder and Claire Davidson

Overview of the performance coach role in elite soccer

Professional soccer structure

A typical professional sports hierarchy (Figure 1.1) consists of a board of directors and investors at the top, supported by the chief executive officer (CEO), the general manager, and/or technical director overseeing the sports staff and office administrators. Generally, the board of directors' main purpose is to increase success and profit within the club, whilst not having an input on day-to-day operations. The CEO will often be in constant contact with the general manager to ensure the operations are on target with the club's mission. The bottom layer of the structure (general manager/technical director, sport staff, and office/admin) is responsible for day-to-day operations with the players and staff.

Sport staff

Amongst the sports staff, there are typically three departments that report to the head coach on a day-to-day basis: assistant coaches, performance department, and medical department. However, in a modern structure, a performance director often speaks on behalf of performance, nutrition, and medical departments (Figure 1.2). The 'sport science' department has become more common in Australia and the United Kingdom. However, remains somewhat of a novel addition in the other countries. Sport scientists often refer to the individuals who manage big data sets that relate to player's health/fitness status. However, the sport scientist title has been applied to those who offer services in strength and conditioning as well as rehabilitation. Due to the lack of certification standards

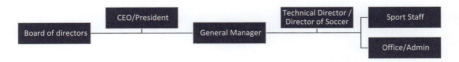

Figure 1.1 Professional soccer hierarchy.

DOI: 10.4324/9781003200420-1

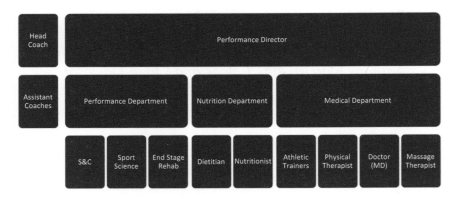

Figure 1.2 Horizontal hierarchy of sports staff in a professional soccer setting.

associated with the sport scientist role (in the United States), the department has become quite broad. For example, the performance director position can be interchangeable with the title 'director of sport science' at some professional organisations, begging the question to what that role oversees. However, in any circumstance, a performance director will filter the necessary information to the coach in order to help drive daily decisions.

Different names/roles/titles

Depending on various aspects within the organisation's structure, the role and title of a practitioner can vary within the working environments. Sometimes the same job description may have different titles, while the same title may also have considerably different job descriptions and requirements. Reasoning for such variability may be due to country, culture, language, club structure, and the number of staff members working at the club. While 'strength and conditioning coach' (S&C coach) may potentially be the most used title in global perspective, other common translations and names used for the positions include fitness coach, performance coach, physical performance coach, physical preparation coach, applied sport scientist, and athletic coach.

In a bigger club, there may be several staff members working in the same department, thus different names may be used for different roles. As mentioned earlier, an example of a club's performance staff structure may consist of the following:

- Performance director:
  - overseeing the departments (performance/medical/nutrition/etc.)
- Fitness coach:
  - Working closely with the coaching staff on the field

- Strength and conditioning coach:
  - Responsible for the work outside of main soccer training on the field, that is, gym-related activities
- Sport scientist:
  - Primarily responsible for the global positioning system (GPS) analysis and data analysis
- End-stage rehab coach:
  - Managing the return to play process after medically cleared for field-related activity

For a performance department to be successful, it is integral that all the above-mentioned performance members are working closely together. In contrast, in a club where such a department may not exist, a practitioner, regardless of working title, may be working with a much wider spectrum of responsibility.

Certifications

With the rapid evolution of sports science in soccer, tertiary courses including undergraduate and post-graduate degrees are developing a direct relationship to performance aspects in soccer (Figure 1.3a). These include degrees being offered both online and in-person setting. Recently in Spain, there has also been growing number of universities offering their own specialised master's-level

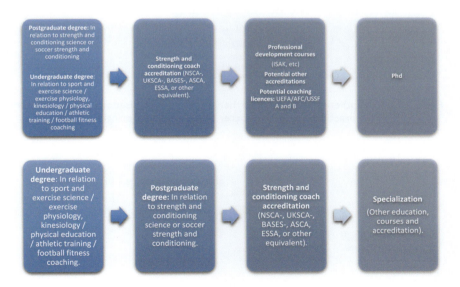

Figure 1.3a A continued professional educational pathway for practitioners in elite soccer (Modified from Springham et al. [1]).

studies with direct relation to soccer performance. However, these studies do not have full official post-graduate accreditation, which is important to note as this is required in the case a practitioner wants to apply for doctorate recognition (PhD) in the future (Figure 1.3b).

In addition to traditional University schooling, many institutions and organisations have begun to offer tertiary education and courses to match the increased interest and demand for sport science in soccer. However, the growing supply of graduates has also highlighted the mismatch between the skill set taught at the university level and the skill set required to work within professional soccer [1]. To close this gap, in several countries, there has been an advance in effort to standardise the requirements in the field with various licences being required or recommended for modern day practitioners to be considered for a job opportunity. Invariably, in most countries, the present-day job descriptions often require the applicant to possess an accreditation from a recognised strength and conditioning/sports science association (UKSCA, NSCA, ASCA, BASES, etc.). However, a lot of variability still exist between countries in the certification process and requirements, as not all nations have an accreditation process for sport science. Additionally, it has become advantageous, for some roles, to obtain a coaching licence (UEFA, AFC, USSF) on top of tertiary education (Figure 1.3b). Practitioners are often required to also possess previous work experience through internships/volunteering, which have become a common prerequisite to obtaining a full-time position in professional soccer (Figure 1.3c).

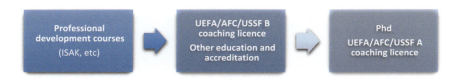

Figure 1.3b A hypothetical pathway of further study and specialisation options for interested practitioners in elite soccer (Modified from Springham [1]).

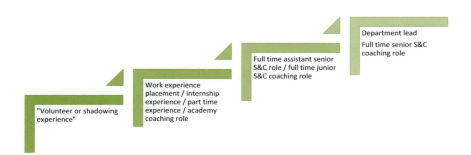

Figure 1.3c A hypothetical continued professional development pathway for practitioners in elite soccer (Modified from Springham [1]).

Value of integration

To integrate effectively within an interdisciplinary team, it is imperative for a modern practitioner to have a basic understanding of operations within a performance team. This means having a crossover of basic knowledge and skill sets in various areas in the field from soccer coaching to weight room, data-analysis, nutrition, and psychology, allowing them to communicate and work effectively as part of the multi-disciplinary team. This is important as maximising the player's and team's performance is a complex and holistic. It could be stated that "S&C coaches in professional football need to be excellent 'generalists,'" referring to this wide spectrum of required knowledge [1]. This does not mean, however, that one should not have one specific area of expertise as this can be very beneficial in certain roles. Such specialisation could potentially be very beneficial when being part of a bigger staff, allowing each member to focus more on certain aspect around player health and performance. Even though required to have wide spectrum of knowledge, a practitioner must also understand their own level of competency and responsibility in different areas and seek support from specialist (nutritionist, psychologist, etc.) when required and advised.

Crossover of competency and knowledge in more than one area related to performance operations has been identified as potentially valuable ability of a practitioner. For example, having knowledge and experience in rehabilitation as well as strength and conditioning can be incredibly advantageous for a performance department and soccer organisation as whole. The value of crossover really becomes evident when there are changes in the personnel, which is extremely common in football, as building trust and understanding among staff members is a pre-requisite for a successful working relationship. At the elite level, time is often very limited, and for this reason, it is common for the head coach to bring their closest staff members to new club (*discussed further in Chapter 11*). However, very rarely full backroom staff are brought in by the head coach, support staff members to quickly adapt to change, in order to enhance cohesion between departments. Having a skill set and knowledge in different areas does not guarantee good communication, but certainly helps in understanding what the coaching staff wants. Furthermore, emotional intelligence in relation to players' health and fitness status is imperative for practitioners to be successful [2, 3].

Contemporary issues

Problems within coaching-orientated staff

From a practitioner's perspective, planning training with the coaching staff can often be a difficult task, depending on the coaching staff. Most head coaches (and assistants) have played the sport, thus having a sense of training was from a player's perspective. This can be advantageous for a practitioner who is trying to provide recommendations on training variables to the coaching staff. On the contrary, these coaches may not be up to date with the evolving aspect of physical preparation. Therefore, if a coach has the mentality of applying what they were exposed to as a player, a practitioner may have issues with training prescriptions. For example, a strength coach may want to prescribe a weight-training session mid-week. However, the coaching staff could refute that weight-training session because they never were exposed to those types of sessions when they played.

Problems within medical/physio staff

It is common for a medical staff and performance staff to clash methods and philosophies. Performance staff, including strength and conditioning coaches, often plan and prescribe training modalities based on a practical approach. However, medical staff members, such as physiotherapists, can potentially have a more conservative, clinical approach. Not one approach is more effective than the other; however, it is imperative that all staff members have the same long-term goal in relation to the player's health status. More specifically, in a return-to-play scenario, it is important that all members of the performance staff are in agreeance of a continuum for personnel involvement. A physiotherapist should be working in conjunction with the strength coach to ensure that appropriate regressions are put in place to create a smooth transition between departments. If this level of communication and collaboration does not occur, the exercise prescriptions may overlap, creating the athlete to be in a non-functional overreaching state.

Limitations with nutritional advice

Without a nutrition department, athletes may be unsure of where to direct nutrition-related questions. Unfortunately, this can be quite a common issue as many performance departments tend to lack full-time nutrition employees. The strength coach often becomes responsible, by default, to answer nutrition-related questions because they are prescribing the recovery strategies to their gym sessions. Strength coaches need to be very cautious in their approach to recommending supplements, as they have limited knowledge in this scope of practice. Specifically, in certain countries, providing detailed nutritional recommendations without appropriate tertiary education and/or certification in the field (dietetic recognition) can have serious repercussions to a practitioner. All strength and conditioning specialists should be certified through the World Anti-Doping Agency (WADA) as well as staying informed as to the banned substance list.

Current issues with professional soccer players

It is common that a team suffers from at least one individual who does not adhere to the requirements of the weight-training programme. It is thought that these players are more common in professional soccer, perhaps stemming from cultural habits. Being that soccer is an aerobically dominated sport, the stereotype regarding physical preparation is running long distances. However, with the evolution of sport-science, it has become clear that soccer has some large strength-power components [4, 5]. Hence, the heavy emphasis on resistance training in the current era [6]. Undesirably, there are some athletes who are still in agreeance with the outdated stereotype. These are the athletes that create unwanted behaviours and attitudes when it comes to the gym sessions. It is certainly challenging, from a practitioner's perspective, to encourage those individuals to adhere to the efforts in the gym to reduce the risk of diminishing the quality of club culture. It is imperative that practitioners display multiple leadership qualities to adhere to the team/club needs and create a winning environment.

Operating as a solo practitioner

While clubs in the highest ranks of soccer have multiple specialists collaborating within a performance department, many clubs below the top-ranks have one practitioner executing all the responsibilities of a performance department.

From designing and implementing training, to monitoring and interpreting training loads, a solo practitioner is responsible for the full spectrum of work within a performance department. Without being afforded the luxury of multiple staff members, operating as a stand-alone department requires a great deal of organisation to get the maximum return from your players. There are multiple factors within one's organisation that will influence what areas to prioritise, but this process is one that must be constantly evaluated and adjusted regularly throughout a season.

Modelling a performance department

Modelling a performance department encompasses a broad spectrum of aspects and should align with the goals set out by the club officials, technical staff, and support staff. When running a performance department individually, a practitioner should strive to build a culture that allows for automation of processes. By automating daily processes, the practitioner can optimise the flow of activity to support organisational goals, create a competitive environment and contribute to building a team culture [7]. To begin this process, a practitioner should analyse the needs of the team from a global perspective when planning. For example, implementing a gym strength-programme focusing on general hamstring injury prevention for the whole team, as opposed to making multiple individual programmes, that share the same goal of building robust hamstrings. Once processes are in place, individualising programmes could be the next logical progression to improving a department, but as a first step, a global programme can address the most important needs for every player. Thus, allowing more time to be spent in other areas that need to be addressed and in essence, permits the practitioner to carefully examine execution of lifting technique.

Once the department model is established, the practitioner must create and promote an environment that allows for the execution and control of processes. This can be achieved by establishing set rules and strict policies to create an environment where athletes hold each other accountable. For example, mandating an athlete to weigh-in prior to training and weigh-out post training. Anyone who fails to do so is disciplined accordingly. Empowering leaders in the locker room to hold this standard can help bridge the gap between staff and players. By giving the players certain responsibilities and autonomy, it can promote a culture of accountability which in turn will help grow the culture of the team [8].

In contrast to structure, other components of the environment could also be less structured in the form of general guidelines or guided practice over time. For example, spending time teaching an athlete proper execution of pre-training movement preparation. Over time the players should understand and be self-sufficient in performing the necessary movements by themselves. As a result, creates accountability while allowing the practitioner to focus on other players or areas. Whether your model encompasses one of these ideas or a combination of both, it is essential that whatever processes are in place allow for consistent execution from the players independent of the practitioner.

Daily obstacles and limitations

Practitioners in a performance department consisting of a well-resourced multi-disciplinary team can specialise in one or two disciplines. The increased manpower allows the focus of each practitioner to play a specific key role that contributes to the whole of the department. Conversely, an obstacle a solo practitioner will encounter is that they will have to simultaneously work across multiple disciplines, limiting the amount of time that can be dedicated to any one aspect of the department. An example of a standard day in-season may be:

- Arrive to work
- Meet with coaches
- Analyse player wellness
- Set up training – field
- Set up training – gym
- Set up monitoring/wearables
- Greet players on arrival
- Have one or two conversations with players/staff pre-training
- Perform movement preparation and on-field warm-up
- Support the field session with technical staff (and rehab session with medical staff)
- Complete necessary on-field conditioning post training
- Collect all RPE's + collect wearables
- Prepare post training nutrition
- Coach gym session(s). Potentially for multiple groups
- Support rehab gym session with medical staff

- Have multiple conversations with players/staff post training
- Analyse and interpret training data
- Deliver filtered training information to all staff
- Meet with coaches/medical staff
- Plan for the following day

It is important to note that this daily outline is not definitive and there will vary depending on factors within the individual's environment.

Along with the multiple considerations, a solo practitioner must have a fundamental understanding of every facet of performance in soccer. To efficiently navigate a day-long workload, the practitioner must be a well-rounded generalist. With limited time and many responsibilities, being a well-rounded generalist will allow practitioners to cover a broad range of needs. It may be difficult to allocate equal time to every area of a performance department so automating as many processes as possible on the front end allows for more interaction with the players. Prioritising needs is not only necessary but also constantly being evaluated and adjusted on a regular basis. If the practitioner can be proficient across all areas of their department, it can give them the greatest return of investment for each component being implemented. If deficient in any area, this will only take away from other areas, thus slowing the daily flow. For example, if the practitioner does not have the GPS report to the coaches in a timely manner, the following day's training plan can be compromised, thus potentially putting the players at risk. Once primary tasks are being consistently implemented, practitioners can identify specific areas that require a higher level of specialisation.

Optimising communication

In a team environment, communication to the players from the performance department and technical and support staff must be clear and concise. A positive aspect to operating as a solo practitioner is every message being sent is filtered by one person. Without multiple lines of communication, messages should be delivered clearly without any miscommunication or misinterpretation from different parties. This is especially important when working in a team with minimal resources. Everyone involved must be aware of the processes across the performance, medical, and technical departments to put the athletes in the best position for success [9]. Proper communication and organisation will allow the team to promote the same messages across the team and in training. Additionally, another positive aspect of operating solo is that there are no competing philosophies or ideas amongst fellow staff members. Without any debate about what should be implemented the practitioner has complete creative control. This control can keep messages consistent which can allow for players to understand and buy-in to the processes across the team. However, the processes put in place by the solo-practitioner won't be challenged by peers, which potentially results in an unfulfilling procedure.

Importance of empowerment

Promoting autonomy amongst the players can be a strategy used to help instil processes that a solo practitioner may not have otherwise have time to dedicate to on a regular basis. It is impossible to do every task operating alone. However, teaching athletes and giving them responsibilities over time can help them to grow as individual problem solvers as well as promote team cohesion that will help drive the culture [8]. It is important to note that not every athlete will have these responsibilities given to them. The responsibilities and level of responsibility will be determined by the practitioner, and dependent on a variety of personality traits of the individuals [10]. Most importantly, practitioner should never leave themselves or an athlete at risk when assigning responsibilities or allocating tasks. Due to high maturity levels, veteran players and team captains are prime candidates who can act as an extension of the department. For example, giving an experienced athlete the permission to cue and correct a younger athlete in the gym can help facilitate the training process. By empowering this experienced player, practitioners will have more freedom to focus attention in other areas that may need focus. When giving responsibility to athletes, it is important that they understand that they are expected to hold themselves and their teammates to a higher standard. Any inconsistencies will create an unclear message and defeat the purpose of entrusting these athletes with a higher responsibility.

Priorities and delegation

Once a needs analysis (see *Chapter 3 for more detail*) is established, a solo-practitioner can decide what testing protocols are most appropriate to implement in their environment. Tests should prioritise the general needs of the sport before looking at specific needs of individuals. With limited time and minimal resources, areas such as player testing must be concise, easy to execute, and provide value while giving actionable information. Once a season has started, finding time to retest every player will be challenging so it is important to emphasise that any tests used hold value and resources required should be minimal, allowing for a valid retest.

Utilising wearable tracking, such as global positioning system (GPS), in training is an example of how a practitioner can perform valid, reliable, and repeatable tests without any extra set up. Tests such as maximum velocity and maximum aerobic speed (MAS) are examples of tests that can be captured within the confines of a training session. Furthermore, physical tests such as a broad jump or vertical jump can be performed quickly as a part of a gym session. The above-mentioned tests are examples of what can be implemented periodically to assess progress for the whole team. Once global needs of the team have been addressed, the practitioner can then focus on additional tests for specific high priority athletes. This could include addressing players seen as a high priority by the club, veteran players who merit special attention, or athletes who are at a greater risk of injury.

Relationships; balance of friendliness and respect

The more face time with your players, the more opportunity there is to build relationships. With limited time each day, it is imperative to capitalise on time available to build trust with the players. These relationships are important ones that help to create and increase buy-in whilst emphasising messages, but this communication goes beyond the sport. Some days you may need to be a coach, other days you may need to lend a friendly ear to a player. Showing your players you care about them as a person, just as much as you care about their success within their career is imperative in building meaningful relationships. However, there is a fine line between creating professional relationships and personal relationships with the players. A solo-practitioner (and any practitioner for that matter) should exclusively focus on creating relationships that are built on trust as opposed to friendships. How those player-coach relationships are built play a crucial role to what a solo-practitioner can implement effectively.

A higher purpose and unwritten laws of the industry

A higher purpose

Whatever one's individual role is within a professional soccer club, evidently, they are only one aspect of a larger organisational structure (Figure 1.2). Within any organisation there exists a higher purpose and each practitioner should be fully aware of what this is and how they positively contribute towards this.

Several key questions should be asked:

- What is the vision, mission and aims of the organisation?
- What are the traditions, culture and heritage within an organisation?
- What are the specific club / organisational values?
- How is success defined within the organisation?
- What are the goals on a macro (organisational) level?

The answers to these questions can be highly varied between clubs depending upon a number of factors such as the size of the club that a practitioner works for, the age and history of the club, and the availability of financial, technological, and human resources, together with the developmental level that a practitioner works within. Greater variety exists at the senior level as organisational aspirations differ between winning titles and trophies, getting promoted, reaching the play-offs, and avoiding relegation. Within the academy environment, the mission and aims of the organisation are generally more consistent, involving the holistic individual development of young people, yet their end goals may differ by way of developing players to play in the club's first team or to sell for a financial profit and future sustainability.

When the answers to the above questions have been determined, the next step is to ensure that the strategies on a micro (departmental) level are aligned to the organisational goals. Key questions involve how these strategies can be measured and key performance indicators (KPI) are generally developed, involving the performance director and other stakeholders to assess the effectiveness of each department. Finally, it is important that as a practitioner performing any role within a performance department (fitness coach, strength and conditioning coach, sports scientist), their work in both the short- and long-term aligns with the departmental strategies, fitting into the multidisciplinary and club-wide organisational approach. This can differ at the international versus the club level, which can be further broken down into a 'club appointed' and 'coach-appointed role.'

Each practitioner that works within high-performance soccer also has an individual higher purpose. This is characterised by an individual set of attitudes, values, and beliefs, together with their own knowledge, skill set, and life experience both inside and outside of soccer. This higher purpose is illustrated by what drives a practitioner on a daily, weekly, and seasonal basis. An in-depth description of motivation is beyond the scope of this chapter but is one of the driving forces behind human behaviour and is typically divided into extrinsic and intrinsic factors. Extrinsic motivation is an external influence that impels people to act in a certain way and may include salary, rewards, bonuses, promotions, or associations with success. Intrinsic motivation refers to an internal form of motivation that occurs as a result of aligning certain actions with values or pleasure for performing and completing a task. In recruiting practitioners into a performance department, the alignment of an individual's higher purpose with those of an organisation can be a method used to identify a person's cultural fit and suitability within a particular organisation.

Different roles within the industry

Club-appointed role

This is a role that is contracted to the club and functions irrespectively of any head coach or managerial change. The role can be within the first team, reserves, or academy environment in either the performance and/or medical department. These positions are generally characterised by permanent contracts with fixed periods of notice and termination for the employer and employee. It should be noted, however, that for these club-wide positions within Major League Soccer in the United States, a number of these positions are 'at will,' involving no fixed notice periods.

Club-appointed roles generally have long-term strategic direction, preventing the organisation from having to replace all members of a performance and medical department in the event of a change of head coach. This provides both a consistency in philosophy and service delivery to players. Nonetheless, the major role responsibilities are to provide a support service to the head coach and technical staff. Club-appointed roles may also have higher education research links to identify 'best-practice' solutions to performance problems, with the ability to implement these consistently over several years.

Coach-appointed role

This is a role recruited by the head coach/manager or appointed as part of their technical staff. In a number of clubs, the head coach/manager personally identifies, selects, and appoints his support staff. These positions generally involve assistant technical coaches but can also involve the head of performance, fitness coach, or medical practitioners. This is a role contracted to the club, but with a fixed-term contract aligned to the length of the head coach/manager's contract. Such fast-paced roles are commonplace in the senior first team setting, with greater emphasis on the day-to-day and short-term approach, given that elite professional soccer is a results-based industry. If results are not as to the owners/board acceptance, then these practitioners may lose their jobs, particularly if there is a change of head coach. Accordingly, these roles can be highly pressured and more volatile, involving a higher reward but associated with greater risk. These roles are more prevalent in larger, and more high-profile elite European clubs.

International role

This is a role that is contracted to work within a country's national federation or governing body, working with the senior or age-group national teams. Practitioners that work within the performance and/or medical department of national federations have historically often also worked for a professional club; however, in recent years, a number of international federations have employed practitioners on an exclusive basis (Figure 1.4). Working within a multi-disciplinary team (MDT) of an international federation requires both short and long-term responsibilities.

In the short-term, there are a number of international friendly matches, competitive qualification matches and tournaments that are characterised by a large number of matches in a short period of time. This requires the practitioner to quickly identify the individual status of players and prescribe an appropriate training and/or recovery stimulus to optimise the preparation and performance of the player during these matches. Following any international camp, appropriate player feedback is generally provided to the respective clubs to allow the player to transition back into the club environment without issue. As there are large periods of time between international fixture periods, it is important that considerable planning takes place to prepare for international camps and tournament scenarios, ensuring that the necessary infrastructure has been identified

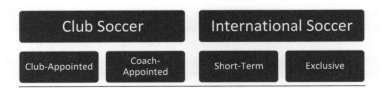

Figure 1.4 Roles within the industry.

and implemented. Furthermore, international staff must communicate, develop relationships and share information with players and their respective club staff to ensure that agreed training and nutritional priorities are being implemented within the club setting and to monitor the programme that the player is conducting from a distance. Finally, the international practitioner may conduct their own 'in-house' research and retrospective analysis to identify the most appropriate ways of operating during the relatively short international periods to increase their opportunity for successful outcomes in the future.

Unwritten laws of the industry

In professional soccer, regardless of the role that is performed within a performance or a medical department, there exists multiple laws/rules that will allow the practitioner to be more successful in both the short- and long-term. These rules are not written down, nor are they taught in undergraduate or post-graduate university courses, rather they are developed with experience once a practitioner has worked within the industry for an extended period of time. It is the hope that these points will provide young and inexperienced practitioners with appropriate information to enable them to better navigate the field of high-performance professional soccer:

- **T.E.A.M.:** Successful soccer performance is multi-disciplinary in nature and involves a number of technical, tactical, physical, and mental disciplines. Within a multi-disciplinary support staff, each service provider needs to appreciate the significance and complementary nature of one another's roles if the preparation and performance of each player is to be optimised.
- **Work in collaboration:** Although successful performance is multi-disciplinary, practitioners are required to work together in inter-disciplinary fashion and collaborate on a daily basis. There is significant power in collaboration and working together for a common goal. Historically, the main critique of strength and conditioning and sports science practice from players and coaches in professional football is that practitioners work independently to the on-field coaching process. This silo approach is often adopted as a result of an inability to align these service deliveries with the goals and game-model of the head coach. This, in turn, can lead to a mis-management of training load and an elevation in injury risk.
- **Know your role:** Understand what your individual role is within the multi-disciplinary team. What are your individual responsibilities that you will be accountable for? Do you have individual KPI's or goals that have been set for you? Focus on doing these to the best of your ability and controlling the factors that you are personally responsible for.
- **Do no harm, but do something:** How can you make a difference and add value to the player, department, or organisation that you are working with?

- **Do not use a reductionist approach:** Please remember that both performance and injury are multi-factorial in nature and affected by many transient and interacting factors. Be very wary of using a reductionist 'cause and effect' nature for more complex occurrences.
- **Power of communication:** We work with people and through people on a daily basis. Appropriate communication across a number of stakeholders within the organisation is vital for success within any role in professional soccer.
- **Educate to innovate:** Educate players if you are attempting to change a particular practice. Explain the reasons for any intervention that you suggest. People don't buy what you do, they buy why you do it. Ensure that the current generation of players do not receive all their sports science information via social media.
- **Don't sweat the small stuff:** Focus your time, effort, and energy on the factors that will transfer to the largest performance or preparation gains. Ensure that the basics are firmly established before attempting to implement the practices that may make a difference. In short, focus on the 99% before chasing the 1%.
- **Treat players as individuals:** Although a squad of players can number more than 20 players, it is important to be aware that players are unique as individuals. They have their own genetics, playing position, strengths and weaknesses, maturation, and training age together with an individual injury history. Do not always use averages, rather manage individuals daily. Furthermore, within the academy setting, it is vital to develop individuals and not teams.
- **Train players, don't chase numbers:** With the rapid growth in technology and the information available to the sports performance and medical practitioner, it is extremely important to remember that our role is to train and rehabilitate players, not chase numbers. Furthermore, leverage data to inform your practice and solve performance problems, but do not be a spreadsheet coach. Ultimately, be data-informed, not data-driven.
- **The research doesn't always apply:** Allowing research to inform your practice is a sensible way of developing your system and philosophy of work to remain current within the industry. It is extremely important to note, however, that searching the internet for soccer-related training, load-monitoring, and recovery interventions will produce a plethora of journal articles across a range of ages, playing standards and research designs. Deciphering this information is a challenge for all practitioners and it is important to critically appraise and filter this information, before adopting it into your practice and scope of work.
- **Be genuine:** The aphorism of 'faking it until you make it' is a strategy of that may serve one well within elite soccer for a very short time, but not throughout a career. Both players and coaches will see through imitation over a prolonged period, thus it is vital that practitioners are genuine and conduct their work with authenticity daily.

Surviving the industry

Staff turnover

Unfortunately, a common characteristic of professional football is high staff turnover. This occurs at both first team and academy levels. There are some key characteristics that practitioners require in order to survive the industry independent of their role; however, there are some bespoke challenges that practitioners will face depending on their type of role and environment they work in (IE. first team vs. academy).

First team

At first team level, the instability of the manager/head coach position primarily dictates the rate of staff turnover. With managerial changes, there will also be changes to coach appointed positions that include coaching staff, medical, and performance staff. Even though these positions are deemed to be shorter-term positions, these types of changes can also alter the structure of departments as well as more longer-term positions that provide direction for long-term strategies, such as a performance director. A practitioner in a club appointed position in first team football needs to be adaptable to different managerial and coaching styles, new strategic direction, and potentially a new game model which will dictate training philosophies. Taking time to learn from a new approach, whilst being authentic and genuine, will pave the way for building strong relationships. Understanding and adopting a new or different language of soccer, as well trying to create a common language will allow a practitioner to communicate how they can add value and provide a support service to the coaching team. It is likely that responsibilities may change with a change in managerial appointments, and therefore being malleable as a practitioner and showing a willingness to change is generally required. Dependent on the circumstances and the situation of the club, a practitioner may look to increase role satisfaction and feeling of impact through seeking new or alternative opportunities. Working within the rehabilitation team, concentrating more on strength, and conditioning process within the gym, or with other squads within the club (such as academy teams), are all viable options to increase value to the organisation and the feeling of making a difference.

In coach-appointed positions, practitioners require an ability to embed quickly into a new club with likely changes in tradition, culture, operations, structure, philosophies, and strategies between clubs. In addition, an ability to understand, accept, and empathise with a new set of staff with a difference in professional opinions, strategies, and working styles are key characteristics.

Academy environments

Within developmental settings, the vast majority of roles will be club-appointed. A high turnover of staff in academies is independent of first team manager changes, with staff transitioning between clubs to seek new opportunities and challenges or to potentially gain a promotion. Staff transition internally within clubs and externally between clubs across all departments and positions. Internally, the coaching staff have frequent changes where coaches tend to move up from younger ages groups to older ones. Performance practitioners, who themselves can transition to older age groups, can find themselves working with coaches who they have previously worked with at younger ages. Alternatively, there will be frequent instances where staff have transitioned in from other clubs, where a different philosophy may be used to develop players. In all scenarios, building strong professional relationships and bonds is therefore a necessity for practitioners. Performance practitioners in academy settings may work across more than one age group and therefore work with multiple coaches and support staff, managed or overseen by a department head (E.G., head of foundation phase U9-U12s). Therefore, creating and managing multiple relationships simultaneously is required in order to be effective. Adopting multiple strategies to apply the same scientific content may be required to cater for the different working and learning styles of coaches, support staff, and players.

Attributes to survive

Although there can be a large amount of staff turnover in the elite soccer environment, there are a number of key attributes required for practitioners independent of their working environment or role orientation. Not only will the below-mentioned attributes aid practitioners in maintaining their role in elite soccer, but also these will help enhance one's mental health and working environment.

Creating and managing relationships

Soccer has often been described by the people that work within it as a 'people business.' Having an ability to create and maintain relationships with all types of staff members are key attributes of interpersonal skills required by practitioners. Building strong relationships with key stakeholders is also a principal requirement to be able to translate scientific knowledge to practice. Recognising, understanding, and managing different personality types is fundamental in establishing rapport with players and staff members (*more detail discussed in Chapter 11*). Having an ability to manage-up is also a desirable characteristic to align and manage expectations of those stakeholders.

Self-care

For a long time, researchers have primarily focused on athletes, their needs, characteristics, and the environment which they require to successfully thrive in. However, since 2008, the attention of investigations has begun to shift to those supporting the athlete and has started to view those around the athlete (the 'team behind the team') as performers in their own right [11–13]. To date the research has primarily centred on managers and coaches, but there are clear and important messages for all those employed in elite sport. We know

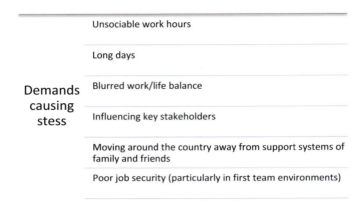

Figure 1.5 Demands of working in elite soccer than potentially cause stress for a practitioner.

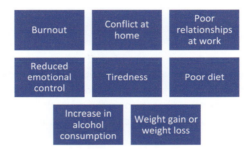

Figure 1.6 Potential long-term negative effects associated with constant stress exposure in the workplace.

in elite sport there are lots and lots of demands that can often leave us feeling stretched (Figure 1.5).

Generally, in the short-term, this stretch is usually something that one can handle. However, research shows that over longer periods of time, it can have negative effects (Figure 1.6) [11–13]. No matter how resilient or tough one perceives themselves, we are all human and we don't have an infinite amount of energy or resource. Therefore, it is imperative that one practices self-care and understands what helps maintain one's best self. Failure to do so will result in a very difficult attempt to help the athletes become the best version of themselves [14, 15]. It is important that practitioners in elite soccer learn how to find a balance between the demands of the job and personal resources so that one can thrive in roles and not just survive each season [16].

Expectancies and working conditions

Working with new staff, especially new line managers or coaches, requires establishing clear responsibilities and expectancies for a harmonious and effective working relationship. Establishing role expectancies will determine role effectiveness and how a practitioner is contributing to the overall aim of the organisation. Some changes and alterations to roles may be less formal in nature to suit the needs of coaching teams. Performing warm-ups and conditioning with or without the ball, providing training load feedback in graphical or a numerical format, conducting formal meetings versus informal conversations, and types of recovery sessions are all examples of small nuances that can accompany changes in managerial changes. Accordingly, this may require flexibility from the performance practitioner.

Communication

Translating knowledge to the end user requires practitioners to be able to communicate complex scientific principles in an easy-to-understand manner. Different end users will require a different type of language from the practitioner. Explaining scientific concepts in an understandable manner will increase buy in from the end user, whether that is a player, a parent, or a head coach. Feedback or explanations must be contextualised to the individual or to how they apply to the team and contribute to the overall strategy of the club.

Continual learning and work ethic

A desire to continually evolve and develop as a practitioner, alongside a dedicated work ethic, is highly regarded values. Sport science in soccer is an ever-evolving field; therefore, maintaining an understanding of the most contemporary research is vital in optimally preparing players for competition.

Conclusion

Overall, the ability to understand that there is more than one way to operate as an applied performance practitioner in soccer is vital. Being open-minded with a continual desire to learn and develop is a vital characteristic to possess as an applied practitioner in elite soccer. There are a variety of roles and responsibilities that a performance practitioner can hold within an elite soccer environment. In order to thrive in an elite soccer setting, a practitioner must understand the knowledge and traits required to operate efficiently within any given environment and circumstance. Staff turnover is often unavoidable in professional soccer; however, there are certain attributes that practitioners can continue to develop to further succeed within in the industry.

References

1. Springham, M., et al., *Developing strength and conditioning coaches for professional football.* Coaching Prof Football, 2018. **50**: p. 9–16.
2. Birwatkar, V.P., *Emotional intelligence: The invisible phenomenon in sports.* European Journal of Sports & Exercise Science, 2014. **3**(19): p. 31–31.

3 Cartwright, S. and C. Pappas, *Emotional intelligence, its measurement and implications for the workplace.* International Journal of Management Reviews, 2008. **10**(2): p. 149–171.
4 McGuigan, M.R., G.A. Wright, and S.J. Fleck, *Strength training for athletes: Does it really help sports performance?* International Journal of Sports Physiology and Performance, 2012. **7**(1): p. 2–5.
5 Wisløff, U., et al., *Strong correlation of maximal squat strength with sprint performance and vertical jump height in elite soccer players.* British Journal of Sports Medicine, 2004. **38**(3): p. 285–288.
6 Suchomel, T.J., S. Nimphius, and M.H. Stone, *The importance of muscular strength in athletic performance.* Sports Medicine, 2016. **46**(10): p. 1419–49.
7 Dumas, M., et al., *Introduction to business process management,* in Fundamentals of business process management. 2013, Springer Berlin Heidelberg: Berlin, Heidelberg. p. 1–31.
8 Halperin, I., et al., *Autonomy: A missing ingredient of a successful program?* Strength & Conditioning Journal, 2018. **40**(4): p. 18–25.
9 Pacanowsky, M., *Communication in the empowering organization.* Annals of the International Communication Association, 1988. **11**(1): p. 356–379.
10 Hersey, P., K.H. Blanchard, and W.E. Natemeyer, *Situational leadership, perception, and the impact of power.* Group & Organization Studies, 1979. **4**(4): p. 418–428.
11 Thelwell, R.C., et al., *Stressors in elite sport: A coach perspective.* Journal of Sports Sciences, 2008. **26**(9): p. 905–918.
12 Olusoga, P., et al., *Stress in elite sports coaching: Identifying stressors.* Journal of Applied Sport Psychology, 2009. **21**(4): p. 442–459.
13 Norris, L.A., F.F. Didymus, and M. Kaiseler, *Stressors, coping, and well-being among sports coaches: A systematic review.* Psychology of Sport and Exercise, 2017. **33**: p. 93–112.
14 Kelly, S., et al., *Psychological support for sport coaches: an exploration of practitioner psychologist perspectives.* Journal of Sports Sciences, 2018. **36**(16): p. 1852–1859.
15 Vijayalakshmi, V. and S. Bhattacharyya, *Emotional contagion and its relevance to individual behavior and organizational processes: A position paper.* Journal of Business and Psychology, 2012. **27**(3): p. 363–374.
16 Wagstaff, C.R., D. Fletcher, and S. Hanton, *Exploring emotion abilities and regulation strategies in sport organizations.* Sport, Exercise, and Performance Psychology, 2012. **1**(4): p. 268.

2 From academy to professional

Alex Berger, Jack Christopher, Nathan Plaskett, Thomas Carpels and Adam Centofanti

The next generation

The journey to becoming a professional soccer player can be a rocky road with many ups and downs. Top prospects are often misguided or lack a certain quality to make it to the next level. As the game has evolved, so has the prerequisite to have elite physical and psychological qualities to play at the professional level. It is no surprise how important good long-term athletic development planning and execution is. Performance practitioners at all levels must have an excellent understanding of the phases of development. This includes each of the key physical qualities required, knowledge of the challenges that youth soccer players may face, how to overcome them, and the overall programming to ensure no key windows of opportunity are missed. Above all, a performance practitioner developing the next generation of soccer players must also understand their responsibility to be an excellent mentor. Someone who develops not only elite athletes, but also exceptional human beings with excellent values, that will carry over into the rest of their lives, and ultimately contribute to a positive performance-driven culture in the first team.

Phases of development

Research and best practice in soccer has begun to increasingly focus on the long-term athletic development (LTAD) pathway and how best to enhance the physical characteristics of the adolescent athlete [1]. The end goal of such programmes is to produce robust resilient players that can withstand the rigours of professional soccer. A key tenet for practitioners to understand, however, is that the developing athlete has differing needs from the fully developed adult athlete, and that there potentially exists windows of opportunity to take advantage of, as the child moves throughout this maturation process. Specifically, the introduction of the Elite Player Performance Plan (EPPP) framework within the UK is centred around these key differences and aims to set out a structured set of principles to guide this process within developmental soccer.

Competition around the world at youth level is centred around a child's chronological age, yet there can be significant differences in a child's needs,

DOI: 10.4324/9781003200420-2

physical abilities, and cognitive development within the same chronological age group [2, 3]. For example, average variations in anthropometric characteristics, such as height and weight, have shown to be as large as 15 cm and 21 kg, respectively, between the least and most mature players within the same chronological age group (i.e. U14's).

The chronological age at which each individual undergoes the most pronounced acceleration in physical development varies greatly from individual to individual, however, tends to be between 11 and 16 years of age, in youth soccer athletes. Termed Peak Height Velocity (PHV), the period of greatest accelerated growth spurt coincides with the commencement of puberty, with players who mature earlier tending to be taller, heavier, and quicker than their later maturing counterparts [4–9]. As a result, a player's level of physical maturity has shown to have relationships with lower leg explosive power, force production capabilities, neuromuscular control, and ability to utilise their stretch shortening cycle efficiently, as well as aerobic endurance capacity, all of which have been shown to be desirable physical characteristics in soccer players [10–12].

It is now commonplace to perform regular testing protocols in youth cohorts, with the aim of highlighting talent and measuring physical performance improvements over time [13]. An important distinction to make is understanding why a high performing athlete within a particular test of athleticism is achieving a high score. For example, is a particular athlete far outperforming others in tests of speed because they are further along in his/her physical development than the rest of the group? What are the implications for that low-scoring athlete, are they ignored in favour of higher performing athletes when it comes to contracts? Whilst the awareness of this concept is becoming better understood globally, players with significant potential and ability can perhaps 'fall through the cracks', because of a lack of understanding of how a youth athlete is achieving their scores in tests of athleticism, at lower levels with limited resources. Ultimately, a player's ability to perform at the highest level is dependent upon performing well in training and competition long-term, as opposed to 'winning' an individual match or performing well in a single test of athleticism in the short term. This philosophical standpoint is key to helping guide a player to fulfil their potential as they move throughout adolescence and should be a key tennet of LTAD programmes.

Several models have been developed to help explain and guide this process, with one of the models describing phases of development and importantly, the focus for training and competition at each phase. Balyi illustrated that it takes roughly 8–12 years for a talented athlete to reach 'elite' levels and describes a model which provides an explanation as to what the main focus of training should be within each phase of development [14]. Table 2.1 outlines phases as either 'Early-Specialisation' or 'Late-Specialisation' and suggests how the focus of training and matches changes as the adolescent athlete undergoes chronological development. It fails, however, to highlight the differences in physical maturation as the athlete moves toward adulthood.

Table 2.1 Early specialisation model vs late specialisation models of development

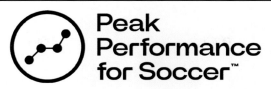

	Early specialisation	Late specialisation
1	Training to train	FUNdamental
2	Training to compete	Learning to train
3	Training to win	Training to train
4	Retainment	Training to compete
5		Training to win
6		Retainment

Resultingly, the research has focused on providing a more in depth understanding of what physiological changes are taking place at each stage of maturation [15, 16]. Structured programmes to enhance physical development at each stage, where practitioners aim to take advantage of 'windows of accelerated development', and have been suggested as the best practice in creating robust professional athletes in the long term [7, 10, 11]. The windows of accelerated development suggest that each phase of development has a period where the type of growth is primarily influenced by differing physiological functions. For example, prior to the onset of puberty, physical development has been suggested to be influenced most greatly by neural adaptations, whereby fundamental motor skills and the creation of neurological pathways responsible for tasks such as running, throwing, and jumping are developed at a greater rate during this time. During puberty, however, the physiological changes occurring at this time have been suggested to be because of a rapid increase in hormonal changes. For the practitioner and athlete, it can be a challenging and critical phase as it encompasses both opportunity and vulnerability in terms of growth and development.

During PHV, bones grow primarily to the musculature, putting added stress on connective tissue and the growth plates where they attach. Flexibility, during the time of accelerated growth, can be compromised through a reduced range of motion, which resultingly has the potential to create abnormal movement patterns, and has been referred to as a period of adolescent awkwardness [17, 18]. Having knowledge of how an athlete moves through the phases of maturation can help practitioners design LTAD models, in order to target the type of adaptations that have been suggested are prevalent at each stage. A physical development programme for a U12 player should focus on developing physical literacy, and proficiency across a variety of movement competencies, providing

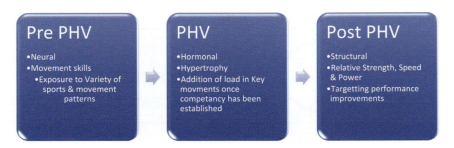

Figure 2.1 Stages of peak height velocity (PHV) and the physical development windows of opportunity.

the U12 player with a range of stimuli to adapt to, both within the confines of the gym space and out on the pitch. By targeting motor learning and exposing the athletes within this phase to a variety of sports, movements, and skills, practitioners can theoretically take advantage of the increased neurological development during this phase [7, 16]. The needs of a U19 athlete will be completely different from the U12 (pre-PHV) athlete. Aims of the programme for the U19 athlete will be to target structural adaptations to training, whether that be through targeting increases in strength and size to developing movement skills that might facilitate success within the athletes given playing position (Figure 2.1).

Developing models that guide the enhancement of a range of physical qualities that lend themselves to successful performance in soccer in adulthood over a long period of time is key. Globally, developmental soccer athletes move through several key phases;

- Foundation phase (U9–U12s)
- Youth development phase (U13–U16s)
- Professional development phase (U17–U18s)
- Performance phase (professional soccer) (should they make the grade)

Considering soccer players can potentially be in academies from U9 to a professional adult (potentially 12+ years), it is crucial that plans aimed at developing a particular player's physicality are diversified from that which would be in place for an adult. Therefore, an important consideration of these LTAD models in soccer is the amount of energy that is put into developing the person, developing a player's understanding for the game, and providing an experience that develops a range of life skills as well as physical qualities.

Athletic development

The modern-day athlete

Firstly, it's important to acknowledge the key characteristics of the modern-day athlete to enable us to relate and communicate with our athletes more effectively. It also allows us to manipulate the training environment to their preferences to help maximise engagement and ultimately athletic development. The industry has seen a cultural shift over the past 15 years which coincides with a shift from millennials to generation Z. So, what do we know about Generation Z? [19].

Who?

Born between 1996 and 2012, it's important to recognise that generation labels aren't completely distinct with some characteristics flowing from one to another. They aren't globally applicable to all individuals within a 'generation'. However, they do provide us with an insight into the product of an ever-changing world and how this has affected our athletes.

Digital natives

Digital natives were born into a more technologically advanced world. They don't know a world without social media and their virtual world is every bit as real as reality. However, they are more astute with their personal data and want more control over where it goes. As coaches, it's important to consider how we share data with players and ensure they get something in return.

Competitive

Individuals in this category are even more competitive than their predecessors and crave constant stimulation. Coaches can embrace this competitive nature by providing players with instantaneous feedback wherever possible. Technological advancements such as Velocity-Based Training have been shown to be very effective at improving intent and could be a great tool for creating competition [20].

Hyper personalisation

In their virtual world, content is tailored to their exact need which drives their desire for personalisation. They tend to be experiential learners and want to be involved in all aspects of their programme: Planning, implementation, and goal setting. Coaches should think of innovative ways to personalise their programmes and utilise coaching techniques bespoke to their preferred style of learning.

9–12s (Foundation phase)

The foundation phase is potentially the most important part of the players' athletic development journey. It's an opportunity to build a broad movement base that sets players up to be agile, robust athletes who can handle the chaotic and random movement demands of the game. The key term is variation. Players need to be exposed to a variety of different movement skills, within a multitude of performance contexts and coached through different practice

Table 2.2 Example of a ten-week training cycle to develop change of direction (COD) qualities in the foundation phase

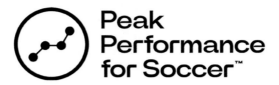

Week	Movement skill	Key coaching points
1–2	Deceleration Rotational Skills	Use of the foot to brake, declined body position Timing of shoulders and hips, how to accelerate rotation – generating momentum
3–4	90°–180° turn	Cross step vs Outside leg push vs Short quick step Use of upper body lean
5–6	Tag Variations	Open practice. Emphasise good practice Attacking – Individuals who use body for deception well Defending – Individuals who can decelerate quickly and turn in response to an opponent's movement
7–8	Deceleration Rotational Skills	Revisit foot contact and body position. Vary exit demands How to initiate and accelerate rotation (e.g. when in the air)
9–10	3v3 Tag Rugby Squash variation	Opportunity to practice good attacking change of direction skills Opportunity to practice deceleration skills and quicker 90° and 180° turns

designs. Utilising a spiral curriculum is a great option. As opposed to a conventional curriculum, whereby you teach topic A, then move on to topic B, a spiral curriculum allows several different skills/topics to be taught at the same time. As the weeks progress, gradually increase depth and complexity until they are ultimately performing the skill as they would in a game (Table 2.2).

The training cycle begins with the fundamentals. Players are exposed to a mixture of open and closed practices. They have a mixture of explicit (how to utilise foot contact to slow down) and implicit learning (how to beat a player in tag rugby) methods (Table 2.3).

Players are taught the skill of deceleration in a multitude of contexts (to react to a squash ball, to beat a player 1v1 when facing an individual, to defend against an attacker). This education is vitally important to help players become more agile movers and more adept at solving the variety of movement challenges the game yields. There is an intentional use of alternative sports to soccer to help teach young players how to move well. Multisport exposure helps to protect against the potential pitfalls of early specialisation which has been associated with reduced motor skill development and overuse injuries and adds more depth when teaching movement skills for soccer [21, 22]. Developing physical capabilities is only part of their development; it's also a vitally important time for development of technical skills and basic tactical understanding. Therefore,

Table 2.3 Implicit vs explicit learning descriptions and example

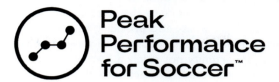

Description	Example
A player practices a skill without conscious thought on how to execute it. The task is set up in such a way that the correct movement strategy will bring about success. The environment is complex enough that the athlete can't rehearse the skill in their head	**Change of direction** Directional tag game Tag rugby **Landing mechanics** Handball Obstacle course time trial
Conscious thought is given on how to perform a skill. Technique can is understood and can be verbalised. The task is potentially more 'closed' and often includes verbal cues from the coach. It gives the player an opportunity to repeatedly rehearse a skill with a high level of support	**Change of direction** 10 m sprint into a 90° turn left **Landing mechanics** Box jumps

programming needs to be flexible to fit in around the training schedule. It's not paramount to stick to the conventional structure of warm-up followed by training. Younger players tend to have a shorter attention span and respond better to short 5–10 minute blocks interspersed within the session, accumulating to 15–30 minutes/session, 2–4x/week. If individuals are really struggling with a particular skill or falling behind the group, the use of additional individual sessions can be beneficial. Generation Z players are very proficient with technology and place a high value on feedback. The use of video feedback can enhance the learning process and allow a continuation of coaching even when the individual is at home. Home programmes can be a great way of increasing contact time and ensuring the player gets the support they need without detracting from their time on the pitch. Certain individuals will inevitably need additional support. Arrival activities can be a fantastic way to achieve this, players will often turn up early for training, utilise this time to work with individuals on specific movement traits they struggle with.

13–16s (Youth development phase)

The youth development phase is potentially the most challenging period for the aspiring soccer to navigate. Players will inevitably experience accelerated periods of growth, for some this can be incremental, for others the rate can be very high which often has negative implications for both movement competency and injury risk as discussed earlier. Players may mature early, providing them with a physical advantage over their less mature peers, or late, providing significant challenges to perform against physically superior opponents.

As players begin to mature and the physical intensity of sessions increases, the importance of physical preparation prior to the session gains significance. Moving athletic development work to the start of the sessions helps ensure contact time is kept high, whilst also providing sufficient preparation for the subsequent session. However, it's important to view these sessions as an athletic development opportunity not solely a 'Warm-Up' and add structure to what and how this is delivered. Contact time should be 15–20 minutes per session, 3–4x/week (Figure 2.2).

As players begin to mature during this phase, if they display good movement qualities, the programme can gradually begin to increase time allocation to developing physical capacities (strength, power, and speed). Ideally contact time should be between 15 and 20 minutes/session (3–5x/week) and is usually placed at the beginning of the session, however, continue to integrate athletic development content within the session where possible.

The spiral curriculum helps to prevent overload or boredom but also ensures structure in the continued development of athletic skills, therefore, preferred over the traditional 'block periodisation'. With strength training, block periodisation is implemented on the premise that developing one physical characteristic (i.e., Strength) will complement the development of the following characteristic (i.e. Power). In the context of skill development, deceleration is needed to change direction efficiently. Many locomotive skills are interlinked, and all complement one another, so it's important to continue to develop them simultaneously.

U17s (Earn the right)

This category refers to a player's transition from a schoolboy programme with reduced training frequency to a full-time programme competing with older players. Not only does training frequency often increase, but sessions also demand greater intensity, the game is played quicker, and there is a gradual shift from a development to performance focus. It is important to give players time to adapt during the early stages of this development phase.

U17+ (Perform)

Players in this category are expected to display good levels of strength and have adjusted to the increased demands of professional soccer, depending on their pathway. Once these things are in place, we can remove the restraint and allow players to compete and push each other to maximise athletic potential. A system-based approach is still appropriate but it's now important to start targeting very specific performance goals and increase individualisation. During this phase, there is more of an emphasis on performance and players are often playing across multiple competitions. Therefore, it's important for programming to have large degrees of flexibility to maximise training opportunities whilst adjusting for fatigue and ensuring players are fresh for games.

Wk	Date	Monday	Tuesday	Wednesday	Thursday	Friday	Saturday	Sunday
		1	2	3	4	5	6	7
	Activity	Rest	Train	Train	Train	Rest	Train	Match
Week 1	Topic	Off	Change of Direction	Running Mechanics	Jumping & Landing	Off	Running Mechanics	Match
	Sub Topic		Deceleration	Foot Contact	Landing Control		Acceleration - Forward Lean	
	Main Points		Aggressive Foot Contact Body Position and COM	Preparing the foot for landing - Dorsiflexion Stiffness of lower limb	Stiffness - Preparing to hit the ground Preventing Knee Valgus		Longer, aggressive foot contacts Push backwards	
	Strength & Stiffness		1. Isometric Wall Hold 2x30s 2. Press Up 2x10 (Tempo) 3. Forward Lunge 2x8es	1. SL RDL 2x8es 2. Lateral Lunge 2x8es 3. Press up - Side pLank 2x6es	1. SL Glute Bridge 2x10es 2. CMJ 2x6 3. Soleus Raise - Lunge Position - 2x12es		1. Isometric Wall Hold 2x30s 2. Pogos 2x12 3. Resistance Band Row 2x10	
	Mobility		Hip Mobility	Ankle Mobility	Thoracic Mobility		General Mobility Challenges	

Figure 2.2 Weekly activation layout example.

Key qualities for development

As part of a young soccer player's journey, there are several qualities that, if trained to maximum capacity, will hold them in great stead as they learn to cope with the increased physical demands of the professional game. To preface, it is not in the purview of this section to discuss the specifics of growth and maturation as they pertain to the training of the qualities listed below. Rather, to provide the 'why' and the 'how' of the key qualities that a soccer player will need from their time as academy players to physically nurture their progression into a first team environment.

Soccer performance for the young player is perhaps best explained using a pyramid model (Figure 2.3) as it illustrates the interaction between physical qualities, e.g., a player benefits from being movement competent before training strength, and a powerful player should see benefits in their acceleration. The pyramid does not attempt to show that certain qualities are more important than others because they are at the bottom of the pyramid or must be trained before others. Of course, it is not that simple and in fact, it's the qualities at the top that are the most specific to the game of soccer. However, beyond movement experience, where we attempt to challenge problem solving and enhance cognitive function, the youth athletic development is about getting improvements from progression. In essence, using the least amount of complexity/intensity as possible. The qualities at the bottom of the pyramid will hold a young player in great stead as they move through the later development phases when the focus shifts from learning, competency and mastering the fundamentals to becoming powerful, fast, and reactive. As we reverse engineer from the game itself to the physical qualities it contains, this chapter answers two fundamental questions:

1 What are the bio-motor qualities in soccer?
2 How do young players train these qualities to become physically prepared for soccer?

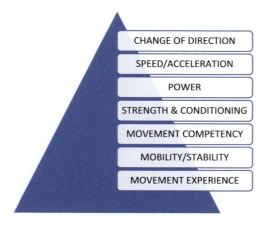

Figure 2.3 Long-term athletic development pyramid.

From a long-term athletic development standpoint, the initial goal is the build a well-rounded athlete, then as they progress, training will become more specific to the physical qualities needed in soccer. While as mentioned, it is important that aspiring players aim to develop all components of the pyramid, including the base, it should be noted that it is not uncommon for some genetically gifted players to be able to maximise certain qualities despite the absence of others. However, as this is not the majority, comprehensive athletic development is integral for the young player.

Beginning with mobility and stability, a critical foundation is required to develop all other physical qualities effectively and efficiently. By having appropriate ranges of motion and stability through and in the end points of that range, it sets the foundation for 'movement competency'. The goal of developing movement competency is to provide athletes with movement options in all three planes of motion – Sagittal, Frontal, and Transverse. This provides the body with a greater ability to adapt and adjust to the chaotic nature of the game as their training and playing age increases. This is a critical part of the pyramid for a young athlete and soccer player as in conjunction with 'movement experience' the process may have important cognitive advantages later into adulthood [23].

Next to movement competency, the development of strength qualities is a critical component of a young soccer players development, as strength underpins many of the qualities listed above (power, acceleration, change of direction). Additionally, strength creates more robust athletes who are less prone to injury [24]. In conjunction with building a strength base, the development of a solid aerobic capacity is fundamental to performance, due to the high aerobic demands of soccer. A high level of aerobic capacity will also improve the athlete's ability to repeat high intensity efforts that are required at the highest level [25], e.g., repeat sprint, power ability, and improve tactical decisions and technical execution [26].

Once adequate strength is established, the next progression is 'power', the expression of as much force in as little time as possible. Training for power will increase rate of force development (RFD) via improved motor unit recruitment and rate coding, leading to improvements in general athleticism [27]. Specifically, the soccer player should see improvements in key physical actions such as jumping, accelerating, and changing direction. These physical actions along with sprinting are some of the more obvious and often indirectly trained in team training. However, in any soccer player, there are benefits to training these qualities in isolation. Strength and power training can lead to improvements in central nervous system activation, facilitating more efficient muscular recruitment when more specific training is completed. Therefore, acceleration training allows for the realisation and transfer of the benefits gained from strength/power training. Furthermore, most high intensity actions in football cover less than 20 m, making acceleration critical to game related outcomes [28].

For both reducing risk of injury and improving on pitch performance, regular maximum velocity exposures are critical [29]. Regular exposure will not only help protect the hamstrings but also improve anaerobic speed reserve, making sub maximal efforts easier and more sustainable. As it relates to soccer, maximal velocity (including acceleration) is the most common physical action prior to a goal being scored [30]. Change of direction, if performed with appropriate intensity, can be considered 'high speed strength training' due to the manoeuvre responsible for a direction change featuring eccentric muscle contraction during braking, followed by concentric contraction, granting propulsive force [31]. This could theoretically assist in the transfer from the gym to the pitch. Specific training in this area provides controlled exposure to more specific contraction speeds, ground contacts, and direction. This has positive implications for both agile performance and ACL risk, as lower level or less experienced athletes experience greater knee valgus moments in unplanned change of direction tasks [32].

Mobility and stability

Does the athlete have movement options in the major joints needed?

Areas needing stability can often be trained via normal progression through strength exercises, especially foot, knee, and lumbar stability (Figure 2.4). On the other hand, mobility is a quality that usually needs to be trained independent of other qualities. There are three common times in which mobility can be trained: sequenced with strength exercises (1A – Back Squat, 1B – Thoracic Mobility), in a pre-activation session prior to team training and in a recovery session.

An example of how to break these down or 'periodise' is to categorise and theme the sessions. Sequencing with strength exercises, focus on either an area that player struggles with or an area that directly impacts the strength exercise.

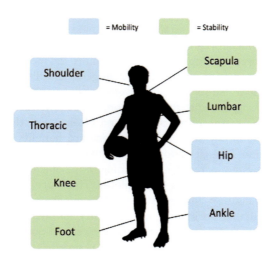

Figure 2.4 Mobility vs stability of joints in the human body.

In a pre-activation session, focus on a more holistic approach – general mobility for thoracic, hip, and ankle, including some strength in range exercises, e.g., no handed 90/90 hip rotation.

Movement competency

It is important to distinguish between movement competency and movement experience. Movement experience is gained in the early (six to ten years) and more unstructured phases for a young person or prospective soccer player. At this stage, free movement, problem solving should be the main priority as this will teach players to be aware of their body and cognitively be able to solve movement problems [16]. Movement competency is mastering the fundamental movement patterns that will underpin the training of key physical qualities. As players move into the older stages of their time in the academy, it is advantageous to have mastered these fundamental movements (Figure 2.5). It is also important to note that part of this process is to create an environment that gives a young player a reason to learn a particular movement pattern.

One of the keys to developing both movement competency and strength is to create progressions that will not only continue to improve a player's movement competency, yet also facilitate strength within that movement. To apply these progressions into practice, it is important that a system is created, one that shows both the player and the coach where they're at. The question to ask here is 'what will determine when a player can progress to the next movement?' Some of the movements will be subjective technical competency, e.g., BW Squat, wall drills, and some will be external loading-based, e.g., 25 kg Goblet Squat for 8–10 repetitions or a 150% BW Back Squat. What these standards are is a conversation to be had within the academy performance department and the

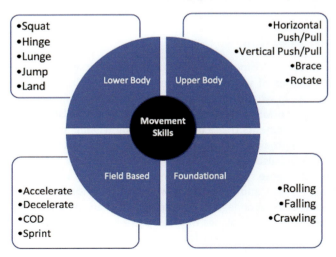

Figure 2.5 Movement skill breakdown.

first team performance department. From a club philosophical standpoint, what condition do the first team staff want academy players to be in if they transition into that environment? What training methodologies do players need to be prepared for? This is by no means a black and white discussion; however, it is important that the entire department is working towards the same physical goals. The gym-based progressions in Figure 2.6 focus on mastering BW before adding load, using load to maximise trunk demands, and then maximising external load to build global relative strength.

Strength

When training for strength, there are a few questions to be asked: What are the main movements? How will intensity be prescribed? How will this be progressed over time?

Overall, the rules that govern these questions should be:

- Technique > Load
- Simple > Complex
- Low Intensity > High Intensity

Strength before the gym

While not at the age where dedicated training in the gym is required, the young athlete can learn to develop whole body strength against external load via wrestling and ball protection drills. Various gymnastic and animalistic movements, e.g., bunny hops, inchworms, and wall climbing, can also help develop coordinated whole body/trunk strength prior to a player's introduction to gym related strength work

Movement selection

Reverse engineering from observation of the sport itself – what are the biomechanical qualities of soccer? Furthermore, how much force is being applied in these actions? In what directions are the forces being applied? In what parts of the range of motion is the force applied? What musculature is responsible? What are the movements that a player should be training to both reduce injury risk and increase physical performance in soccer? When considering movement selection, we must also consider injury history, equipment access, and logistics. Soccer is a 360-degree sport and contains movements in all three planes of motion (Sagittal, Frontal, and Transverse) with high joint forces that are often unevenly dispersed between legs (e.g., running and changing direction) As such, it is important that all three planes of motion are trained, overloaded to prepare the relevant tissues for the high forces and a range of bilateral and unilateral exercises utilised. To aid in programming and progression, these movements can be prescribed in patterns (Table 2.4).

From academy to professional 35

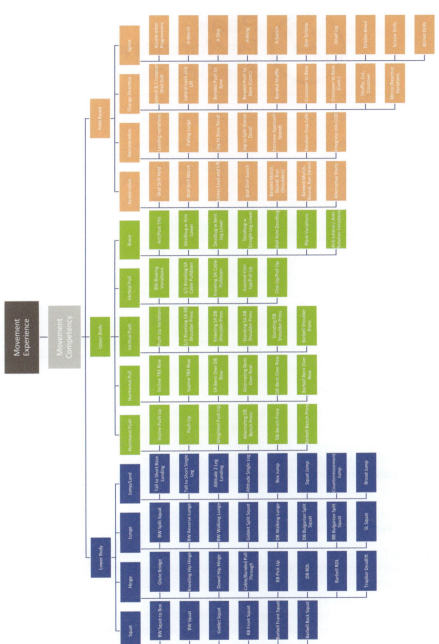

Figure 2.6 An example of progression system for key movements.

36 Alex Berger et al.

Table 2.4 Movement patterns and examples

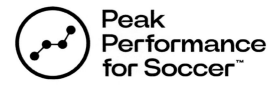

Movement pattern	Movement example
Lower body	
Bilateral knee dominant	Barbell back squat
Bilateral hip dominant	Barbell Romanian deadlift
Unilateral knee dominant	Rear foot elevated split squat
Unilateral hip dominant	Single leg hip thrust
Isolated accessories – commonly injured areas in soccer	
Hamstring	Nordic curls
Adductor	Copenhagen's
Quadricep/rectus femoris	Reverse nordic
Calf/soleus	Seated & standing calf raises
Upper body & trunk	
Horizontal push/pull	Barbell bench press/single arm dumbbell row
Vertical push/pull	Barbell shoulder press/chin ups
Anti-rotation	Pallof Press
Anti-lateral flexion	Suitcase carry
Anti-extension	Deadbug
Rotation	Standing cable rotation

Prescription options

For most young players, working through exercise progressions will provide enough overload to induce strength gains and advanced prescription methods aren't necessary. Beyond this, there are certain methods that can be employed to continue strength gains once they have achieved an appropriate level of movement competency. Such methods include: % 1RM, Reps in Reserve (RIR) and Velocity-Based [33].

Periodisation options

During the younger phases of development, periodisation beyond linear progression is considered unnecessary as the focus should be on fun, engagement, and appropriate development vs. games or competition related outcomes. However, when discussing periodisation in the later stages of academy development, often there can be a large gap between theory and application. Especially in season when intensity/volume is high, programming needs can become more reactive. When prescribing strength training, there are several popular methods to periodise (*Note:* these are not with respect to other physical qualities and as such options such as conjugate or agile are not relevant), including constant, reverse linear, rep accumulation, set accumulation, and undulating.

Power

From its role in acceleration, to its role in jumping, optimising power output will provide a significant advantage to any soccer player – young or old. Due to the inverse relationship of force and velocity during concentric contractions, we can manipulate external load and target a specific adaptation. For example, a 3RM deadlift will produce high amounts of force but move at a slow velocity. Conversely, a barbell countermovement jump would produce low amounts of force but move at high velocity. Due to the nature of the power equation (Power = Force × Velocity) (see Chapter 4), an increase in either force or velocity should lead to greater power outputs. However, to only train for strength is likely to reduce a player's ability to produce force in times specific to the sport. Therefore, the goal of a strength and power programme is to be able to produce larger amounts of force at quicker speeds. Because of an increase in Rate of Force Development, a more explosive player is the result.

As aforementioned, direct power training is not necessary for the foundation- or youth-phase soccer player, rather a form of training more commonly utilised by the professional development phase player. However, there are two important components of power training that young players can learn and develop while progressing through the youth development phase. Firstly, developing technical competency in the movements associated with this form of training will create a strong foundation and enhance the effectiveness of this training in the future. Secondly, learning to perform strength movements with maximum intent will have excellent transfer to the intent required to augment outputs in direct power training [34]. General recommendations when training for power: 3–6 sets, 2–5 repetitions, 3 min + rest between sets. Beyond these general recommendations, more well-trained soccer players, typically in the professional development phase, may benefit from some more advanced methods when training for power. Such methods include Band Resisted, Band Assisted (Overspeed) Post-Activation Potentiation, French Contrast, and Cluster Sets. These methods are designed to manipulate the force velocity curve and nervous system to further enhance explosive power (see Chapter 4).

Plyometrics

Plyometrics are defined as quick and powerful movements that utilise the stretch shortening cycle (SSC), with 'true' or 'fast' plyometrics having a ground contact time of less than 250 ms [35]. Appropriate progression of plyometric training is of the utmost importance as the ground reaction forces accepted by the body's joints can exceed 3–4x bodyweight (BW) for more advanced progressions (Figure 2.7) [36]. If a player is going to produce large amounts

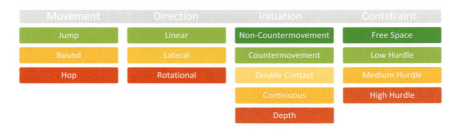

Figure 2.7 Plyometric progression system.

of force and express it in times specific to the sport, then they must have the ability to accept the consequences – the higher the jump, the harder the landing. If a player cannot safely absorb forces in a slow controlled environment, being injured by fast, high force changes in direction and landings in game play, is much more likely. Consequently, technical mastery of landing drills to improve eccentric force absorption is critical, especially in young soccer players. Landing training can be implemented early in a player's development, typically at the start of the youth development programme (YDP). Stiff landings while having the same vertical ground reaction force increase knee flexion/compression forces. Conversely, 'soft' landings will help dissipate forces, reduce knee flexion/compression forces and ultimately injury risk [37].

Despite their effectiveness and most common utilisation in building a foundation prior to more intense drills, landing training is a beneficial injury reduction tools at all stages. Specifically, utilising more challenging options via perturbations, load and obstacles can help prevent ACL injuries (Figure 2.8) [38]. The use of extensive plyometrics not only serves to progress intensity of ground reaction forces but also improves coordination, rhythm, and timing. Continuous sub maximal jumps and hops for higher repetitions are a great way to build tissue resilience.

Some recommendations when prescribing plyometrics: count ground contacts – as a basic rule, the lower the intensity of the plyometric, the higher ground contacts can be tolerated. Later in an academy players career, the intensity and volume of plyometrics will likely need to be manipulated around training/playing schedule as these elements become more intense and frequent. Although limited evidence, general recommendations for recovery time of a plyometric training session is 48–72 hours [39].

Acceleration

One of the easiest ways to improve acceleration is to practise accelerating. When the opportunity to accelerate (in closed conditions) presents itself, such as the warm-up or training drill, perform it with maximum intensity and good technique. Simply practising the skill will contribute towards better projection, rhythm, and coordination, three vital components of acceleration. Greater relative strength and power will maximise the effect of this rehearsal more than just rehearsal itself [40]. This is perhaps the most effective way for the young soccer player to develop acceleration – technique, repetition with intent, and off-field progression.

A crossbridge between accelerating itself and strength/power training is the use of tools such as sleds, prowlers, and adjustable training lines (such as Exergenie). These pieces of equipment can be very effective at overloading key acceleration positions and qualities. This is significant as players will see better transfer to acceleration performance if exercises mimic the motor pattern and contraction type of the movement [41]. When determining sled or Exer-genie resistance, loads resulting in a 75% max velocity loss produce the greatest improvements in 0–5 and 0–10 m performance [42]. Additionally, using different percentages of velocity loss may represent different training zones as per the force velocity curve and helpful prescriptive tool [43]. Alternatively, sled loading of 75% BW seems to optimise peak power output, while loads of up to 130% BW are still effective [43]. Overall, acceleration with any weight has been shown to be better than unresisted for improving acceleration performance [44].

Maximum velocity

The best strategy to improving max velocity is to run at maximum velocity [41]. While there are variations of running drills and specific gym-based exercises that can be done to support this goal, ultimately, all will fall short in the absence of regular sprint training. However, there is an injury risk to doing too much and too little maximum velocity training [45]. As such, it is generally recommended in team sport that there is a minimum of six exposures >85% and a maximum of ten, ensuring one to two bouts at maximum velocity per week to decrease risk and improve sprint performance [46–48]. Outside of sprinting itself, there are a number of other modalities that can positively contribute, such as non-sprint training, sprint training, technical mastery/re-enforcement, and non-linear sprint training. The strong relationship between back squat strength and sprint performance might be explained by the fact that individuals exhibiting greater lower-body strength are able to produce a higher peak ground reaction force (pGRF), impulse, and RFD during each foot strike while running. It is clear from the scientific literature that an individual's overall sprint performance or ability to express higher sprint velocities is impacted by his ability to express high pGRF and impulse.

Non-linear sprint training

Soccer is not played in a straight line and consequently, maximum velocity will not always be required in a straight line [49]. Utilising curvilinear running can help provide a more specific training stimulus. Examples such as arc and s-shaped runs can help replicate the true non-linear running paths seen in gameplay while building resiliency to the ankles and hamstrings as they react to the internal and external rotation moments. Building on this, integrating these runs into game play situations and drills can further assist with the transfer of speed to gameplay, e.g., strikers changing their running path.

Technical mastery

Technique is a critical aspect of running fast and doing it safely [50]. Building timing, coordination and rhythm are key factors when it comes to adapting sprinting speed to the chaos of game play. The drills used must replicate the key technical elements of sprinting to ensure any crossover effect, already limited due to lower movement velocities [41]. All the above can be achieved via technical drills and constraint-based running. Examples of technical drills include A & B Skips/Pops/switch variations, straight leg bounds, and a mixture of all into runs/bleeds. Constraint running can include the use of dowels/aqua bags overhead or in front, integrated into technical drills, linear running, and curvilinear running. Perhaps most common is the use of 'wickets' (cones or mini hurdles) to encourage front-side mechanics, specifically cyclical heel recovery, limb exchange, and direction of foot strike while also manipulating stride length and frequency.

For the young player, it is critical that these sub-components of sprinting performance are not rushed in the name of 'transfer'. Build technical proficiency and training experience in the running patterns, plyometric, and strength training foundations as per previous sections. One of the most effective ways of programming maximum velocity and all its constituents is 'Micro-dosing'.

Microdosing

The realities of sport training are that sometimes dedicated 15–20-minute speed blocks aren't possible, so it is important to find strategies to circumvent the issue; therefore, microdosing is a very effective strategy. The method consists of mini sessions that are high intensity, low volume, and done frequently. In application to maximum velocity, including a maximum effort sprint at the end of a warm-up on two to three occasions throughout a training week is a great way to maintain (and increase) robustness. This can also be done with technical speed drills, non-linear sprinting, and plyometrics, incorporating them as part of a team warm-up to not only prepare for training but to also reinforce key sprinting constituents.

Change of direction

Change of direction (COD) drills can be effectively utilised in a warm-up setting both as session preparation or a training intervention. It is important to recognise that players are exposed to large volumes of direction change during technical drills, team training and games [51]. For the early developing athlete, COD should be trained via free play and games. For example: team evasion games, Cat & Mouse, and 1 v 1 tag games. As players mature, COD training can begin

From academy to professional 41

to capitalise on the dedicated learning of COD postures /positions, translating into closed skill drills to help ingrain these patterns. As a closed skill, two of the fundamental ways to train and improve change of direction are to manipulate the entry velocity and the cutting angle. Both will increase the intensity of the impact at the knee, hip, and ankle and have significant influence over knee valgus moments generated [52]. To progress COD drills, it is suggested to start with slow entry velocity and gradually progress to fast entries (accelerations). Start with small cutting angles and progressively increase the dimensions (Figure 2.9). Ultimately, progressing from planned to unplanned with the inclusion of different auditory and visual stimuli to create a reactive component. The inclusion of a reactive component for young players is of particular benefit in developing a player's cognitive ability to react to stimuli [53].

Ways to progress Y-drill

- Increase cutting angle – cone colour (Red = hardest), increase approach distance and velocity consequently.
- Random call of 'left' or 'right', use person at black triangle to point in direction, use person at black triangle to move in opposite direction.
- Add 2 more cones to the traditional drill, e.g., green and yellow. Then add back pedals, additional cuts, or figure 8s could be used in conjunction with the reactive progressions above (Figure 2.8).
- Use combinations of the above with technical components, e.g., bounce pass off player at black triangle.

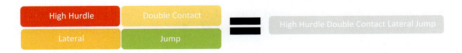

Figure 2.8 An example of exercise selection and how it relates to progression system.

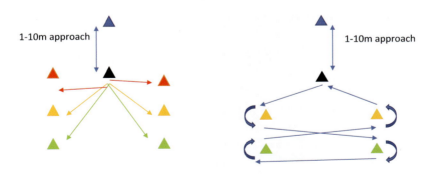

Figure 2.9 Y-drill progressions.

Conditioning

As aforementioned, younger academy players programmes (9–14 years) should not contain specific conditioning interventions, rather, developing qualities via free play, games, team training, and variations. As players progress through the ages and especially into the professional development phase, specific conditioning methods can be implemented to further support players in preparing for the demands of the professional game. Such methods can include low-intensity steady state (time- or distance-based), maximum aerobic speed (MAS) and tempo running (<75% Maximum velocity). In conjunction with such methodologies, small-sided games can begin to be manipulated via pitch size, playing numbers, etc. to emphasise certain physical qualities and global positioning system (GPS) metrics. Governing any conditioning method should be knowledge of work intervals and work:rest ratios. Figure 2.10 provides an outline of recommended durations and work:rest ratios for each energy system and its power and capacity elements. Traditional on-pitch 'conditioning' will focus on the aerobic and glycolytic energy systems, while alactic conditioning is developed via previously discussed qualities (power, speed, etc.). Different ratios will lead to different adaptations; therefore, it is important that a specific goal is thought about prior to the programming of a session, be it small-sided games or running based conditioning.

Programming

The purpose of an academy athletic development programme is to create an environment that provides talent with the best possible chance of progressing. Programmes need to be adaptable and personalised to ensure players maximise their athletic potential and avoid 'survival of the fittest'. An academy benefits from a more stable environment than that of a first team, subsequently contact time can be high.

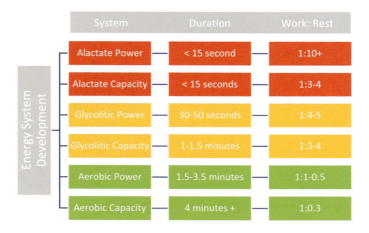

Figure 2.10 Energy system development guide.

With professional soccer getting faster, teams are playing more fixtures with less breaks in the calendar to rest and recover [54]. Consequently, time for athletic development can be limited with staff prioritising technical and tactical sessions in preparation for games [55]. In addition, the life of a soccer player is always changing, players may change clubs, affected by team selection, changes in style of play or position. Therefore, it is vitally important to recognise their time in the academy as precious and utilise it effectively. In addition, a programme needs to ensure players have a level of self-awareness and autonomy to be able to adjust their preparation, training, and recovery to their current situation and thrive in any environment. Athletic development programmes need to strike an appropriate balance between surrounding players with a safe space to develop, whilst ensuring they can be comfortable with chaos and instability.

On-field conditioning

Implementing training models which reflect the environment that youth players are attempting to join, such as the first team, allow for an easier transition when players are called-upon. An academy environment will typically have a much higher number of training sessions due to less competition demands, which provides a great opportunity to isolate conditioning, and optimally develop energy systems and position specific conditioning. Players are exposed to a concurrent training stimulus with on-field conditioning and off-field strength development.

Training models

There are many training models utilised at first team level (see *Chapter 10*) including: 5-Day, 2-Game Week and Midweek Recovery. Including various models on a regular basis in the academy setting helps ensure players are adaptable and helps prepare them for their transition from academy to first team or loan. It is important to establish your training model based on development, environment/culture, and realities of first team soccer. There are various examples of training models in an academy, such as the following.

- **5-Day Training Model:** This model places the toughest training days at the start of the week and reduces volume and intensity towards the game. This works well in an academy setting as it provides the most training opportunities for technical, tactical, and physical adaptation. Within this model, players can be exposed to a high gym load Monday to Wednesday with plenty of opportunities for additional physical sessions.
- **2-Game Week:** It's so important players are exposed to this model within the academy system as players are frequently required to play games with limited recovery. The two games should be separated by two to four days and if competition demands don't allow this to occur, it should be artificially replicated through 11v11 in training or the arranging of friendlies. This training model is fantastic for conditioning and allows players to develop their own recovery techniques to cope with these demands. However, it

does limit opportunities for physical development in other areas with the focus switching to recovery. This is a really important point to emphasise with young academy players. Once their careers begin in the adult game it is unlikely, they will get another situation whereby they are exposed to so many training opportunities to work on aspects of their game away from the match.
- **Midweek Recovery:** This model separates the two toughest training session with a recovery day in between. It is a great alternative to the five-day model and helps protect against training monotony. There is still ample opportunity for physical development off the field throughout the week between Monday and Thursday. It also allows a mental down day midweek for players to focus primarily on schooling.

Types of training days

Training needs to provide a sufficient stimulus to prepare players for the demands of the game. Practitioners should strive to achieve this through soccer-based practices wherever possible to support training specificity. However, isolated running practices do serve a purpose within the training day as they allow a practitioner to target an energy system with more specificity. Isolated running drills are also a good opportunity to practise correct running mechanics. Physical recommendations need to be flexible enough to support the technical and tactical theme of the session outlined by the technical coach. By providing coaches with an adaptable framework, we can ensure players are exposed to all physical aspects of the game within a training week and can ensure optimal physical development alongside their progression as soccer players.

The physical themes below allow practitioners to provide training sessions with a specific emphasis but aren't intended to act as a one-size-fits-all approach. For an in-depth look at training days, see *Chapter 10*.

Intensive days

- High in accelerations & decelerations
- High intensity
- Shorter work periods
- Smaller spaces

Extensive days

- High in total distance
- High in high-speed running and sprint distance
- Max velocity sprinting
- Longer work periods
- Larger spaces

Hybrid (intensive/extensive) days

- Combination of intensive/extensive principles
- Commonly performed four days out from match if middle day in week is given off

Reactive speed days

- Quality over quantity approach
- Reduced high speed and sprint distance
- Work periods short
- If performed coming off a day off, this session can incorporate max velocity sprinting exposure

Pre-match days

- Low total distance
- Non fatiguing reactive and potentiation physical work
- Work periods short

Second-day recovery ('re-entry') days (MD+2)

- Low intensive actions
- Adaptable day depending on individual recovery status
- Moderate work periods
- Small to medium spaces

Avoiding monotony

With a high number of training sessions, it's imperative to avoid training monotony as this can lead to a plateau in athletic development and increased injury risk. Strategies to mitigate against monotony include:

- **Order of Session:** Vary the placement of your most intense practices within the session. The first five minutes of a game is often the most intense, so place intense periods at the start of training from time to time.
- **Rest Periods:** During a game, rest periods would only occur due to stoppages in play and players are expected to play continuously for 45 minutes. Consider rest periods both within and between practices to provide variation.
- **Training Models:** Regularly include various training models. Where possible, arrange fixtures mid-week or replicate a 2-game week with a high training stimulus.
- **Time of Day:** Vary training times between morning, afternoon, and evening. This may also provide an opportunity to prescribe strength training before training with less fatigue.

Creating the right environment

It is imperative to create an environment that supports the modern-day player and allows them to challenge themselves to maximise athletic potential. Finding the appropriate balance between an enjoyable, sociable space where individuals feel comfortable, whilst also aspiring to create a challenging environment for players to grow. It's important to start with non-negotiables and ensure these are clearly communicated and agreed. These will be specific to your environment but centre around respect for each other and the facility, appropriate clothing and footwear, punctuality, and willingness to work.

To encourage healthy competition, simple additions such as large leader boards are a great way to get players thinking about their efforts and is where technology can make a huge difference. For example, provision of instantaneous feedback when performing max velocity squat jumps has shown to support athletes in maintaining a greater jump intensity throughout the training intervention. Subsequently they showed greater improvements in horizontal jump and 30 m sprint performance [20].

Limitations and challenges

A player's development pathway typically involves multifactorial challenges caused by changes in different areas (i.e. athletic, psychological, psychosocial, and academic) which he or she needs to cope with in order to progress [7, 16]. Simultaneously, players mature from childhood into adolescence into adulthood; transitions that are characterised by accelerated changes in non-sport specific areas such as social and cognitive functioning. Considering such changes, it can be argued that the overall development process, in addition to his or her soccer education, has a profound impact on both the player as well as the individual. Therefore, the aim of this section is to highlight some of the main concerns regarding the holistic development of young players that should be addressed appropriately by practitioners and any stakeholders with a direct involvement in player development.

Biological maturation and physical development

One of the biggest and most common challenges young players face early on in their career are those linked to biological maturation and physical growth and development. Ironically, while maturation is an individual biological process, it is the environment that is created by others that often has the biggest impact on the physical development of young players, which will ultimately shape their formative years. Key concepts that should be acknowledged and considered when designing a nurturing and effective development strategy include chronological age, biological age, and training age. Chronological age refers to the exact age of a player at one moment in time relative to his or her date of birth. A player's biological age indicates the progress to a physically mature state,

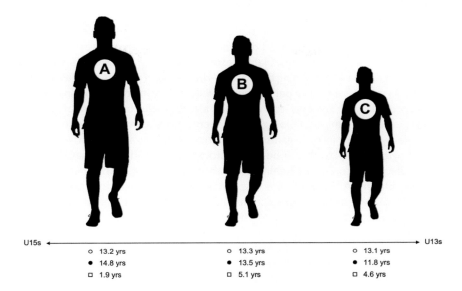

Figure 2.11 Chronological (o), biological (●), and training age (□) of hypothetical U14s players A, B, and C.

irrespective of chronological age, while training age refers to the number of years that a player has been participating in structured and deliberate practice. While they all represent an area-specific age, a linear relationship between all three concepts cannot be assumed. Consequently, academy players within the same squad who have a similar chronological age can vary significantly in terms of biological and training age (Figure 2.11).

As is quite common in any other educational setting, academy players are traditionally categorised into training groups according to their chronological age. However, such categorisation may not always be the most suitable means of classifying children and adolescents involved in competitive sports. Research on the relative age effect has investigated the presence of significant anthropometric differences between players, following skewed birth-date distributions and meaningful chronological age differences within the same age groups [56]. However, when chronological age differences between players within the same selection year are eliminated or deemed negligible, adolescents still grow and mature at a different rate. Therefore, players of the same chronological age can differ greatly in biological maturity, resulting in significant physical (dis)advantages compared to their peers [57, 58]. Such a relative superior or inferior physical capacity during developmental stages can have a massive impact on individual performance and selection [3, 59, 60]. Consequently, it could deny young talents equal opportunities and quality attention, ultimately affecting their chances to progress and maximise their potential. Moreover, a chronological categorisation could present detrimental effects on physical fitness as players within the same age group who differ in biological maturity are subject to the same loads during generic team-based training sessions, while potentially being less robust to cope with imposed demands. This ultimately can result in an increased risk of injury. When available resources enable practitioners to do so, they are urged to tailor training sessions to the needs of players as effectively as possible to maximise soccer performance while mitigating the risk of injury [61].

As chronological age fails to represent a meaningful indication of physical maturity, the assessment of biological age seems more appropriate when grouping academy players in an organised competitive environment. Relative to their chronological age, players can be either biologically ahead (early maturing), 'on time' (average maturing) or behind their chronological age (late maturing). For example, players A, B, and C are respectively early, average, and late maturing (Figure 2.10). An effective approach that has been adopted extensively to assess and track biological maturation is through regular anthropometric measurement [62]. A consistent collection of somatic data (i.e. stature, seated height, leg length, and body mass) allows practitioners to identify and monitor sensitive periods of accelerated growth by providing valuable estimates on the predicted age of PHV and maturity offset (i.e. time prior to or following PHV) [63–65]. For example, by calculating maturity offset as a numerical value relative to a player's chronological age at the time of measurement, the age at which PHV occurs can be determined as the difference between chronological age and maturity offset (Figure 2.12). More recently, rather than using 'maturity offset' as a key variable, it has been argued that the application of a 'maturity ratio' (i.e. chronological age relative to age at PHV) presents a more reliable and accurate indicator of the non-linear growth process [65].

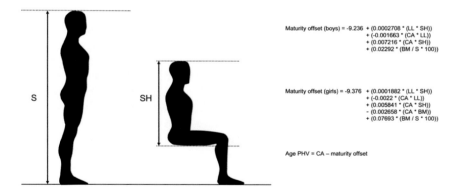

Figure 2.12 Anthropometric measurement and calculation to determine predicted maturity offset and age at peak-height velocity (PHV). S = stature, SH = seated height, LL = leg length (= S-SH), CA = chronological age, BM = body mass (Adjusted equations for predicted maturity offset by Kozieł, S.M. and R.M. Malina [64]

Identifying these periods is key when developing young talent, as it has been evidenced that players approaching PHV are at an increased risk of developing acute and chronic injuries [61, 62]. The time spent at PHV is often characterised by an increased rate of bone growth disproportionate to muscle lengthening, resulting in a phenomenon often referred to as 'adolescent awkwardness'. Imbalances between bone growth and muscle lengthening can impede neuromuscular function and cause structural damage [66, 67]. Muscular integrity is usually compromised following the exposure of soft tissue to superior stress and repetitive loads when participating in untailored performance-driven sessions. Logically, the most common injuries include muscle tears and ligament sprains (see Chapter 9). Other overuse injuries can be attributed to reductions in the regulation of overall body control, such as proprioception, flexibility, and stability [61].

Quantifying biological maturity will allow appropriate interventions to be taken sooner rather than later. The overall volume and specific content of training for 'at-risk' players (e.g. players within 6 months of their PHV, before or after) should be monitored closely. Avoiding excessive loads and high-explosive actions will reduce the risk of injury, as sudden rapid and repetitive eccentric contractions can cause severe strain on the tendons and ligaments of muscles that are already 'playing catch-up' with the growth rate of a developing body. In addition to a reduction in cumulative training load, special attention to re-optimise technical movement patterns and to enhance mobility and strength to facilitate neuromuscular function and control is recommended. While proportionally less time is usually allocated to strength training, this might be the perfect window to increase the volume and time spent in the gym. To answer the need for a more maturity-appropriate environment on the pitch, bio-banding has become an established approach in academy soccer in recent years [68, 69]. The concept of bio-banding focuses on grouping players during training and games based on physical attributes associated with their individual growth and maturation, rather than chronological age. From a physical development perspective, bio-banding can enable players to engage in a challenging and competitive format with their similar-mature peers, while avoiding regular exposure to superior physical demands they are not ready to cope with yet, allowing an appropriate and undisrupted growth process.

Like biological age, training age can vary amongst players within the same squad. Someone with a greater training age is more able to cope with an increased complexity of training compared to someone of a lower training age. Therefore, practitioners need to consider both biological and training age when planning and designing training programmes and aim to tailor their sessions to the significant differences and needs of players, to maximise development and performance while mitigating the risk of injury and increasing player availability.

Education

School and soccer can clash with increased regularity as young players progress through the development stages, most commonly due to inefficient time management or conflicts of interests. Therefore, understanding the role of education and the way it can be presented and experienced is crucial in finding an appropriate balance that offers the best of both. It is important to note that schools and soccer clubs are both educational institutes. Soccer academies are in fact soccer schools where players are students. As such, both offer a high level of interaction with educators and exposure to a social environment that is characterised by a wide variety of age groups, personalities, and sociocultural backgrounds. All these factors shape psychosocial development. While schools initially focus on general knowledge and academic performance to prepare students for a professional career that could span a lifetime, soccer academies target an education in a very specific industry where athletic performance is key for survival in a career that could just span up to 15 years. Taking these considerations into account, clubs and their academies are urged to encourage and support school education while also nurturing and fuelling the passion for soccer, regardless of where the player's initial priorities may lie.

Considering the low retention rate in soccer due to drop-out or deselection – only 0.5% of the number of registered youth players worldwide are listed as professional soccer players – it is in everybody's best interest that the quality of both development plans is of the highest level [70]. Only when a balanced collaboration in terms of time and educational content is achieved, will all three stakeholders (player, school, and academy) benefit the most. Some great initiatives that offer an effective school-soccer balance include performance schools. Talented young players are enrolled in (online) educational programmes which are aimed to give them the opportunity of sufficient daily soccer practice within an academic environment without having to sacrifice valuable school time. Another example are partnerships between schools and academies where tutors are deployed to improve the student-athlete's study time and increase individual attention.

More and more clubs are acknowledging their role as an educational institute, by intensifying their investment in coach and player education that specifically focuses on soccer-specific topics to maximise development and performance. Coach education through courses aimed at continuous professional development (CPD) should be a key pillar in the development strategy driven by any club/academy management. Given the amount of overall contact time they have with players, coaches are often in the best possible position to deliver soccer-relevant interventions and reinforce key messages that promote learning and maximise functional capacity and cognitive development. Creating better coaches leads to better mentoring, which leads to better player development. While many opportunities for CPD are already offered externally by national federations and governing bodies, clubs should look to provide their coaches with as much support as possible, either by organising quality educational interventions themselves, or by funding courses outside of the club. Player education in key areas such as training principles, lifestyle, recovery, nutrition, and sleep will help players develop valuable attributes such as increased self-awareness and the ability to make informed decisions autonomously. Most importantly, it will empower them to take ownership and responsibility for their own career as a soccer player. Considering the time players spend away from the club and the abundancy of factors with an immediate impact on performance, lifestyle training is a key development area that offers insights on how players can develop good habits and build an effective daily routine, to support optimal short- and long-term performance levels. It is important that internal education courses are given with consistent regularity (e.g. monthly presentations, workshops, etc.) and that these emphasise the meaning and consequences of training and lifestyle principles (i.e. understanding the 'why' and 'how') rather than on practicing the principles themselves (i.e. knowing the 'what') to increase competence and to avoid nurturing a dependency culture.

Psychological wellbeing and performance mindset

From an early age, young players typically show high motivation levels to play soccer, which in addition to genuine passion for the game ties into a strong sense of belonging. Common risks that can have an impact on motivation include deselection following a performance-driven philosophy, bullying, and injuries. Failure and/or pressure to perform can further increase insecurity and harm an already fragile state of mind. Players who fail to successfully cope with such experiences will eventually drop out of the club and potentially the sport, as they have lost all desire to continue to pursue a career in soccer. To prevent such outcomes, investing in a long-term strategy of handing players effective coping mechanisms and thus building mentally resilient players should be a key priority for academies. Following an increased awareness to safeguard and promote psychological wellbeing, practitioners should strive to ensure an academy environment that always protects principles such as respect and equality regardless of personality, ability, and background. Additionally, a mental health officer and sports psychologists can be appointed to further maximise mental support.

One contemporary threat that seems to present itself with increased regularity among gifted young players is a lack of relentless determination. One of the main barriers between academy teams and a first team is the consistency in performance output. Being the best for one day is insignificant to being the best every day. While moving up through the age groups, youth players try to mimic and mirror themselves to senior players as much as possible in terms of behaviour and style of playing. However, a potential turning point in their development occurs when they start focusing more on the perceived benefits of being a first-team player, rather than on the sacrifices that are required to make the first team in the first place. This misconception breads a potential mismatch between their expectations and their reality: they confuse what they believe the life of a player is like (e.g. the minute proportion of a player's life that appears on television and social media) for what a player needs to do (i.e. adopt a full-time performance lifestyle and mindset). Unfortunately, in some cases, this mismatch is intensified by the increased support (e.g. better facilities and equipment, and improved contracts) and attention players are given (e.g. media exposure and player agents) while progressing through the ranks. This has the potential to create an unrealistic perception of their own status and an inappropriate sense of entitlement that is toxic for the team culture and their own development. As a result, some senior talents develop a lack of urgency to prove themselves, consequently failing to deliver consistent high-level performances and denying themselves the opportunity to bridge the gap between academy and senior soccer. While a lack of intrinsic motivation will never lead to a durable career, practitioners are urged to inspire rather than motivate their players, by leading by example and reinforcing the message that talent will only get a player in the club, whereas consistency will get a player in the team. Additionally, media training and mentoring programmes linking senior players to academy talents, to increase a sense of awareness and reality, might be effective strategies in installing a performance mindset.

Conclusion

Developing the modern-day professional soccer player requires deep understanding of the phases of development, as well as the key physical qualities required to excel at professional level. Practitioners must be aware of the various challenges players will experience along the way including maturation, psychological wellbeing, and balancing education. Putting it all together from a programming perspective is key to the long-term athletic development of each player in the developmental pathway. Finally, ensuring that developing players goes beyond just the field and gym, as overall development as a person will help them pre, during, and post career as a professional soccer player.

References

1. Varghese, M., S. Ruparell, and C. LaBella, *Youth athlete development models: a narrative review.* Sports Health, 2022. **14**(1): p. 20–29.
2. Deprez, D., et al., *Relative age, biological maturation and anaerobic characteristics in elite youth soccer players.* International Journal of Sports Medicine, 2013. **34**(10): p. 897–903.
3. Malina, R.M., et al., *Maturity-associated variation in the growth and functional capacities of youth football (soccer) players 13–15 years.* European Journal of Applied Physiology, 2004. **91**(5): p. 555–562.
4. Philippaerts, R.M., et al., *The relationship between peak height velocity and physical performance in youth soccer players.* Journal of Sports Sciences, 2006. **24**(3): p. 221–230.
5. Di Mascio, M., et al., *Soccer-specific reactive repeated-sprint ability in elite youth soccer players: maturation trends and association with various physical performance tests.* The Journal of Strength & Conditioning Research, 2020. **34**(12): p. 3538–3545.
6. Hammami, R., et al., *Associations between balance and muscle strength, power performance in male youth athletes of different maturity status.* Pediatric Exercise Science, 2016. **28**(4): p. 521–534.

7 Lloyd, R.S., et al., *Long-term athletic development-part 1: a pathway for all youth.* The Journal of Strength & Conditioning Research, 2015. **29**(5): p. 1439–1450.
8 Lovell, T., et al., *Factors affecting sports involvement in a school-based youth cohort: implications for long-term athletic development.* Journal of Sports Sciences, 2019. **37**(22): p. 2522–2529.
9 Meylan, C.M., et al., *Adjustment of measures of strength and power in youth male athletes differing in body mass and maturation.* Pediatric Exercise Science, 2014. **26**(1): p. 41–48.
10 Deprez, D., et al., *Characteristics of high-level youth soccer players: variation by playing position.* Journal of Sports Sciences, 2015. **33**(3): p. 243–254.
11 Fransen, J., et al., *Modelling age-related changes in motor competence and physical fitness in high-level youth soccer players: implications for talent identification and development.* Science and Medicine in Football, 2017. **1**(3): p. 203–208.
12 Wing, C.E., A.N. Turner, and C.J. Bishop, *Importance of strength and power on key performance indicators in elite youth soccer.* The Journal of Strength & Conditioning Research, 2020. **34**(7): p. 2006–2014.
13 Unnithan, V., et al., *Talent identification in youth soccer.* Journal of Sports Sciences, 2012. **30**(15): p. 1719–1726.
14 Balyi, I., R. Way, and C. Higgs, *Long-term athlete development.* 2013: Human Kinetics.
15 Ford, P., et al. *The developmental activities of elite international soccer players aged 16 years.* In *16th Annual ECSS-Congress*, Liverpool. 2011.
16 Lloyd, R.S. and J.L. Oliver, *The youth physical development model: a new approach to long-term athletic development.* Strength & Conditioning Journal, 2012. **34**(3): p. 61–72.
17 Quatman-Yates, C.C., et al., *A systematic review of sensorimotor function during adolescence: a developmental stage of increased motor awkwardness?* British Journal of Sports Medicine, 2012. **46**(9): p. 649–655.
18 Wachholz, F., et al., *Adolescent awkwardness: alterations in temporal control characteristics of posture with maturation and the relation to movement exploration.* Brain Sciences, 2020. **10**(4): p. 216.
19 Schwieger, D. and C. Ladwig, *Reaching and retaining the next generation: adapting to the expectations of Gen Z in the classroom.* Information Systems Education Journal, 2018. **16**(3): p. 45.
20 Randell, A.D., et al., *Effect of instantaneous performance feedback during 6 weeks of velocity-based resistance training on sport-specific performance tests.* The Journal of Strength & Conditioning Research, 2011. **25**(1): p. 87–93.
21 Mostafavifar, A.M., T.M. Best, and G.D. Myer, *Early sport specialisation, does it lead to long-term problems?* BMJ Publishing Group Ltd and British Association of Sport and Exercise Medicine. 2013. p. 1060–1061.
22 Carter, C.W. and L.J. Micheli, *Training the child athlete: physical fitness, health and injury.* British Journal of Sports Medicine, 2011. **45**(11): p. 880–885.
23 Curlik, D.M., et al., *Physical skill training increases the number of surviving new cells in the adult hippocampus.* PLoS One, 2013. **8**(2): p. e55850.
24 Pichardo, A.W., et al., *Integrating models of long-term athletic development to maximize the physical development of youth.* International Journal of Sports Science & Coaching, 2018. **13**(6): p. 1189–1199.
25 Strøyer, J., L. Hansen, and K. Klausen, *Physiological profile and activity pattern of young soccer players during match play.* Medicine and Science in Sports and Exercise, 2004. **36**(1): p. 168–174.
26 Chamari, K., et al., *Endurance training and testing with the ball in young elite soccer players.* British Journal of Sports Medicine, 2005. **39**(1): p. 24–28.
27 Prue, P., M. McGuigan, and R. Newton, *Influence of strength on magnitude and mechanisms of adaptation to power training.* Medicine & Science in Sports & Exercise, 2010. **42**: p. 1566–1581.

28 Loturco, I., et al., *Maximum acceleration performance of professional soccer players in linear sprints: is there a direct connection with change-of-direction ability?* PLoS One, 2019. **14**(5): p. e0216806.
29 Edouard, P., et al., *Sprinting: a potential vaccine for hamstring injury.* Sport Performance & Science Reports, 2019. **1**: p. 1–2.
30 Faude, O., T. Koch, and T. Meyer, *Straight sprinting is the most frequent action in goal situations in professional football.* Journal of Sports Sciences, 2012. **30**(7): p. 625–631.
31 Castillo-Rodríguez, A., et al., *Relationship between muscular strength and sprints with changes of direction.* The Journal of Strength & Conditioning Research, 2012. **26**(3): p. 725–732.
32 Lee, S.J., et al., *Effects of pivoting neuromuscular training on pivoting control and proprioception.* Medicine and Science in Sports and Exercise, 2014. **46**(7): p. 1400.
33 Shattock, K. and J. Tee, *Autoregulation in resistance training: a comparison of subjective versus objective methods.* Journal of Strength and Conditioning Research, 2022. **36**(3): p. 641–648.
34 Kawamori, N. and R.U. Newton, *Velocity specificity of resistance training: actual movement velocity versus intention to move explosively.* Strength and Conditioning Journal, 2006. **28**(2): p. 86.
35 Turner, A.N. and I. Jeffreys, *The stretch-shortening cycle: proposed mechanisms and methods for enhancement.* Strength & Conditioning Journal, 2010. **32**(4): p. 87–99.
36 Wallace, B.J., et al., *Quantification of vertical ground reaction forces of popular bilateral plyometric exercises.* The Journal of Strength & Conditioning Research, 2010. **24**(1): p. 207–212.
37 Verniba, D., et al., *The analysis of knee joint loading during drop landing from different heights and under different instruction sets in healthy males.* Sports Medicine-Open, 2017. **3**(1): p. 1–9.
38 Herrington, L.C. and P. Comfort, *Training for prevention of ACL injury: incorporation of progressive landing skill challenges into a program.* Strength & Conditioning Journal, 2013. **35**(6): p. 59–65.
39 Davies, G., B.L. Riemann, and R. Manske, *Current concepts of plyometric exercise.* International Journal of Sports Physical Therapy, 2015. **10**(6): p. 760.
40 Wisløff, U., et al., *Strong correlation of maximal squat strength with sprint performance and vertical jump height in elite soccer players.* British Journal of Sports Medicine, 2004. **38**(3): p. 285–288.
41 Haugen, T., et al., *The training and development of elite sprint performance: an integration of scientific and best practice literature.* Sports Medicine-Open, 2019. **5**(1): p. 1–16.
42 Cahill, M.J., et al., *Sled-push load-velocity profiling and implications for sprint training prescription in young athletes.* The Journal of Strength & Conditioning Research, 2021. **35**(11): p. 3084–3089.
43 Cross, M.R., et al., *Optimal loading for maximizing power during sled-resisted sprinting.* International Journal of Sports Physiology and Performance, 2017. **12**(8): p. 1069–1077.
44 Cahill, M.J., et al., *Influence of resisted sled-push training on the sprint force-velocity profile of male high school athletes.* Scandinavian Journal of Medicine & Science in Sports, 2020. **30**(3): p. 442–449.
45 Haugen, T., *The role and development of sprinting speed in soccer.* 2014: Universitet i Agder/University of Agder.
46 Tønnessen, E., et al., *The effect of 40-m repeated sprint training on maximum sprinting speed, repeated sprint speed endurance, vertical jump, and aerobic capacity in young elite male soccer players.* The Journal of Strength & Conditioning Research, 2011. **25**(9): p. 2364–2370.

47 Malone, S., et al., *High-speed running and sprinting as an injury risk factor in soccer: can well-developed physical qualities reduce the risk?* Journal of Science and Medicine in Sport, 2018. **21**(3): p. 257–262.
48 Malone, S., et al., *High chronic training loads and exposure to bouts of maximal velocity running reduce injury risk in elite Gaelic football.* Journal of Science and Medicine in Sport, 2017. **20**(3): p. 250–254.
49 Nicholson, B., et al., *Sprint development practices in elite football code athletes.* International Journal of Sports Science & Coaching, 2021: p. 17479541211019687.
50 Colyer, S.L., et al., *How sprinters accelerate beyond the velocity plateau of soccer players: waveform analysis of ground reaction forces.* Scandinavian Journal of Medicine & Science in Sports, 2018. **28**(12): p. 2527–2535.
51 Harper, D.J., C. Carling, and J. Kiely, *High-intensity acceleration and deceleration demands in elite team sports competitive match play: a systematic review and meta-analysis of observational studies.* Sports Medicine, 2019. **49**(12): p. 1923–1947.
52 Dai, B., et al., *The effects of 2 landing techniques on knee kinematics, kinetics, and performance during stop-jump and side-cutting tasks.* The American Journal of Sports Medicine, 2015. **43**(2): p. 466–474.
53 Lloyd, R.S., et al., *Considerations for the development of agility during childhood and adolescence.* Strength & Conditioning Journal, 2013. **35**(3): p. 2–11.
54 Barnes, C., et al., *The evolution of physical and technical performance parameters in the English Premier League.* International Journal of Sports Medicine, 2014. **35**(13): p. 1095–1100.
55 Rønnestad, B.R., B.S. Nymark, and T. Raastad, *Effects of in-season strength maintenance training frequency in professional soccer players.* The Journal of Strength & Conditioning Research, 2011. **25**(10): p. 2653–2660.
56 Gil, S.M., et al., *Relationship between the relative age effect and anthropometry, maturity and performance in young soccer players.* Journal of Sports Sciences, 2014. **32**(5): p. 479–86.
57 Malina, R.M., et al., *Biological maturation of youth athletes: assessment and implications.* British Journal of Sports Medicine, 2015. **49**(13): p. 852–859.
58 Towlson, C., et al., *One of these things is not like the other: time to differentiate between relative age and biological maturity selection biases in soccer?* Science and Medicine in Football, 2022. **6**(3): p. 273–276.
59 Helsen, W.F., J. Van Winckel, and A.M. Williams, *The relative age effect in youth soccer across Europe.* Journal of Sports Sciences, 2005. **23**(6): p. 629–636.
60 Parr, J., et al., *The main and interactive effects of biological maturity and relative age on physical performance in elite youth soccer players.* Journal of Sports Medicine, 2020: p. 1–11.
61 Towlson, C., et al., *Maturity-associated considerations for training load, injury risk, and physical performance in youth soccer: one size does not fit all.* Journal of Sport and Health Science, 2021. **10**(4): p. 403–412.
62 Mirwald, R.L., et al., *An assessment of maturity from anthropometric measurements.* Medicine and Science in Sports and Exercise, 2002. **34**(4): p. 689–694.
63 Moore, S.A., et al., *Enhancing a somatic maturity prediction model.* Medicine & Science in Sports & Exercise, 2015. **47**(8): p. 1755–64.
64 Kozieł, S.M. and R.M. Malina, *Modified maturity offset prediction equations: validation in independent longitudinal samples of boys and girls.* Sports Medicine, 2018. **48**(1): p. 221–236.
65 Fransen, J., et al., *Improving the prediction of maturity from anthropometric variables using a maturity ratio.* Pediatric Exercise Science, 2018. **30**(2): p. 296–307.
66 Davies, P.L. and J.D. Rose, *Motor skills of typically developing adolescents: awkwardness or improvement?* Physical & Occupational Therapy in Pediatrics, 2000. **20**(1): p. 19–42.

67 Sheehan, D.P. and K. Lienhard, *Gross motor competence and peak height velocity in 10- to 14-year-old Canadian youth: a longitudinal study.* Measurement in Physical Education and Exercise Science, 2019. **23**(1): p. 89–98.
68 Malina, R.M., et al., *Bio-banding in youth sports: background, concept, and application.* Sports Medicine, 2019. **49**(11): p. 1671–1685.
69 Romann, M., D. Lüdin, and D.-P. Born, *Bio-banding in junior soccer players: a pilot study.* BMC Research Notes, 2020. **13**(1): p. 1–5.
70 Carpels, T., et al., *Youth-to-senior transition in Elite European Club Soccer.* International Journal of Exercise Science, 2021. **14**(6): p. 1192–1203.

3 Needs analysis and testing

Jarred Marsh, Alex Calder, Jordan Stewart-Mackie and Martin Buchheit

Overview of testing

Systematic testing of human physiology has been used for decades to determine the physical state of athletes and their readiness to train or compete in their chosen sport. Historically, the pursuit of understanding how our bodies function under exercise began in the early 1900s when Nobel Prize winner and experimentalist August Krogh began investigating the active role of capillaries during muscle contraction and exercise [1]. Similarly, published work assessed muscle activity and running performance to determine the secrets behind elite runners' success [2, 3]. However, while the early work has been criticised almost 90 years later [4], the research of these early pioneers created a need to understand the physiology of the human body and its response to exercise.

Over the next ten decades, investigation of the human physiology and physical capacities has evolved significantly. From early analysis of anaerobic work and recovery [5], predicting VO_{2max} through the Beep test [6], and Yo-Yo test [7], to most recently the development of the 30-15 Intermittent Fitness test (30-15$_{IFT}$) [8]. As our understanding of physiology, and our response to exercises, evolve, so too must the exercise tests that are designed to determine our physical state. While many of these early testing protocols were originally designed to assess members of the general population, the desire to improve physical performance in professional athletes has created the need for more sport-specific testing procedures. It is through these procedures that we can develop performance baselines for our athletes and teams.

Developing the performance baselines of athletes allows practitioners and coaches alike to more accurately prescribe training programmes to develop major physiological qualities. However, it is important to determine what testing procedures can and should be used, and which key areas should be assessed within the testing and training environment.

Performance, monitoring, and injury risk

Understanding the principal role of physical testing is important when outlining the best practical approach. Historically, the testing procedures have evaluated players' physical fitness through assessing isolated physiological categories, such as aerobic capacity, strength, agility, speed, and power. Traditionally, coaching staffs would assess how effective players were within isolated tests, and, in turn, use this performance data to establish individual performance benchmarks and tailor training programmes.

However, with the advancement in sport science and medical assessments, these tests have evolved to evaluate both performance and injury risk [9]. Understanding the individual player's capacity can also highlight their physical limitations at that stage of the training programme. For example, if a player scores lower on the preseason Yo-Yo IR2 test, than the mean value for the squad, should they train differently? If so, should they train more or less than the rest of the squad for the preseason period? Lower physical capacity might reveal that the player is unable to compete at the same level as their teammates and therefore will need to be managed until their capacity improves. In the same manner, a player who presents a significant asymmetry or imbalance in various tests can potentially have an increased risk of injury [10]. This should be considered when planning the individual training load.

Through assessing training load, we can determine an individual player's readiness to train. This refers to a player's current physical state and is used to determine their training load for the upcoming session. Assessment procedures and measurements such as Counter Movement Jump (CMJ) height, wellness questionnaires, hamstring and adductor strength, and biomarkers such as heart rate variability, *IgA*, and cortisol can all show an athlete's level of residual fatigue and their readiness to train [11–14]. These testing data can allow coaches and practitioners to make more informed decisions around training sessions and individual player involvement.

Preseason testing

Historically, teams have opened their preseason training period with physical testing. While competition calendars vary across the globe, most teams would generally have a minimum two to four week 'off-season' where players would be able to rest and regenerate physically and mentally. Players are often issued with training programmes to complete on their own in a bid to stay ready for the upcoming preseason training period. Some players could potentially hire practitioners within their respected club, or more commonly, consult externally to coach them through their off-season period. However, with more competitive games being scheduled (i.e. international duty, cup games, tours, etc.), into an already-congested calendar, the off-season period inherently becoming shorter. Players may then choose to rest completely in a bid to avoid burnout [15]. As a result of undertraining, players may return to preseason training in a detrained state and, therefore, have an increased risk of injury [16]. Additionally, coaches and practitioners need to investigate whether it is safe to conduct testing on the first day of training or spread the testing procedure out over different periods of the pre-season phase.

Specifically, scheduling testing across the first few weeks of the preseason period allows players to get back into training first and build some chronic load (tolerance), prior to maximum testing.

When to test

Spreading testing protocols across the pre-season poses a dilemma to a technical team. The coaching and performance staff will be eager to know the physical state of the players, in order to appropriately design and implement training prescriptions in the short preparation period prior to the commencement of the season. By performing submaximal testing and screening on the first day of pre-season (e.g. anthropometrics, submaximal aerobic assessment, etc.), the performance staff are able to determine some baseline data while identifying and addressing injury risk. Furthermore, conducting fitness and strength and power tests that require maximal effort may aid practitioners in initial prescriptions. Conducting maximal fitness tests, such as the Yo-Yo and repeat sprint ability tests, give practitioners knowledge of specific cardiovascular and muscular capabilities of the players [17, 18]. Therefore, early knowledge of maximal output tests can help practitioners gather insight to individual players' maximal thresholds, such as maximum heart rate (HR_{max}), maximum oxygen uptake (VO_{2max}), and maximum velocity (V_{max}). With maximum thresholds, specific prescriptions can be put in place (based of a percentage of the maximum output), to enhance likelihood of desired adaptations. Similarly, conducting maximal strength tests can also help practitioners prescribe exercise variables via percentages of their 1-repetition max (%1RM). Practitioners will be able to effectively programme throughout the entirety of the pre-season phase with early knowledge of submaximal and maximal testing protocols. However, conducting a battery of tests within the first week of pre-season has its limitations.

Delaying the commencement of pre-season tests that require maximum efforts from players provides many benefits in the long term. The above-mentioned maximal tests, such as the Yo-Yo and repeat spring ability tests, offer many useful pieces of data, however, need to be scheduled with caution. As mentioned previously, scheduling maximally demanding tests on within the first week of pre-season comes with potential risks, due to the unknown fitness status of players post off-season. For instance, a lack of off-season training compliance could result in players arriving to the first day of pre-season in a detrained state. As an example, exposing players to maximum outputs, such as V_{max}, without the presence of a high-chronic workload (accumulated sprint distance over four weeks), could increase the risk of injury [19]. Thus, maximum testing procedures need to be scheduled with consideration to players' training and injury history, as well as the proposed pre-season loads and objectives. While this process may seem drawn out, allowing more time for testing reinforces player safety by reducing injury risk, thereby enhancing player availability at a key stage in the preparation period. While maximal-output testing can still take place in the pre-season, it is recommended that submaximal-demanding tests are completed first, with adequate time for players to adapt to the initial pre-season training stimulus prior to the remainder of the testing battery.

Testing for injury risk

Another important aspect is the ability to interpret data to establish individual injury baselines. Inevitably, players may sustain injuries or illness throughout the season and these baseline data is used as a guideline to help the medical and performance staff build the conditioning of the player back to their pre-injury baseline values (*see Chapter 9*). These data will also help practitioners in accurately determining the fitness status of players through the season. The performance staff should plan for retesting periodically throughout the season. It is important to use the initial baseline data as a starting point in building the players' physical capacity and robustness over the coming months. Assessing the players' progress from this initial baseline will determine the success of the strength and conditioning programme and need for potential adjustments, should the players not achieve the desired outcomes. The performance staff will need to determine the most appropriate time to retest the team. For example, certain tests may warrant weekly monitoring (assessing anthropometrics and readiness to train), six-week intervals (i.e., post-preseason), or three-month intervals (i.e. quarterly). There are, of course, different aspects to consider when scheduling the testing procedures, as not all tests need to be conducted in the same period. However, targeting the correct physical testing process at the right time is integral in achieving the desired outcome and actionable data.

Performance tests

The approach

Once establishing the needs analysis of the cohort, positions and individuals, practitioners can make clear judgment in test exercise selection. It is important to approach the test exercise selection with a systematic process (Figure 3.1). As aforementioned, practitioners need to carefully select testing protocols that are measurable and that can appropriately transfer to the performance of the team. Hence, outlining the overall objective of the exercise chosen to test. For example, practitioners should ask the following questions;

− Why are we conducting this test?
− What are the metrics being collected and what does that mean for performance and/or injury risk?

Practitioners should understand the validity and reliability of the chosen tests, to ensure accurate data collection is taken place. Allowing the same practitioner(s) to conduct allocated testing exercises increases the likelihood of validity,

Needs analysis and testing 61

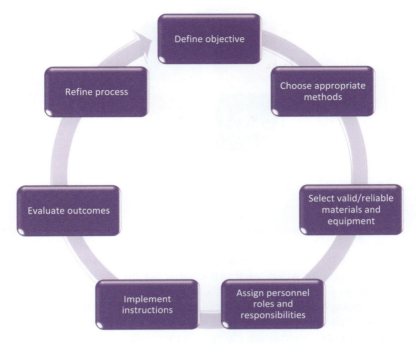

Figure 3.1 A systematic approach to solving problems and questions within a performance department of an elite soccer organisation.

via a decrease in user error. However, the department should all be observant of the implementation, in the circumstance that someone else must conduct the testing protocol. Furthermore, practitioners should feel confident that the interpretation of the results is concise, allowing for appropriate delivery to coaching staff and other stakeholders. Developing a testing battery that is valid, reliable, and re-testable allows practitioners to effectively analyse the results, but more importantly, prescribe appropriate interventions. The ability to re-test, with similar (if not, same) environments and procedures, re-affirms practitioners of the effectiveness of their training prescriptions.

The parameters

Fundamental principles of testing performance parameters should reflect five key components:

Relevant | reliability | representative | real | relatable

All these components will dictate the level of specificity and sensitivity a test has and how conducive that test is to determine what matters.

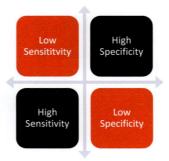

Figure 3.2 The sensitivity-specificity quadrant.

Specificity and sensitivity are inversely proportional which means the higher the level of specificity a test has the less sensitivity a test will have and vice versa (Figure 3.2). As a prerequisite of a testing battery design, we must have a clear understand of where each test chosen lies on the range of specificity and sensitivity.

Understanding how test sensitivity can be affected over time will be an important consideration for practitioners to ensure testing protocols are optimised to meet the objective outcomes. Multiple factors such as training periodisation, training status, and maturational influences will impact the sensitivity to detect meaningful changes in testing parameters. Understanding the sensitivity element of a test may influence how practitioners choose to utilise different tests throughout different stage of a calendar year.

Some tests may provide high levels of efficiency during pre-season, as opposed to in-season and, as a result, practitioners may choose to select tests that have varied levels of sensitivity to detect changes overtime.

The reliability of the numbers produced represents the ability to provide similar outcomes from day to day without any external interventions. Understanding the importance of maintaining some level of control of variables, when testing within a high fluid environment, is essential. In the elite soccer environment, not everything can be controlled to meet the standards of best practice. However, we must strive to deliver the highest degree of reliability by controlling the controllable that can minimise variability within our testing environment. The quality and accuracy of sport performance testing will always carry some level of instability, due to the condition in which testing data is obtained. If we as practitioners can ensure the conditions remain somewhat similar, even within a highly fluid environment, data provided will still be informative and applicable relative to the specific environment.

The accuracy and reproducibility of a testing battery will be dependent on the level of competence the practitioner has in conducting, analysing, and extrapolating testing data. The consistency and quality of the testing data is only as good as the practitioner performing the tests and therefore its importance to consider the feasibility of delivering certain tests based on staffing technical competencies and experience. There are also a number of limiting factors in reproducibility and accuracy tests based on the athletes themselves. Athletes training age, gender, training status all can affect both the reproducibility and accuracy of testing data.

The reporting and visualisation of testing data will ultimately be highly varied across organisations, based on the processes and systems in place. The key piece in dissemination information is clarity and consistency of data and output. Streamlining players' performance profiling and benchmarks into readily accessible and user-friendly constructs will facilitate more effective discussions on how the data can influence training inventions and periodisation models.

Developing a testing battery with performance markers with target objectives should not only optimise transfer from training to game performance but also help gain 'buy-in' from players and coaching staff. Performance markers that have great relevance to specific soccer actions will facilitate engagement and understanding from the key stakeholders.

Test exercise selection

When investigating specific physical parameters, test exercise selection is integral. Each test will present different data which should be used to develop a baseline data set for the individual player. The results will also illustrate their comparison to the rest of the squad, comparison to their positional group, the potential risk of injury, and current physical progression. Consideration for timing and specificity of tests is vital. Some examples of various testing categories are below.

- Anthropometric Profile [20]
- Isokinetic Testing [21]
- Muscular Strength [22]
- Power Output [22]
- Change of Direction [23]
- Blood Markers [24]
- Speed Testing [22, 25]
- Repeat Sprint Ability [18, 26]
- Submaximal Aerobic Capacity [24]
- Maximal Aerobic Capacity [27, 28]

The testing procedure, test exercise selection, and coordination of which of the players will be involved in testing needs to be carefully planned. It is also advisable to take into consideration which tests result in altered/greater variance or reliability during any given time of the season. Hence, the importance for scheduling and execution of tests in relation to the periodisation model. Discussion within the performance and medical departments is paramount to ensure the overall training process is not affected, as well as all players being cleared to participate.

To determine the individual targets for these tests, practitioners must understand the physical demands for each player. There is a myriad of factors that can determine what the general target for the squad should be, such as league match demands and the club's desired playing style. However, there are also individual targets that we should aim for, such as position requirements and individual player characteristics, such as age and injury history.

Needs analysis

The game of soccer has evolved significantly at its highest levels, and the physical and technical demands of professional football matches have increased dramatically [29–31]. Between 2006/2007 and 2012/2013, there was a significant increase in high intensity running outputs during matches of the English Premier League. Comparing the 2012/2013 season to the 2006/2007 seasons, positions ranged anywhere between 24% and 36% increase in high intensity running distances. The greatest differences were identified in defenders (central and full-backs) and central midfielders, with a range of 30%–36% increases [30, 31]. Furthermore, other explosive outputs, such as sprint distances increased ~50% between the 2006/2007 and 2012/2013 seasons, with full-backs illustrated the greatest observation with a 64% increase [30, 31]. Although the physical outputs of the sport have shown increases, so have some technical elements. In both World Cup final, and English Premier League matches, increases in the number of passes were observed [29–31]. It has been indicated that these trends may have been due to the enhanced physical preparation (resulting in improved physical capacities), as well as players entering the top divisions of soccer with higher levels of physical fitness [31]. Thus, with the speed and technical demands of the game increasing yearly, the testing battery should be designed around enhancing players' physical attributes to meet the needs of the sport.

With the subsequent increase in match intensity and inherent physical demands, there has also been some fluctuation in the rate of non-contact injuries. Although hamstring injuries have increased at a rate of roughly 4% over a 13-year period of European soccer seasons (2001–2014) [32], a further investigation was made and suggested that overall injury rates in European soccer has decreased slightly [33]. However, these findings specifically highlight a decrease in ligament injury rate and re-injury rate, whereas no decrease was noted in muscle injuries [33]. Therefore, it was suggested that injury rate reduction strategies may be effective given the understanding of how the modern game is played.

With the increase in the number of sprints being performed, there is an inherent risk to the hamstring muscle [34]. Historically, muscle and tendon injuries are the most common type of injury [35] (see *Chapter 9*). Specifically, the thigh is the most common injury site in soccer [36–38], of which the hamstring has been the most common injury site [35, 36, 39–41]. Understanding the relationship between high-speed running volumes and the injury risk in the hamstring muscle group creates the need for practitioners to evaluate the variety of testing protocols for posterior chain tolerance [42, 43]. Thus, the increased physical demand is directly linked to increased risk of injury. Practitioners should include tests that evaluate both high-speed running demands as well as localised injury risk in elite soccer.

With an identified physical evolution of soccer, establishing match demands that are specific to our respective leagues is important. The physical requirements of various national leagues, around the globe, vary dramatically. The technical, tactical, and physical aspects of each league, along with the character type of the players involved, all have an impact on the match demands of each league [44]. For example, the English Premier League is renowned for being one of the most physically demanding leagues in the world [44]. The playing style in English soccer is one of taller, more physically robust players who can dominate the ball at high match speeds, resulting in a fast paced, aggressive competition. On the contrary, the Spanish leagues are classified by players who control the game through individual technical quality and more ball possession [44]. However, players in some African leagues generally may not be as technically astute as their European counterparts due to the lack of grassroots development, but are more mobile and possess more speed and power [45, 46]. This may create a faster, more transition-based style of play due to possession being turned over more frequently.

Each league around the world will have differences in the overall style of play. This will have an impact on the game model of the teams' managers, which, in turn, will have an impact on the physical demands of the players in the teams. Each playing position has specific physical demands, that are influenced by various facets, such as tactical formation [47, 48]. For example, manager A may want to play a 4-3-3 system with his full-backs advancing high up the pitch in the build-up phase to support attacks. The head coach/manager may also want them to recover at speed back to their defensive shape during a defensive transition. This circumstance would require the full-backs to have a strong aerobic capacity to recover quickly, as well as formidable speed endurance to be effective on multiple transitions [48]. Conversely, manager B may play with a 4-2-3-1 formation with his team playing a lone striker and a high line press. This situation would require the striker to be able to make repetitive, short sprints to squeeze the opposition defenders and force them to concede possession or play a long pass.

Categories and rationale

A manager or club's playing philosophy and game model will ultimately dictate the physical qualities that will need to be trained (see *Chapter 11*). Once we

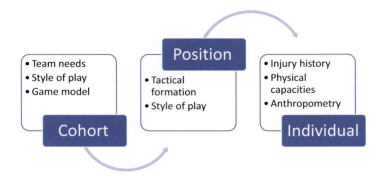

Figure 3.3 Testing categories with associated influential attributes.

understand the physical demands of the game model, we can break the testing categories down into the following sub-groups:

- Cohort
- Position
- Individual Player

Cohort

The cohort or group testing should address the needs of the sport, organisation and group, fitted to the environment (Figure 3.3). Within the cohort, the players can be categorised into more medium-sized, positional groups – Goalkeepers, Defenders, Midfielders, and Attackers. Positional categorisation will aid practitioners in programming specific test exercises for the demands of each group. To understand the Cohort testing procedure, practitioners need to align with the physical requirements of the game model set out by the manager and/or club (see *Chapter 11*). For example, Manager B may want to play with a four-man defensive line who are both physically strong in both aerial duels and one-on-one defensive situations. As a result, it would be important for the defensive cohort to perform maximal strength testing to determine their baseline values. It is important to note, that in this above-mentioned scenario, it is not suggested that the defensive cohort be the only group subjected to a specific type of testing. More so, the suggestion is made that given the style of play taken into account, some performance benchmarks should be set for different cohorts within the organisation, based on the club/manager's game model.

Positional

In the same manner, the cohort can be broken down into position-specific testing. Using the above-mentioned example, Manager A wants to use his full-backs in both attack and defence, requiring them to excel in multiple physical attributes. These players will not be assessed in the same manner as a centre-back or defensive midfielder, as they will potentially result in less total distance or high-speed running (HSR) distances covered compared to the full-backs, during match-play. Therefore, allowing practitioners to compare the data collected in terms of positional group targets and the group mean values.

Individual

Finally, testing should take individual traits and attributes into account when allocating variables and testing protocols. There are a number of key considerations when assessing the player in isolation and comparing them to the team or their position. Firstly, it is important to know the physiological status of the player and what may limit their testing performance or participation in the testing. A player's age can have an important impact on their ability to produce speed or power [49, 50]. Older age can also pose a non-modifiable injury risk, specifically for the hamstring group in elite soccer players [51, 52]. An older player, though potentially technically and tactically well-versed, may not be able to reach their previous best in a variety of performance-based tests, such as repeat sprint ability [50, 53]. In a similar manner, a younger player may not be able to produce power due to the maturation process [54, 55] (see *Chapter 2*). Genetics and ethnicity may also have a similar impact on the anthropometric profile of a player. As such, we need to look at the player in isolation (age, genetics, ethnicity, etc.), and compare them to their own previous testing data to assess them effectively [56].

Knowing a player's training history is necessary for practitioners to apply effective and safe prescriptions. Players may be acquired by the club in transfer windows or have via free agency prior to joining the team. Incoming players may have recently been exposed to adequate training stimulus or, conversely, neglected training due to a variety of reasons. Therefore, practitioners should prescribe with caution, as neglecting training history information, could place the player at a higher risk of re-injury and result in poor testing data. On the contrary, players arriving to new clubs with a desired training history allow for practitioners to accurately allocate a testing battery and immediately prescribe a progressive training stimulus. In any scenario, it is highly suggested that practitioners carefully assess players' training history prior to prescribing testing protocols (Figure 3.4).

Lastly, when assessing an academy player who has recently been promoted, they may not excel in the testing battery, compared to the senior members of the team. While academy/youth player may be accustomed to the testing procedure, they may not produce the same results due to maturity, strength deficits or mental stress caused by moving into the new environment. Having a database of the testing data from their time in the academy will be a better reference point than older, more experienced players in their position.

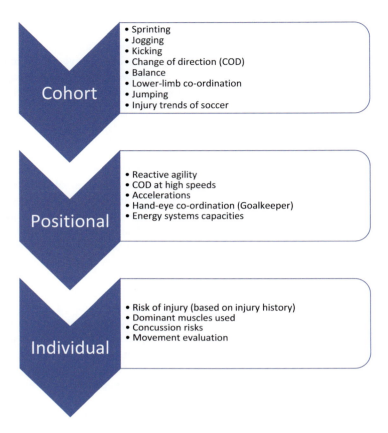

Figure 3.4 Needs analysis based on the groups: cohort, positional, and individual.

Therefore, it is imperative that practitioners working within an academy environment align testing procedures with the first team to allow for an easier transition when players are called upon.

Limitations

As the quest for greater understanding of how to make athletes perform better grows, so too does our assessment and criticism of previous 'common practices'. As many of the common understandings of physiology, such as VO_{2max} and plateau, have been criticised, so have many field-based fitness tests [4, 57]. Specifically, it was suggested that the Modified 505 (M505) test and Change of Direction Deficit (CODD) have limited practicality in assessing the change of direction ability in youth footballers [25]. Further research has challenged change of direction assessments, as movements are seen as pre-planned, and not taking sport-specific movements into consideration [58]. Investigators also found that Beep test performance can significantly be affected by only 30 minutes of cognitive work, questioning it's true validity [59]. In relation to soccer, testing batteries have been challenged due to its lack of transference to actual technical performance on the pitch [60]. Instead, practitioners should be assessing physical qualities that will have relevance in a training setting and provide the coaching and performance staff with informative data to help improve overall performance of the team.

Ultimately, the how, what, when, and why of testing needs to be a collective decision, made by the coaching and performance staff. Practitioners' understanding of players, the characteristics of their respective league, and desired match model, will provide a clear understanding of the physical testing processes.

Types of tests

The types of tests can be broken down in a variety of ways. In the attempt to simplify the rationale for exercise selection, the testing protocols can be categorised by objective and group (Figure 3.5). The categories that tests will be identified in this chapter as either injury-risk or performance tests. Furthermore, the groups for categorisation are as aforementioned: cohort, positional, and individual.

Cohort

Whilst is seems evident that soccer is an aerobic-dominant sport, there is a great emphasis on testing the aerobic capacity to develop a physiological profile (Figure 3.6) [61, 62]. However, during the early 1990s, researchers identified the need to test players' endurance performance via intermittent exercise protocols [63]. The overall objective of testing endurance performance in soccer players it to measure individuals' VO_{2max} in a field-based setting. The gold standard of VO_{2max} measurements is obtained via a laboratory, however, in an

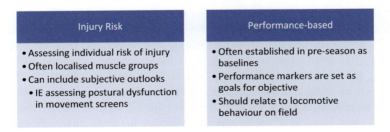

Figure 3.5 Types of tests based on the objective. Injury risk tests assess the likelihood of injury risk within a player. Performance-based tests assess output-related qualities of a player.

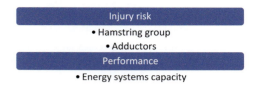

Figure 3.6 Cohort considerations when selecting tests from the outlined objectives: injury risk and performance-based tests.

Injury risk	Nordic force	
	Adductor squeeze	
	Various hand-held dynamometer	
Performance	Aerobic capacity fitness test	Yo-Yo
		30-15
		Beep tests
		Time trials

Figure 3.7 Examples of tests with cohort-related benchmarks.

elite soccer environment, this procedure is not feasible. Therefore, a variety of field-based intermittent tests were introduced, including the Beep test, Yo-Yo test, and 30-15$_{IFT}$ (Figure 3.7) [6, 8, 17, 57, 63].

After decades of applying the Yo-Yo intermittent tests, researchers were able to collate the results and establish differences between sports and levels of competition [17, 64]. Thus, creating some overarching, cohort performance benchmarks for practitioners. Similarly, a variety of 'Beep tests' were applied, with the same objective, to differentiate results between levels of competition [65]. The most common versions of the 'Beep tests' are the Maximum Multistage 20m Shuttle Run Test (MMSRT) and the Interval Shuttle Run Test (ISRT), both resulting in a predicted VO_{2max} for individuals [65]. Recently, the 30-15$_{IFT}$ has been popularised in a team-based setting to obtain individuals' VO_{2max} [66]. Likewise, with the Yo-Yo and 'Beep test' variations, the 30-15$_{IFT}$ shows to be valid and applicable in a team-setting environment with established benchmarks for a variety of sports [8, 57, 67]. Although the Yo-Yo, 3015$_{IFT}$, and 'Beep test' variations are effective for collecting various fitness markers from players, simple time trials can be prescribed to obtain maximum aerobic speeds (MAS) [28]. Specifically, time trails for any distance between

1200 and 2200 m has indicated to be effective in a team setting [68]. Applying a five, six, or seven-minute time trial is a simple and quick method to obtain individual MAS results in a team environment. Additionally, the reproducibility of simple time trials is high. Furthermore, normative data for MAS results, across a variety of sports and levels of competition, is readily available in current literature [69]. Therefore, time trial tests may be more appealing to those practitioners with lack of time and/or resources. Without exhausting the test exercise selection process for practitioners, the main identified cohort (team-based) testing protocols to date are the Yo-Yo variations, 'Beep test' variations, various time trials, and the 30-15$_{IFT}$. The determining factor for practitioners during the selection process is purely dependent on their environment and organisation's objectives.

In terms of testing for injury risk in elite soccer, it is evident that the number one injury site is the hamstring group [32, 33]. Therefore, it is imperative to test localised hamstring strength on a team level. Research indicated that elite soccer players illustrating below 337N of eccentric knee flexor force (via the NordBord) are at a significantly greater risk of hamstring injury [70]. Additionally, the same notion applies to the adductor muscle group. Research concluded that a hip abduction imbalance favouring the preferred kicking limb, along with high levels of hip adductor and abductor strength (measured in pre-season) significantly reduce the risk of hip/groin strains [71]. Similar to assessing knee-flexor strength outputs, practitioners should assess adductor and abductor force outputs and establish desired thresholds based on the norms outlined in current literature [72].

Positional

Additional tests, outside the well-established field-based protocols, can be implemented with the desired outcomes altered based on the positional groups (Figure 3.8). As identified decades ago, positional roles have different work

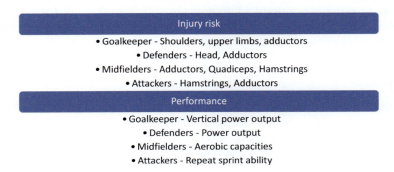

Figure 3.8 Positional considerations when selecting tests from the outlined objectives: injury risk and performance-based tests.

Injury risk	Shoulder isokinetic force	
	Concussion tests	
Performance	Vertical power output	*Countermovement jump*
		Reactive strength index (RSI)
	Repeat sprint ability	*Time trials sprints for distance. Various work:rest ratios*

Figure 3.9 Examples of tests with positional-related benchmarks.

rates during match-play, therefore, it seems as though some testing should occur that considers these various work rates [73]. Although some of the physiological profiles of positional groups show little-to-no differences, it is important to note that the outputs of match-play remain different positionally, at all age groups [47, 48, 74]. Due to the noted differences in physical outputs during match-play, such as high-speed running and/or sprinting, positional benchmarks can be put in place for a variety of tests. Specifically, when implanting a repeat sprint ability test, it would be suggested that practitioners expect players who sprint more throughout the game, to excel in a sprint-related testing protocol [75]. Other results obtained from a repeat sprint ability test, such as fatigue index, will vary dependant on the position, training stimulus, and desired playing style [75]. Other testing protocols, such as strength/power testing, have shown to result in positional differences [76, 77]. Therefore, it is strongly recommended that positional benchmarks, in relation to the club's game model, are implemented when investigating additional testing protocols (Figure 3.9).

Individual

If a particular test provides no valuable information regarding physical profiling to influence training programmes or establish baselines to work from in the return to play process, then it has no purpose. This is especially important when it comes to individual testing and how results are monitored throughout the season (Table 3.1).

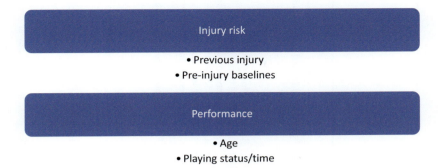

Figure 3.10 Individual considerations when analysing test results from the outlined objectives: injury risk and performance-based tests.

In individual cases, particular tests may closely relate to previous injury, and close monitoring becomes increasingly important to minimise the risk of re-injury (Figure 3.10). Specifically, knowing the previous injury is an important risk factor for injury, individual benchmarks need to be established for those with previous injury history [78] (*see Chapter 9*). For example, a player with a history of hamstring strain injury (HSI) would be carefully monitored in objective markers and integrity of movements, such as Nordics. Although strength may not need to be fully restored when returning to training, it is suggested that exceeding pre-injury results will best prepare the athlete for competition and reduce the likelihood of injury [79–81]. Furthermore, frequency for testing and monitoring a player with recent injury history will be increased.

In conjunction with injury risk, individual test results will aid practitioners in developing appropriate training prescriptions to address the individual's weaknesses. When interpreting testing results on an individual level, it is important that practitioners assess non-modifiables (outside of injury risk) that potentially inhibit performance outcomes. Specifically, age can be a non-modifiable factor that relates to decreases in performance outputs [49, 50, 82]. Therefore, practitioners must interpret results with caution when identifying players' weaknesses. For example, as players age, their maximum velocity outputs may show a gradual decrement from season to season. Additionally, players that are not being exposed to playing time (for a variety of reasons) may show decrements in performance tests. Increased involved of playing time has shown to favour the increase (and maintenance) of strength and sprint testing abilities in soccer players [83]. In these circumstances, practitioners must account for these decrements when analysing testing results.

Sample pre-season testing battery

Table 3.1 Example of testing battery in elite soccer

Type	Category	Test	Description	Benchmark	Re-test	Notes
Anthropometric	Individual profiles	Body fat, height, weight	This testing is for preseason, in season and post season to monitor changes in body tissue related to performance and health.	Body fat <10%	2-3 times	Requires additional staff, including nutrition
Injury risk	Lower limb	NordBord	Localised muscular testing for hamstring group. Ability to categorise injury risk players.	337 N	When needed	Useful tool for minimising hamstring issues. Highly recommended moving forward
Injury Risk	Lower Limb	Groin squeeze/pull (Force Frame)	Localised muscular testing for adductor groups. Ability to categorise injury risk players.	Add: 370 N Add: 385 N	When needed	Useful tool for minimising adductor issues. Highly recommended moving forward
Performance	Aerobic	30-15$_{IFT}$	This sub-max fitness test is designed to evaluate individual maximum aerobic speeds (MAS).	V_{IFT}: 19.5	every 3+ weeks	Positional outcomes should be set
Performance	Anaerobic	RSA phosphate recovery test	Assessing the ability to recover between sprints as well as reproduce the same amount of metabolic power required.	<15% Fatigue index	every 6+ weeks	Will need to be max effort to minimise pacing strategies
Performance	Horizontal Power	Broad Jump	This test is an assessment of posterior chain power output. The distance (cm) will be measured for test and retest.	>240 cm	Every 3+ weeks	Establish individual power profiles
Performance	Vertical power	Vertical jump	Measure of vertical power output. Three reps completed, with the best score being recorded.	>50 cm	Every 3+ weeks	Establish individual power profiles

Coach's insight

Martin Buchheit

Soccer specific tests – the overwatered plants of sports science

> *I remember testing one of our best South American players one day. We were doing CMJs as part of the pre-season screening. As my colleagues were explaining the protocol to the squad, he stopped us straight and said: 'you guys don't understand football, we never jump from two feet like this, this is just good for volleyball!! Did you see my last header and the incredible goal I scored? I jumped from one foot!!'*

An anecdote from the field, and true that in soccer you often don't jump from both feet, so why perform CMJs? Explaining the reasons as to why the testing protocol is approached in a certain way to some players is imperative to creating increased 'buy in'. However, despite a practitioner's best efforts, the player may still not give 100% for a given test as they may lack belief in the process.

For this reason and others mentioned below, sport-specific testing, and even training, has become a trend in the performance science and soccer strength and conditioning worlds. Tests that replicate the key movements of players in their soccer context are believed to provide more motivation to players and more relevant information to practitioners. Specifically, training mimicking the match demands is believed to be superior to generic training in the name of better transference of the expected physiological adaptations. However, practitioners must understand their real value, and keep in mind the true objectives of testing and training. Testing is about profiling players first, to then provide the most relevant training stimulus (prescribe and orientate training contents) in relation to this profiling. Training is first about improving the overall physical performance of soccer players, which can be achieved by improving physical capacities, but also increasing technical/tactical efficiency, and increased robustness to minimise injury risk. The impact that changes in fitness can have on performance is also highly contextual and player dependent.

> *Take locomotor patterns during a football match, how long do they walk for? 70% of the time? So based on this, your specific testing should examine walking patterns, and training should include a lot of walking, right? Over reliance on sport-specific testing and training may in fact derail us from achieving our goals.*

Soccer-specific testing

In 2013, an editorial from Martin Buchheit and Alberto Mendez-Villanueva was published, in which the limitation of soccer-specific testing was discussed [60]. The provocative title was 'Football-specific fitness testing: adding value or confirming the evidence'. The example of people getting overly excited to test 5–10 m performance only and using the Yo-Yo or other protocols even including the ball as a proxy of acceleration capacity and soccer specific high intensity running performance capacity, was used respectively. The new technology used to perform non-specific tests today can in fact help us to improve our capacity to profile players and, in turn, offer better individual training plans.

Testing for speed

The first point in the editorial was that when testing speed, using only 5–10 m performance in the name of specificity (player doesn't always reach max speed and conversely repeat >100 accelerations during matches), did not allow for a complete profiling of a player's potential [60]. In fact, the 5–10 m test on its own may only confirm what coaches already know (and see every weekend when the player is or isn't able to overtake opponents over short spaces). The 5–10 m test may be only useful when used in combination with other speed measures including maximal velocity and/or further profiling (F/V). In short, since all players may not run 40 m at full speed very often (or never, for some) during matches, 40 m sprints are rated as poorly specific by a lot of practitioners. In contrast, using split times or advanced modelling techniques, this type of test can provide an incredibly valuable level of information, such as prioritising the type of training required for each player, i.e., more oriented towards force vs velocity development. Also, assessing maximal sprinting speed is imperative when analysing external demands during matches (i.e. to express running demands in relation to maximal velocity when using global positioning system [GPS]).

Testing for strength

While there are hundreds of tests available to sport scientists to assess strength and power [84], jump tests are probably those that carry the greatest level of variations and opinions [85] about how they should be performed. Is it more insightful to measure the height of a one-legged jump ending with a header, that coaches and players can already examine during matches, or uncover precise neuromuscular performances using a dual force plate? While the first provides only anecdotal evidence that may motivate players to execute the test with full intention, the second likely provides a myriad of crucial information on how the jump is performed, and in turn, about the lower limb muscle characteristics. This includes many variables from explosive concentric capacity, to braking and landing force and of course all the possible asymmetries of those parameters. Tested regularly, CMJs (and many other types of tests using force plates) can be used as incredibly powerful and useful fatigue monitoring tools [86]. The one-legged jumps still have a place in the testing batteries of course, but again, the absolute performance (height or length of the jump) in itself is meaningless – it's only by comparing both limbs performance that some information can be gained – and if all this can be measured on a force plate, this opens the door for greater insights of for the CMJs.

As for speed, any strength/power tests should be viewed as tools to profile players; very often moving away from sport specificity is the best way to achieve this.

Testing for fitness

Similarly, if considering soccer-specific fitness evaluations such as the Hoff test or the FootEval (which both consist in repeating high-intensity actions with the ball) [87–89], what is the actual information that could be derived from the results? And what is new information in comparison to what coaches, again, can see every weekend from the bench? More importantly, the performance on these tests is multifactorial, and likely includes a mixed contribution of aerobic function, anaerobic capacity, recovery abilities, changes of direction, neuromuscular capacities, and technique. Therefore, since the same overall performance can be achieved while taxing all the above-mentioned capacities to a different extent, players with completely opposite profiles can in fact reach the same performance on the test. A highly technical player may compensate for his lack of fitness and outperform a fit, but less skilled player, for example. This makes it impossible to uncover which of these capacities would need to be improved and which are already sufficient. From that, what are we prescribing for training?

It seems, therefore, that removing the technical component is the first step for more relevant fitness assessment. While numerous incremental tests without the ball such as the Yo-Yo tests or the 30-15$_{IFT}$ are popularised for various reasons, such as the effort looks specific to the sports, and performance can be used as a proxy of overall high-intensity running performance, only the 30-15$_{IFT}$ provides simultaneous information about a players' locomotor profiles and training prescription [8, 66, 90]. Importantly however, the above-mentioned critiques about the limits of tests with multifactorial determinants apply for the 30-15$_{IFT}$ too (i.e. the same performance can be achieved while taxing different determinants to different extents). Therefore, to further improve player fitness profiling, the 30-15$_{IFT}$ can be completed with measures of maximal aerobic speed (using an incremental continuous test such as the Vam-Eval or a 2 km all out run); in this case, the comparison of the 30-15$_{IFT}$ performance with MAS helps to isolate the high-intensity/supramaximal and change of direction components from the aerobic power measure (with the greater the difference in speed between both tests, the greater this latter capacity).

Further than allowing profiling players to guide training priorities, fitness tests should also be able to be used for training prescriptions. Using MAS only is insufficient to accurately prescribe high-intensity interval training (HIIT), and other measures such as lactate thresholds may only be appropriate to programme submaximal intensity runs, which represent very little (or sometimes even nothing) of conditioning programming practices in soccer. The final performance at the Yo-Yo, even if converted into a running speed, cannot be used for training prescription since its relationship with MAS is not proportional. In contrast, the speed reached at the of the 30-15$_{IFT}$ is the perfect reference running speed when prescribing HIIT with short intervals within the anaerobic speed reserve range, since is directly related to both player's maximal aerobic speed and maximal sprinting speed.

Finally, as for speed and strength/power testing, the more relevant approach to fitness testing is to use tests that have as few as possible physical determinants (first exclude all technical aspects), or at least, it's important to know them well enough so that the test can be completed with others to fine tune the profiling (e.g. adding a measure of MAS to the 30-15$_{IFT}$). Finally, since HIIT requires it to be tightly individualised, tests that allow prescription in addition to profiling should also be preferred [91].

Conclusion

While trying to replicate the sport when testing, is it possible to provide more information than what the sport is already providing us with? Whenever it is about speed, strength, power or fitness, tests should be viewed as tools to profile players – and not to confirm the evidence; very often moving away from the so-called sport specificity is the best way to achieve this. The current writing piece, of course, only is aimed at describing the overall idea of favouring non-specific testing; the choice of the actual tests should always be left to the practitioners, who may select them based on their 'specific' context.

References

1. Krogh, A. and J. Lindhard, *The regulation of respiration and circulation during the initial stages of muscular work.* The Journal of Physiology, 1913. **47**(1–2): p. 112–136.
2. Furusawa, K., A.V. Hill, and J. Parkinson, *The dynamics of 'sprint' running.* Proceedings of the Royal Society of London. Series B, Containing Papers of a Biological Character, 1927. **102**(713): p. 29–42.
3. Hill, A.V., *The physiological basis of athletic records.* The Scientific Monthly, 1925. **21**(4): p. 409–428.
4. Noakes, T.D., *How did AV Hill understand the VO2max and the 'plateau phenomenon'? Still no clarity?* British Journal of Sports Medicine, 2008. **42**(7): p. 574–580.
5. Dill, D., et al., *Analysis of recovery from anaerobic work.* Arbeitsphysiologie, 1936. **9**(3): p. 299–307.
6. Leger, L.A. and J. Lambert, *A maximal multistage 20-m shuttle run test to predict max.* European Journal of Applied Physiology and Occupational Physiology, 1982. **49**(1): p. 1–12.
7. Bangsbo, J. and F. Lindquist, *Comparison of various exercise tests with endurance performance during soccer in professional players.* International Journal of Sports Medicine, 1992. **13**(02): p. 125–132.
8. Buchheit, M., U. Dikmen, and C. Vassallo, *The 30-15 Intermittent Fitness Test – two decades of learnings.* Sport Performance & Science Reports, 2021. **1**(148): p. 1–13.
9. Chalmers, S., et al., *The relationship between pre-season fitness testing and injury in elite junior Australian football players.* Journal of Science and Medicine in Sport, 2013. **16**(4): p. 307–311.
10. Fousekis, K., E. Tsepis, and G. Vagenas, *Multivariate isokinetic strength asymmetries of the knee and ankle in professional soccer players.* The Journal of Sports Medicine and Physical Fitness, 2010. **50**(4): p. 465–474.
11. Watkins, C.M., et al., *Determination of vertical jump as a measure of neuromuscular readiness and fatigue.* The Journal of Strength & Conditioning Research, 2017. **31**(12): p. 3305–3310.
12. Thomas, K., et al., *Etiology and recovery of neuromuscular fatigue after simulated soccer match play.* Medicine & Science in Sports & Exercise, 2017. **49**(5): p. 955–964.

13 Budgett, R., *Fatigue and underperformance in athletes: the overtraining syndrome.* British Journal of Sports Medicine, 1998. **32**(2): p. 107–110.
14 Minetto, M.A., et al., *Changes in awakening cortisol response and midnight salivary cortisol are sensitive markers of strenuous training-induced fatigue.* Journal of Endocrinological Investigation, 2008. **31**(1): p. 16–24.
15 Carfagno, D.G. and J.C. Hendrix, *Overtraining syndrome in the athlete: current clinical practice.* Current Sports Medicine Reports, 2014. **13**(1): p. 45–51.
16 Girardi, M., et al., *Detraining effects prevention: a new rising challenge for athletes.* Frontiers in Physiology, 2020. **11**: p. 588784.
17 Bangsbo, J., F.M. Iaia, and P. Krustrup, *The Yo-Yo intermittent recovery test.* Sports Medicine, 2008. **38**(1): p. 37–51.
18 Rampinini, E., et al., *Repeated-sprint ability in professional and amateur soccer players.* Applied Physiology, Nutrition, and Metabolism, 2009. **34**(6): p. 1048–1054.
19 Maupin, D., et al., *The relationship between acute: chronic workload ratios and injury risk in sports: a systematic review.* Open Access Journal of Sports Medicine, 2020. **11**: p. 51.
20 Joksimovj, M., et al., *Anthropometric characteristics of professional football players in relation to the playing position and their significance for success in the game.* Pedagogics, Psychology, Medical-Biological Problems of Physical Training and Sports, 2019. **23**(5): p. 224–230
21 Delvaux, F., et al., *Preseason assessment of anaerobic performance in elite soccer players: comparison of isokinetic and functional tests.* Sports Biomechanics, 2020: Published online. p. 1–15.
22 Turner, A., et al., *A testing battery for the assessment of fitness in soccer players.* Strength & Conditioning Journal, 2011. **33**(5): p. 29–39.
23 Lockie, R.G., et al., *Reliability and validity of a new test of change-of-direction speed for field-based sports: the change-of-direction and acceleration test (CODAT).* Journal of Sports Science & Medicine, 2013. **12**(1): p. 88.
24 McMillan, K., et al., *Lactate threshold responses to a season of professional British youth soccer.* British Journal of Sports Medicine, 2005. **39**(7): p. 432–436.
25 Taylor, J.M., et al., *The reliability of a modified 505 test and change-of-direction deficit time in elite youth football players.* Science and Medicine in Football, 2019. **3**(2): p. 157–162.
26 Wragg, C., N. Maxwell, and J. Doust, *Evaluation of the reliability and validity of a soccer-specific field test of repeated sprint ability.* European Journal of Applied Physiology, 2000. **83**(1): p. 77–83.
27 Marcos, M.A., P.M. Koulla, and Z.I. Anthos, *Preseason maximal aerobic power in professional soccer players among different divisions.* The Journal of Strength & Conditioning Research, 2018. **32**(2): p. 356–363.
28 Darendeli, A., et al., *Comparison of different exercise testing modalities to determine maximal aerobic speed in amateur soccer players.* Science & Sports, 2021. **36**(2): p. 105–111.
29 Wallace, J.L. and K.I. Norton, *Evolution of World Cup soccer final games 1966–2010: game structure, speed and play patterns.* Journal of Science and Medicine in Sport, 2014. **17**(2): p. 223–228.
30 Barnes, C., et al., *The evolution of physical and technical performance parameters in the English Premier League.* International journal of sports medicine, 2014. **35**(13): p. 1095–1100.
31 Bush, M., et al., *Evolution of match performance parameters for various playing positions in the English Premier League.* Human Movement Science, 2015. **39**: p. 1–11.
32 Ekstrand, J., M. Waldén, and M. Hägglund, *Hamstring injuries have increased by 4% annually in men9s professional football, since 2001: a 13-year longitudinal analysis of the UEFA Elite Club injury study.* British Journal of Sports Medicine, 2016. **50**(12): p. 731–737.

33 Ekstrand, J., et al., *Injury rates decreased in men's professional football: an 18-year prospective cohort study of almost 12000 injuries sustained during 1.8 million hours of play.* British Journal of Sports Medicine, 2021. **55**(19): p. 1084–1091.
34 Small, K., et al., *Soccer fatigue, sprinting and hamstring injury risk.* International Journal of Sports Medicine, 2009. **30**(08): p. 573–578.
35 López-Valenciano, A., et al., *Epidemiology of injuries in professional football: a systematic review and meta-analysis.* British Journal of Sports Medicine, 2020. **54**(12): p. 711–718.
36 Waldén, M., M. Hägglund, and J. Ekstrand, *UEFA Champions League study: a prospective study of injuries in professional football during the 2001–2002 season.* British Journal of Sports Medicine, 2005. **39**(8): p. 542–546.
37 Falese, L., P. Della Valle, and B. Federico, *Epidemiology of football (soccer) injuries in the 2012/2013 and 2013/2014 seasons of the Italian Serie A.* Research in Sports Medicine, 2016. **24**(4): p. 426–432.
38 Lu, D., et al., *Injury epidemiology in Australian male professional soccer.* Journal of Science and Medicine in Sport, 2020. **23**(6): p. 574–579.
39 Jones, A., et al., *Epidemiology of injury in English professional football players: a cohort study.* Physical Therapy in Sport, 2019. **35**: p. 18–22.
40 Ekstrand, J., M. Hägglund, and M. Waldén, *Injury incidence and injury patterns in professional football - the UEFA injury study.* British Journal of Sports Medicine, 2011. **45**(7): p. 553–558.
41 Ekstrand, J., M. Hägglund, and M. Waldén, *Epidemiology of muscle injuries in professional football (soccer).* The American Journal of Sports Medicine, 2011. **39**(6): p. 1226–1232.
42 Tokutake, G., et al., *The risk factors of hamstring strain injury induced by high-speed running.* Journal of Sports Science & Medicine, 2018. **17**(4): p. 650.
43 Duhig, S., et al., *Effect of high-speed running on hamstring strain injury risk.* British Journal of Sports Medicine, 2016. **50**(24): p. 1536–1540.
44 Yi, Q., et al., *Differences in technical performance of players from 'the big five' European football leagues in the UEFA Champions League.* Frontiers in Psychology, 2019. **10**: p. 2738.
45 Tendonkeng, J.F., et al., *Physical and physiological characteristics of Cameroon professional soccer players according to their competitive level and playing position.* International Journal of Sports Science and Physical Education, 2021. **6**(1): p. 8.
46 Clark, J.R., *Higher log position is not associated with better physical fitness in professional soccer teams in South Africa.* South African Journal of Sports Medicine, 2007. **19**(2): p. 40–45.
47 Abbott, W., G. Brickley, and N.J. Smeeton, *Physical demands of playing position within English Premier League academy soccer.* Journal of Human Sport and Exercise, 2018. **13**(2): p. 285–295.
48 Calder, A. and T. Gabbett, *Influence of tactical formation on average and peak demands of elite soccer match-play.* International Journal of Strength and Conditioning, 2022. **2**(1): p. 1–10.
49 Tanaka, H. and D.R. Seals, *Endurance exercise performance in Masters athletes: age-associated changes and underlying physiological mechanisms.* The Journal of Physiology, 2008. **586**(1): p. 55–63.
50 Allen, S.V. and W.G. Hopkins, *Age of peak competitive performance of elite athletes: a systematic review.* Sports Medicine, 2015. **45**(10): p. 1431–1441.
51 Verrall, G., et al., *Clinical risk factors for hamstring muscle strain injury: a prospective study with correlation of injury by magnetic resonance imaging.* British Journal of Sports Medicine, 2001. **35**(6): p. 435–439.
52 Timmins, R.G., et al., *Short biceps femoris fascicles and eccentric knee flexor weakness increase the risk of hamstring injury in elite football (soccer): a prospective cohort study.* British Journal of Sports Medicine, 2016. **50**(24): p. 1524–1535.

53 Trombetti, A., et al., *Age-associated declines in muscle mass, strength, power, and physical performance: impact on fear of falling and quality of life.* Osteoporosis International: A Journal Established as Result of Cooperation between the European Foundation for Osteoporosis and the National Osteoporosis Foundation of the USA, 2016. **27**(2): p. 463–471.
54 Keiner, M., et al., *Differences in squat jump, linear sprint, and change-of-direction performance among youth soccer players according to competitive level.* Sports, 2021. **9**(11): p. 149.
55 Sal de Rellán-Guerra, A., et al., *Age-related physical and technical match performance changes in elite soccer players.* Scandinavian Journal of Medicine & Science in Sports, 2019. **29**(9): p. 1421–1427.
56 Mattsson, C.M., et al., *Sports genetics moving forward: lessons learned from medical research.* Physiological Genomics, 2016. **48**(3): p. 175–182.
57 Bok, D. and C. Foster, *Applicability of field aerobic fitness tests in soccer: which one to choose?* Journal of Functional Morphology and Kinesiology, 2021. **6**(3): p. 69.
58 Young, W., R. Rayner, and S. Talpey, *It's time to change direction on agility research: a call to action.* Sports Medicine-Open, 2021. **7**(1): p. 1–5.
59 Macmahon, C., Z. Hawkins, and L. Schuecker, *Beep test performance is influenced by 30 minutes of cognitive work.* Medicine and Science in Sports and Exercise, 2019. **51**(9): p. 1928.
60 Mendez-Villanueva, A. and M. Buchheit, *Football-specific fitness testing: adding value or confirming the evidence?* Journal of Sports Sciences, 2013. **31**(13): p. 1503–1508.
61 Bangsbo, J., *Energy demands in competitive soccer.* Journal of Sports Sciences, 1994. **12**(sup1): p. S5–S12.
62 Mangine, R.E., et al., *A physiological profile of the elite soccer athlete.* Journal of Orthopaedic & Sports Physical Therapy, 1990. **12**(4): p. 147–152.
63 Bangsbo, J. and F. Lindquist, *Comparison of various exercise tests with endurance performance during soccer in professional players.* International Journal of Sports Medicine, 1992. **13**(2): p. 125–132.
64 Schmitz, B., et al., *The yo-yo intermittent tests: a systematic review and structured compendium of test results.* Frontiers in Physiology, 2018. **9**: p. 870.
65 Lemmink, K., R. Verheijen, and C. Visscher, *The discriminative power of the Interval Shuttle Run Test and the Maximal Multistage Shuttle Run Test for playing level of soccer.* Journal of Sports Medicine and Physical Fitness, 2004. **44**(3): p. 233–239.
66 Buchheit, M., et al., *Cardiorespiratory and cardiac autonomic responses to 30-15 intermittent fitness test in team sport players.* The Journal of Strength & Conditioning Research, 2009. **23**(1): p. 93–100.
67 Stanković, M., et al., *30–15 intermittent fitness test: a systematic review of studies, examining the VO2max estimation and training programming.* Applied Sciences, 2021. **11**(24): p. 11792.
68 Bellenger, C.R., et al., *Predicting maximal aerobic speed through set distance time-trials.* European Journal of Applied Physiology, 2015. **115**(12): p. 2593–2598.
69 Baker, D. and N. Heaney, *Review of the literature normative data for maximal aerobic speed for field sport athletes: a brief review.* Journal of Australian Strength and Conditioning, 2015. **23**(7): p. 60–67.
70 Timmins, R.G., et al., *Short biceps femoris fascicles and eccentric knee flexor weakness increase the risk of hamstring injury in elite football (soccer): a prospective cohort study.* British Journal of Sports Medicine, 2016. **50**(24): p. 1524–1535.
71 Bourne, M.N., et al., *Preseason hip/groin strength and HAGOS scores are associated with subsequent injury in professional male soccer players.* Journal of Orthopaedic & Sports Physical Therapy, 2020. **50**(5): p. 234–242.
72 O'Brien, M., et al., *A novel device to assess hip strength: concurrent validity and normative values in male athletes.* Physical Therapy in Sport, 2019. **35**: p. 63–68.

73. Reilly, T., *A motion analysis of work-rate in different positional roles in professional football match-play.* Journal of Human Movement Studies, 1976. **2**: p. 87–97.
74. Yildirim, A., et al., *Physiological profiles of soccer players with respect to playing positions,* in Science and Football VI. 2008, Routledge: London. p. 396–399.
75. Kaplan, T., *Examination of repeated sprinting ability and fatigue index of soccer players according to their positions.* The Journal of Strength and Conditioning Research, 2010. **24**(6): p. 1495–1501.
76. Śliwowski, R., et al., *The isokinetic strength profile of elite soccer players according to playing position.* PLoS One, 2017. **12**(7): p. e0182177.
77. Wik, E.H., S.M. Auliffe, and P.J. Read, *Examination of physical characteristics and positional differences in professional soccer players in Qatar.* Sports, 2018. **7**(1): p. 9.
78. Hägglund, M., M. Waldén, and J. Ekstrand, *Previous injury as a risk factor for injury in elite football: a prospective study over two consecutive seasons.* British Journal of Sports Medicine, 2006. **40**(9): p. 767–772.
79. N, V.A.N.D., et al., *Similar Isokinetic strength preinjury and at return to sport after hamstring injury.* Medicine & Science in Sports & Exercise, 2019. **51**(6): p. 1091–1098.
80. Ithurburn, M.P., et al., *Knee function, strength, and resumption of preinjury sports participation in young athletes following anterior cruciate ligament reconstruction.* Journal of Orthopaedic & Sports Physical Therapy, 2019. **49**(3): p. 145–153.
81. Kim, S.-H., et al., *Low rate of return to preinjury tegner activity level among recreational athletes: results at 1 year after primary ACL reconstruction.* Orthopaedic Journal of Sports Medicine, 2021. **9**(1): p. 2325967120975751.
82. Ganse, B. and H. Degens, *Current insights in the age-related decline in sports performance of the older athlete.* International Journal of Sports Medicine, 2021. **42**(10): p. 879–888.
83. Silva, J.R., et al., *Individual match playing time during the season affects fitness-related parameters of male professional soccer players.* The Journal of Strength & Conditioning Research, 2011. **25**(10): p. 2729–2739.
84. McGuigan, M.R., S.J. Cormack, and N.D. Gill, *Strength and power profiling of athletes: selecting tests and how to use the information for program design.* Strength & Conditioning Journal, 2013. **35**(6): p. 7–14.
85. Klavora, P., *Vertical-jump tests: a critical review.* Strength and Conditioning Journal, 2000. **22**(5): p. 70–75.
86. Claudino, J.G., et al., *The countermovement jump to monitor neuromuscular status: a meta-analysis.* Journal of Science and Medicine in Sport, 2017. **20**(4): p. 397–402.
87. Hoff, J., et al., *Soccer specific aerobic endurance training.* British Journal of Sports Medicine, 2002. **36**(3): p. 218–221.
88. Manouvrier, C., J. Cassirame, and S. Ahmaidi, *Proposal for a specific aerobic test for football players: the 'Footeval'.* Journal of Sports Science & Medicine, 2016. **15**(4): p. 670.
89. Manouvrier, C., J. Cassirame, and S. Ahmaidi, *Sensitivity of the footeval test to different training modes.* The Journal of Strength & Conditioning Research, 2020. **34**(5): p. 1440–1447.
90. Buchheit, M., *The 30-15 intermittent fitness test: accuracy for individualizing interval training of young intermittent sport players.* The Journal of Strength and Conditioning Research, 2008. **22**(2): p. 365–374.
91. Buchheit, M., C. Vassallo, and M. Waldron, *One box-to-box does not t all-insights from running energetics.* Sport Performance & Science Reports, 2021. **1**(136): p. 1–11.

4 Strength, power and injury prevention

Mike Beere, Christian Clarup, Cody Williamson and Adam Centofanti

Importance of strength and power in soccer

There is great variance in the physical qualities required for successful soccer performance [1, 2], and the increasing physical requirements in elite soccer [3, 4] suggest that the inclusion of strength and conditioning (S&C) practices would be beneficial to help players cope with this demand. Research indicates that soccer performance requires a level of contractile strength which can be improved through S&C practices. Lower limb strength training has been shown to have a positive influence on soccer specific movements such as sprint speed and jumps, therefore, seen as important factors in physical success [5–7]. The basic demands of many sports require athletes to rapidly exert high forces to accelerate, decelerate, or change direction [8–10]. During these events, greater force is applied to the ground and greater velocity is generated [11, 12]. Physical qualities such as strength and speed have been shown to be a highly impactful capacity that can transform soccer performance [13]. Therefore, the development of lower limb strength, is critical to improving athletic development and underpins both individual and team sport performance [9]. As such, in elite soccer, strength development is frequently prioritised by practitioners aiming to improve performance and prevent injuries [14, 15]. It has been highlighted that 86% of practitioners working in senior male professional soccer determine strength training to have a "very important" or "important" benefit to improving soccer performance, with all practitioners including lower limb strength training in their respective programmes [15]. Elite soccer players compete over long competitive seasons, with multiple games per week [16, 17]. Given that decisive games with larger consequences, such as play-offs, knockout stages of competitions or cup finals often take place at the end of the season, it is vital that key physical qualities are maintained, performance is high, and injuries are minimised throughout the entirety of a competitive season. Practitioners must therefore strike a difficult balance between training to improve performance capacities and providing adequate rest and recovery to ensure optimal performance on a weekly or bi-weekly basis.

The influence of injuries in professional soccer is significant, with relationships between reduced injury rates and improved team performance (*increased average points per game and higher league ranking*) being evident [18]. Due to the negative effects that injuries have on team performance [18], the large

DOI: 10.4324/9781003200420-4

financial cost (whereby the average cost of a hamstring injury can be €500,000 per month [19]), and long-term player health [20, 21], injury prevention strategies are seen as an essential part of sports performance [22]. Additionally, many practitioners are judged on injury rates and keeping players available for match selection, hence it is of paramount importance. Moreover, the majority of coaches, staff, and players (>90%) questioned in a recent research suggest that it is the fitness coach's responsibility to ensure "injury prevention programmes" are implemented [23–25]. Although the cause of injury is not always known and can be multi-factorial in cause, there are several potential factors that may increase its incidence [26]. Injuries are often related to non-modifiable and modifiable, and intrinsic and extrinsic factors. Non-modifiable factors are those that cannot be regulated or altered by the practitioner, such as athlete age, sex, and injury history [27]. Modifiable factors that include player training load, warm-up preparation, muscular imbalances, and neuromuscular strength deficits can all be targeted with interventions and regulated by the practitioner [28, 29] (see Chapter 9).

The role of muscle strength and muscle imbalances as risk factors for lower limb injuries has been widely discussed [30–33]. In fact, muscle imbalances have previously been ranked as the third most important intrinsic risk factor for injury in elite soccer [32, 33]. Adequate training to improve muscular strength has been reported as the main measure for reducing these imbalances and reducing injury risk in soccer players [34, 35], and has been shown to reduce injuries to less than 1/3, and over-use injuries almost halved [36]. A recent study into professional practices in soccer has shown that the main focus of S&C programmes was to "prioritise performance enhancement strategies" rather than "prioritising injury prevention or reduction strategies" [15]. The physical demands of professional soccer are continually increasing [3, 4]. Consequently, improving the ability not only to tolerate these demands but also to enhance performance can bring significant benefits to the club. It could be noted that reducing a player's risk of injury could, in turn, be a performance enhancement strategy. Specifically, if a player spends more time training and available for match-selection, due to a reduction in their injury risk and increase in work capacity, then this should be seen as a performance enhancement strategy. Whilst the reduction of injuries is an important factor in success, pushing the boundaries of physical performance to meet the growing demands should be a key focus of performance practitioners in any sport, including soccer.

Strength – injury prevention and availability

Success of a soccer team is underpinned by a multitude of interrelated factors, one of the most important is undoubtedly player availability. Availability is one of the primary goals of the high-performance team (strength and conditioning coaches, physiotherapists, sports medicine physicians, and alike) (see Chapter 1). Low injury rates within a season would be looked upon favourably when determining the success of an overall programme; however, it is important to consider the underpinning factors which determine availability. Durable and resilient players keep themselves on the pitch, week in, week out. We can gain insight into the durability and resilience of the player by analysing training exposure, missed sessions, and modified sessions. Match-minute exposure across seasons can also provide vital information. With easy access to such information in the modern era, clubs can analyse match exposure when looking at potential signings as a part of their overall screening process.

It is imperative clubs have a holistic and objective framework for player recruitment. This will help the coaching staff, in collaboration with the performance team, to determine the relative risk profile of a given player. This objective framework for player recruitment can also incorporate data on the physical demands of player positions, the style of play, and the league(s) that the team is competing in. It is worth noting that although there will be some crossover between case profiles, certain leagues may expose athletes to different physical demands [37]. An in-depth analysis of what the key performance indicators (KPIs) are for each position, from a physical standpoint, may help guide programming and also determine whether a given player is the right 'fit' for the club. High-performance staff can also identify key performance inhibitors which may hinder an athlete's ability to undertake the desired role within the team, and prevent 'square peg, round hole' scenarios. Therefore, communication between coaching staff, leadership, and the high-performance team is a vital component to the delivery of the holistic and objective framework.

It is well-established in the scientific literature that age and prior injury history are strong risk factors for future injury [38–40]. These non-modifiable risk factors should be expressed to the coaching staff when developing a risk profile of a given player. Chronological age is straight forward; however, injury history can be identified via a thorough subjective assessment performed by the performance team's medical staff. An extensive injury history (soft tissue, recalcitrant problems, chronic injuries etc.) in conjunction with retrospective analysis of a player's exposure to games and minutes across several years can help gain insight into player durability. Therefore, the medical staff can identify any deficits or areas of concern and present a player risk profile to the club's stakeholders. This can aid the recruitment decision-making across the season and assist with prospective player signings.

Internally, there is an equally unique range of considerations for the coaching staff and performance team. With the emergence of elite academy systems, integration of developing players into first team environments also needs to be discussed. Assessment of biological maturation and identifying the early versus late maturing players can help assess their preparedness for the transition, and how coaching and performance staff can safely manage the player's integration [41]. Strengths and weaknesses, individual characteristics, and idiosyncrasies should be documented also. In recent research, soccer players with a fast muscle fibre typology displayed a 5.3-fold higher risk of experiencing a new hamstring strain injury compared with slow typology players [42]. Fibre type profiling as a novel risk factor may help the sports medicine community better manage explosive athletes with unique muscle performance qualities. Although the focus of this chapter is on strength, recruiting a list of players, that do not have the capacity to deal with the stressors of the competition, will result in difficulty to maintain low injury rates, regardless of the injury mitigation strategies put in place by the performance team [43].

We must acknowledge the importance of load management in maintaining low injury rates. There has been an explosion of methods used in professional sport to track and manage load [44, 45]. Such methods include but are not limited to; wearable technology and survey analysis (see *Chapters 6 and 7*). To keep injury rates low, special considerations to these metrics can highlight acute or unprecedented spikes in load which may put an athlete at heightened risk [46]. This is especially important in the presence of congested match fixtures for players with increased minute exposure, as well as monitoring and maintaining loads of those who are not playing regularly via top ups and on-pitch extras (see *Chapter 10*). Meticulous planning of training sessions with clear objectives can also help reduce training related injuries because of programming errors and will avoid creating excessive fatigue leading into games.

Understanding the physical requirements of each position, which may change with formation and tactical style, is of paramount importance [47]. Within the soccer-medicine community, there is a plethora of research analysing the common injuries seen within the sport [48–50] (see *Chapter 9*). This understanding of physical stressors associated with the game, and injury analysis, can help triage assessments and interventions that are driven by the performance staff. Considerations to specific injuries that a player has suffered across their career should also be noted; when incomplete rehab occurs, compensations develop as players continue to train and play with injuries.

Perhaps one of the most important tools to identify potential issues, and/or highlight deficits, is via a targeted soccer specific screening process commonly performed at the beginning of pre-season (see *Chapter 3*). Identifying deficits in muscle groups and side-to-side asymmetries can provide vital information for the high-performance team to help guide programming and identifying target areas for individual players. Pre-season testing also provides baseline objective data which can aid the rehabilitation process when injuries do occur as mentioned above. Although general programmes have been shown to be effective in reducing time lost due to injury [51], at the elite level, it is evident that individualised programmes will have better outcomes and promote athlete adherence to prescribed interventions. Similarly, it is now common practice for practitioners to prescribe individualised conditioning interventions, based on a players' fitness status to help mitigate overall risk of injury [52, 53] (see *Chapter 5*).

Eccentric hamstring strength [40, 54], adductor:abductor strength ratios [55], and quadriceps strength [56] are examples of potential muscle strength measures that may provide useful data for the performance team. It is pertinent to acknowledge that clubs and respective clinicians will have access to varying degrees of resources and technology, which will impact the testing battery which the performance team decides to implement (see *Chapter 3*). Even with limited resources, it is possible to develop an effective pre-season screening between the medical team and performance staff. Testing options that require little equipment could involve the single leg bridge test [57] and/or hip muscle strength assessment using a sphygmomanometer which has been shown to be valid and reliable [58]. Additionally, various testing procedures (e.g. performance and field tests) can provide quantitative and qualitative information for the clinician (see Chapter 3). Filming specific movement tests in the sagittal and coronal plane can provide useful information for potential energy leaks and movement inefficiencies, such as excessive anterior pelvic tilt during sprinting [59]. Utilising strategies that address lumbopelvic deficits and promote efficient mechanics during high-velocity locomotive activities is developing promising research; however, it is recommended to approach with caution [60]. Movement mechanics, and their interdependent relationship with fitness-fatigue continuum, should always be considered when determining the aetiology of new or recurrent injuries [61]. To avoid 'paralysis by analysis', it is imperative that the testing performed is relatable to soccer and ensures that the information gained from the testing directly influences programming. If timing and resources permits, it is useful to have additional targeted testing for identified high-risk players who have been hampered by injuries or a specific injury in the past. It is crucial for baseline testing to be performed, and the medical team has an in-depth understanding of the player's injury history. A comprehensive programme can be developed to address identified deficits and target desired muscle qualities in-or-around previously injured tissues. Exercise selection should also address the multiplanar nature of athletic movement in soccer.

Individualised programmes to address target areas should be the cornerstone of injury mitigation interventions, although the influence of a structured strength and conditioning programme, that aims to promote athlete development, will often address many of these issues anyway. Periodising speed work and exposure to maximum velocity is a potent intervention for altering hamstring muscle architecture, alongside isolated hamstring strength exercises [62–64]. Therefore, the perennial interplay between performance training and injury mitigation strategies is self-evident. It is imperative that the performance staff work collaboratively when designing the overarching programme that aims to drive performance metrics, combat injury prevalence, and promote player availability.

Assessing strength

Assessments of basic physical components, such as strength and power, are considered highly important within sports that require high amounts of accelerations and change of directions [65, 66]. Therefore, an appropriate and relevant testing battery for strength and power should be established and used in elite soccer clubs. Various test types, like repetition max (RM), isokinetic dynamometry, handheld dynamometry, variations of jump testing (e.g. the countermovement jump, CMJ), and isometric testing of maximum strength (e.g. the isometric mid-thigh pull, IMTP) have all been established and described in the literature as methods used for assessments (Figure 4.1) [65, 67, 68].

Strength & Power Tests	Repetition max (RM)	Back squat
		Trapbar Deadlift
	Isokinectic dynanometry	Biodex
	Isometric mid-thigh pull (IMTP)	
	Jump varations	CMJ
		Broad Jump
	Hops	Triple hop
		Crossover hop
	Isolated strength protocols	Adductor (groin squeeze)
		Hamstring (Nordic force output)

Figure 4.1 Example of common strength and power tests performed in professional soccer.

The different tests can be helpful for the practitioner, due to different reasons such as, monitoring of an acute response to training, measuring, the chronic response to a training stimulus, identifying individual weakness and strength, comparing data to normative data, and planning individualised training programmes. It is critical for the practitioner to select a test that is appropriate and relevant when assessing the athletes. High levels of strength have been associated with lower risk of injuries [9, 66], and high levels of power have been associated with improved speed and change of directions [69]. Therefore, appropriate testing of these variables could give useful insights of relevant physical qualities of the elite soccer player. The 1-RM back squat test is often recommended as a useful tool for testing maximal strength in soccer players [10, 67]; however, from a practical and technical aspect, some soccer players can struggle with the back squat exercise due lack of powerlifting skills or mobility [70]. Additionally, other testing forms might give useful information regarding levels of maximum strength.

Isometric testing or a different selection of exercises could be an alternate solution to test maximum strength. For example, multiple movements in team sports, like sprinting, jumping and change of directions, are often performed unilaterally and should be taken into consideration when designing a strength testing battery. Therefore, one should always find a test that suits the specific group of athletes, as opposed to selecting only one, out of habit/tradition. Upon determining if a test is useful, the practitioner must establish the validity, reliability, and sensitivity of the selected test methods [71]. It is of high importance that tests are valid and adequality sensitive to detect meaningful and systematic changes at both group and individual level [71, 72]. When the practitioner is ready to implement testing, it is important to avoid testing just for the sake of testing. A practitioner working in elite soccer should ask the following questions when deciding on strength-testing parameters:

- Is it practical to do conduct the testing under question?
- Are the results meaningful for the players and technical staff?
- Will the data be used for programming?
- Is retesting feasible throughout the season?
- Is the selected test assessing relevant data regarding match performance?
- Will testing outcomes have a substantial positive effect on athletic performance?

Proceeding the strength-testing selection process, practitioners must evaluate the athlete's physical capacities to establish baselines, strength profiles and detect possible deficits. Strength profiles like the Dynamic Strength Index (DSI) provide a ratio of the peak force the athlete can produce in both isometric and ballistic testing. The DSI provides a strength and power profile of the athlete, informing practitioners of individual's force-velocity capabilities [68, 73]. Establishing a sound strength-power profile of individuals can eliminate the simplistic notion that "stronger is always better". Even if the athlete has sufficient levels of strength, this might not be the inhibitor of performance. Therefore, a more holistic approach to the strength training should be implemented. It must be noted that soccer players can be fast, with-out being powerful, which might not be desirable.

As aforementioned, high levels of muscular strength have a positive effect on the rate of injuries, thus emphasising the importance of relevant strength and power testing. With the current understanding of muscle injuries in elite football (*see Chapter 9*), relevant testing and consistent training for isolated areas, such as eccentric hamstring exposure, is highly recommended [74, 75]. Specifically, key metrics to aim for have been thoroughly discussed in the literature to date [54, 76–78]. Identifying isolated strength deficits allows practitioners to create strength profiles, alongside other relevant data. Establishing strength-power profiles, paired with locomotive profiles (game data), can aid practitioners when determining training interventions, altering priorities, and designing individual training programmes. This holistic approach will result in an efficient prescription for the individual player, resulting in overall increases in physical performance.

In elite soccer environments, with a high frequency of competitive matches, limited periods for strength and power training must be taken into consideration when planning for desired adaptations. Therefore, when testing, a time-efficient and practical approach is necessary. Relevant strength testing data provide proficient information to the practitioner, when it comes to designing training programmes, both on-and-off the pitch. Additionally, the results obtained from strength testing will aid the practitioner in adjusting the modifiable aspects within the training schedule. With the chaotic nature of soccer, unexpected events can occur. Therefore, it is necessary for a practitioner to be adaptable when planning any strength training or testing. Establishing baselines and collecting various strength-power data is extremely valuable, helping practitioners make effective and efficient decisions when considering the status of a player.

Modules of strength-power (force-velocity curve)

The force–velocity curve is a physical representation of the inverse relationship between force production and velocity of movement (Figure 4.2) [79, 80]. Understanding the interaction between force and velocity, and their influences on exercise selection, is vital for any practitioner. For example, it is essential that practitioners understand the physiological and biomechanical differences between prescribing a 1RM deadlift and 5RM jump squats – as one will produce higher forces and lower velocities than the other. Failure to understand the relationship and its importance will likely lead to less-than-optimal training prescription. Dynamic, explosive, powerful qualities such as rate of force development (RFD) and explosive strength have been suggested to better predict athletic performance [81]. Training modalities to develop RFD should be targeted by practitioners working in soccer. Developing the neuromuscular system, to enhance the capabilities to produce force, is one of the most important goals of a strength and conditioning programme.

Strength is typically viewed as the ability to lift heavy objects, quantified as the peak force or torque, measured during isometric testing or rep max testing [82]. Maximal strength has a strong correlation with rate RFD and power, and is a vital component in producing the high levels of force needed in sport [83–85]. Strength is therefore an important, trainable skill that needs to be expressed during competition. Strength is not only the ability to generate force, but also a vehicle that carries with it other abilities such as RFD, impulse, momentum, velocity, and power. Different levels of strength exist ranging from submaximal to maximal, with maximal strength being a major factor influencing performance [85]. Heavy load resistance exercise results in an increase in the isometric peak force and can cause a shift in the force-velocity curve in untrained individuals [8, 86]. However, although heavy resistance training can increase the athlete's strength reserve and positively impact the RFD, it is likely that with stronger more experienced athletes, the optimisation of the RFD and subsequent power development is better achieved with the incorporation of explosive or ballistic

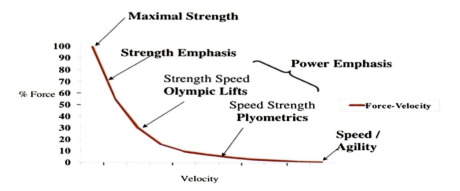

Figure 4.2 Force–velocity relationship applied to training methodologies.

exercises [8, 87]. Therefore, various training methods have the potential to impact different parts of the force-time and force- velocity curves. For example, heavy resistance training can significantly increase the ability to generate peak force and the RFD when compared with untrained individuals [88, 89]. Conversely, ballistic, or explosive training can result in increases in the overall RFD that is greater than what can occur with heavy resistance training or during an untrained state. However, ballistic training cannot increase the overall maximal strength levels to the same extent as heavy resistance training. Therefore, a mixed training approach is often recommended when attempting to maximise the RFD and power output [87]. Protocols containing both high velocity and high force training produce better results than training each aspect alone, but a proper sequencing must be used to maximise mixed training stimuli [90, 91]. Research has shown that training maximal strength before maximal velocity provides the most beneficial adaptations, and this may be due in part to delayed gains in performance and shortening velocity [91].

Power prescription

The implementation of power-based exercises within a professional soccer setting can be executed in a multitude of ways. As aforementioned, training different areas of the force velocity curve can be advantageous towards athletic development, injury reduction and overall performance. Plyometric-based exercises can be prescribed during on field warm-ups (see Chapter 5), however can also be utilised during gym-based sessions either pre or post training [15]. It is recommended to perform plyometrics when players are in a rested state; however, logistically this may not be possible and some plyometrics may be performed following field sessions or in the later part of the training week. Ideally, plyometric based activities are appropriately progressed over time during the season, yet when performing in a team setting, athletes may be at different levels, so caution is advised with regard to the intensity of plyometric prescription. Certain players may have existing pathologies that prevent them from performing more intense plyometric progressions on-field, so careful consideration is needed when prescribing for the team and allowing simple regressions for individual players. Additionally, fixture congestion, player fatigue/readiness play a crucial role in the prescription of plyometrics and may need to be more gradual in design than an individual training in an off-season period. Alternatively, prescribing plyometric work during pre-or-post training during gym settings may be more appropriate for the individual, as well as enabling more appropriate rest times that may not be possible on field (Table 4.1).

Other power-based exercises such as step-up jumps, squat jumps, lunge jumps and Olympic lifting derivatives etc. are examples of exercises that can be implemented into gym sessions, either exclusively or as part of a contrasting sequence with a particular strength exercise [80]. Depending on the goals of the holistic strength and conditioning programme, individual objectives, and phases of training, power-based exercises can be incorporated into gym sessions to achieve the desired adaptations for specific areas on the force velocity curve.

Table 4.1 Example of an on field plyometric prescription

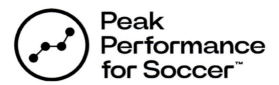

Plyometric exercise
Double leg pogos forwards and backwards 2 × 10 Single leg pogos forwards 1 × 10 each side Broad jump single effort 2 × 3 Counter movement jump single effort 2 × 3 Skip bound for height 2 × 20m Skip bound for distance 2 × 20m

Exercise selection in soccer

Key exercises

There are a variety of exercises at a practitioner's disposal when it comes to strength development. Understanding which exercises are essential, and have the most positive affect on strength adaptations, is important for any elite soccer team. The demands of the game, common injury sites, and individual characteristics assist in mapping out what each strength session will look like. There is a plethora of content to be found online with regard to strength training for soccer players, however understanding what is commonly used in professional soccer settings and why certain exercises are used over others is key. A recent survey of 51 practitioners working in elite soccer (the UK and the USA) highlighted the most common exercises used in professional soccer (Table 4.2) [92]:

- *Trap Bar Deadlift (TBD) (hex bar deadlift)* is most used exercise (51%): Research has demonstrated that the use of a TBD results in greater force, power, and RFD and has a greater correlation with vertical jump due to similar body positions when compared to traditional squat or deadlifts [93]. Hex bar jumps have been shown to elicit greater jump height, peak force, power, and peak RFD across varying loads when compared to jump squats. In the authors' experience, soccer players also struggle with hip and ankle injuries and subsequent lack of range of motion, that often lead to a poor technical ability in the traditional barbell squat exercise. These limitations can often be reduced by utilising the TBD exercise.
- *Split stance exercises* such as rear foot elevated split squats (RFESS) were frequently reported exercise utilised in soccer practitioners programmes (n = 20, 39%)

Table 4.2 Key exercises frequently utilised in professional soccer

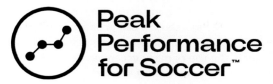

Exercise	
Strength	Plyometrics
Trap bar deadlift (TBD)	Multiple hops/jumps
Split stance (e.g. RFESS, lunges, step ups)	Box drills
Romanian deadlifts (RDL + derivatives)	Reactive jumps in place
Nordic hamstring exercise (NHE)	Bounding
Copenhagen adductor holds	Vertical jumps
Hamstring eccentric slide outs	Horizontal jumps
Calf raises	Depth jumps

- While Olympic lifting exercises have a great value in improving athletic qualities, they are not often incorporated in soccer practices, and less used than previously reported in other sports such as Rugby Union (used by 90% of practitioners) [94], Rowing (87%) [95], NFL (88%) [96], and NHL (91%) [97].
- Other frequently used exercises included the *Romanian or stiff leg deadlift* variations (n = 22, 43%), *Nordic hamstring* curls (n = 15, 29%), and *hip thrusts* (n = 13, 25%). Numerous other exercises were also ranked in coaches main five exercises, including

    - eccentric hamstring curls,
    - calf raises,
    - lunge patterns,
    - isometric hamstring holds,
    - step ups,
    - Copenhagen adductor holds,
    - single leg jumps, and
    - derivatives of Olympic weightlifting, such as jump shrugs, hang cleans, and drop snatches.

- In addition, plyometrics are frequently and commonly prescribed in strength and conditioning sessions, for improving RFD, improving reactive strength, improving stiffness, and preventing injury.
- In this research, 45 out of 51 (88%) coaches reported using eccentric exercises, with 40 (78%) using eccentrics for preventing injuries. These results support those previously reported in the literature where 85% of practitioners believe that eccentric exercises can help prevent lower limb injuries in soccer players [24]. Eccentric muscle actions involve the active

lengthening of muscle tissue against an external force or load [98], in contrast to isometric and concentric muscle actions which involve no change in muscle length or the shortening of muscle tissue, respectively [99]. It has been reported that skeletal muscle can produce more relative force during eccentric muscle actions compared to isometric and concentric actions [100], and as such, the use of many eccentric exercises are gaining popularity during strength and conditioning sessions.

Injury prevention exercises

Eccentric exercises have previously been ranked as the most effective way to prevent non-contact injuries in soccer players [32]. It has been suggested that eccentric exercises may prevent injury by improving the muscles' ability to absorb more force before failing [101]. While research and practice-based evidence back up the idea that eccentric exercises are important for injury prevention in professional soccer players, the uptake of the Nordic hamstring exercise protocol is surprisingly often poor in elite soccer teams competing in the UEFA Champions League [35]. Ultimately, the range of exercises utilised demonstrates that there is a requirement for athletes to be competent in several exercises to assist in performance and reduce the most common injuries that occur in soccer. However, what is also clear is that fundamental exercises such as TBD, RDL, and squat patterns are consistently reported in many practitioners' sessions.

Application of strength and power training

Scheduling

Scheduling appropriate strength and power sessions for a soccer team can be a complex task, with multiple factors influencing when, what, and how much strength training is prescribed. There are various ways in which strength sessions are implemented by clubs around the globe. However, commonly team sessions are performed on a match day-4 (MD-4) or match day-3 (MD-3), which falls in line with the acquisition phase of field-based training (heaviest loads of the week) during a seven-day microcycle (see *Chapter 10*). With each club and player having their own history of strength training or culture around strength development, practitioners often must adapt to achieve the greatest compliance. Therefore, selecting the most important exercises to achieve the minimum effective dose will be required. Depending on the quantity of sessions during the week or best opportunities based around fixtures, it may be advisable to micro-dose a strength stimulus prior to field training spread across the week (Table 4.3).

The content for each gym session often changes, with teams either opting for a total body gym session, on both days incorporating upper and lower body, or separate sessions of upper body and lower body exclusively. Additionally, when incorporating total body-based gym sessions, selecting exercises that suit the type of field work completed or alternatively, in preparation for the proceeding

Strength, power and injury prevention 95

Table 4.3 Gym session scheduling example for a seven-day microcycle

Peak Performance for Soccer™

	Recovery	Key acquisition day	Key acquisition day	Taper	Taper	GAME	Recovery
Day Code	MD+2	MD-4	MD-3	MD-2	MD-1	MD	MD+1
Session Type	OFF	Intensive	Extensive	Reactive speed	Pre-match	Match day	Recovery/top up
Field Physical Target		ACC/DEC	Max velocity + high speed running	Coordination + agility	Priming		Regeneration
Individual prep prior to activation		Individual preparation	Individual preparation	Individual preparation	Individual preparation	Individual preparation	
Pre training themes		Glute + adductor	Glute + hamstring	Mobility + core stability	Reactions + priming	Match day preparation	
Gym themes		Anterior chain focus	Posterior chain focus				Optional gym or top up group gym

training session, is advisable. For example, prescribing anterior-chain dominant exercises (e.g. squat patterns) on the MD-4 aligns with intensive nature of the field sessions. Furthermore, posterior-chain dominant strength exercises (e.g. RDL and Nordics) prescribed on MD-3 overload the muscle regions associated with high-speed running (extensive) [102]. When prescribing exclusively isolated body-region gym sessions during the week (i.e. lower body and upper body), allocating the lower body gym session could be problematic. There is no right or wrong answer, with varied preferences for MD-4 and MD-3. Performing the lower-body gym session on MD-4 allows the longest time between resistance training and the match, potentially minimising the chance of fatigue leading into match-play. However, the immediate onset of residual fatigue (24-hours post-session) may compromise field-based work on the proceeding day (MD-3). On the contrary, scheduling the lower-body gym session on MD-3 may be preferred. However, unlike MD-4, there is a greater chance of players exhibiting delayed muscle soreness closer to match-day. Understanding the implications of both options is imperative in the decision-making process and may help the performance team decide which approach suits their respective cohort of players and environment. Ultimately, the intensity and response of soccer-specific training (field sessions) may limit practitioners with options in scheduling. Therefore, it is recommended that practitioners are flexible and agile when constructing gym sessions.

In addition to main team gym sessions, individual strength prescriptions may be scheduled throughout alternate days (other than MD-4 or MD-3). For example, players demonstrating undesired levels of localised muscle soreness, from resistance training, may require an individualised micro-dosing scheme. Specifically, some of the key exercises (Table 4.2) can be prescribed at the desired intensity, with varied volumes throughout the week. Alternatively, performing individual strength work post game or on an MD + 1 can prove to be an effective solution to strength development. However, it must be noted that fatigue from match play, decreased player motivation, or coach preference may not allow this to occur. Educating all stakeholders in the rationale for specific strength prescription post game may be required to ensure additional work to be completed.

Fixture congestion

Practitioners may be limited with time to allow for adequate adaptation from strength training during congested-game periods. Fatigue from games and minimal time between games can be challenges that the performance team will encounter when looking to provide a strength stimulus for their cohort of players. The lack of strength stimuli during these congested phases may result in detraining of strength qualities, thus emphasising the importance of desired strength prior to the commencement of fixture congestion. However, there may be windows of opportunity for practitioners to micro-dose strength stimuli, to minimise the likelihood of detraining (Table 4.4).

Table 4.4 Example of a strength-training prescription during fixture congestion

	Taper	Taper	GAME	Recovery	Taper	GAME	Recovery
Day Code	MD-2	MD-1	MD	MD+1	MD-1	MD	MD+1
Session type	Reactive speed	Pre-match	Match day	Recovery/top up	Pre-match	Match day	OFF
Strength option post training/field	Adductors (Copenhagen's)	Upper Body	Nordics or single leg hamstring sliders	Unilateral quad (split squat)	Upper body	Nordics or single leg hamstring sliders	

Content

The content of gym sessions in microcycles varies greatly amongst clubs, as resources, environment, and equipment play a key role in determining what limitations practitioners are dealt with. It is also worth mentioning that there are many performance coaches across the world that have differing views of strength training. However, well-researched exercises for developing strength and power, as well as being valid for performance enhancement, will be identified in further examples. Although multiple variations of the outlined examples exist, as well as the inclusion of differing accessory exercises, the aim is to provide a simple, effective, and minimal approach to prescribing strength-training in elite soccer. The prescriptions detailed are general and must be adapted to the environment of a practitioner, such as the goals of the organisation, phase of season/training, individual players and cohort, and readiness amongst other variables.

Two-day split – total body

MD-4

1A – Trap bar deadlift 3 × 5
1B – Bench Press 3 × 5
2A – Rear foot elevated split squat 3 × 6
2B – Dumbbell shoulder press 3 × 6
3A – Lateral lunge 3 × 6
3B – Copenhagen's 3 × 20sec

MD-3

1A – Single leg RDL 3 × 6
1B – Pullups 3 × 8–10

2A – Nordics 3 × 3
2B – Dumbbell single arm rows 3 × 6
3A – 45 degree back extension 3 × 12
3B – Single leg calf raise 3 × 15

Two-Day split – upper and lower body

<u>MD-4</u>

1A – Bench Press 3 × 5
1B – Pullups 3 × 8–10
2A – Dumbbell shoulder press 3 × 6
2B – Dumbbell single arm rows 3 × 6
3A – Hanging leg raises 3 × 8
3B – 45-degree back extension 3 × 12

<u>MD-3</u>

1A – Trap bar deadlift 3 × 5
1B – Single leg RDL 3 × 6
2A – Rear foot elevated split squat 3 × 6
2B – Nordics 3 × 3
3A – Copenhagen's 3 × 20sec
3B – Single leg seated calf raise 3 × 15

The above two-day split programmes emphasise key areas to address from a holistic standpoint. In many cases, programmes and exercise selection can be smaller or bigger depending on a myriad of aforementioned factors. The primary objective to a comprehensive strength programme is the proper execution of all movements with adequate load to elicit positive change (strength adaptations). Too often, social media is littered with 'strength' alternatives which emphasise increased complexity, as well as 'specific' exercises to transfer to field, and on-field circuits which lack the load to change muscle architecture and physiology. It is highly recommended that exercise selection and gym-based strength sessions be evidence-based and address key areas of physical performance and injury reduction. With little time and opportunities dedicated to strength training during the season, practitioners must decide on the most effective exercises to increase player availability whilst improving performance.

Considerations

Limitations

It is well-known that soccer schedules are often congested, chaotic, and at constant threat of changing due to several factors, such as television coverage, and progression in one or several knockout tournaments. Issues around fixture congestion are impossible to change, as the nature of the sport can require teams to play two to three games per week for much of the season [34, 103]. This is the case for not only the elite teams playing in European competition, but also in many domestic leagues around the world, due to involvement in multiple cup competitions on top of a 38–46 game league seasons. It becomes difficult to periodise, manage training load, and avoid accumulated fatigue, while ensuring that players remain at an optimal level of physical fitness during the season [103, 104].

A recent survey of 51 S&C working in elite soccer (the UK and the USA) highlighted most common barriers towards strength training prescriptions [15]:

- Time availability is the biggest challenge facing the implementation of S&C practices.
- Importance of winning matches overshadows the ability to push the boundaries of S&C development.
- Lack of staff and lack of or poor facilities are third- and fourth-ranked barriers to S&C practice.
- It is concluded that employing qualified staff and providing adequate training facilities should be of high importance to senior club staff. Lack of staff has previously been highlighted as a substantial barrier to the effectiveness of any training load monitoring practices in soccer [105].
- In agreement, Weldon et al. (2020) also found that [14]:
- Time/schedule/fixtures were the biggest barrier to practice in elite soccer.
- With lack of equipment/staff/facilities also highly ranked.
- Coach relationships and difference in opinions were also a barrier to practice.

Cultural differences

Although sound strength and conditioning principles of prescription have been well documented to improve performance and minimise the risk of injury, there are also many alternative views to achieve strength stimuli. Across the globe, different cultures may perceive strength in their own way, which leads players potentially being misled and adapting to habit. When, or if, these players transfer to different leagues/clubs across the world, they may find themselves exposed to valid and robust strength prescriptions as discussed throughout. However, if exposed to alternate approaches, practitioners may be initially faced with decreased levels of compliance. Misconceptions of strength and power training allows for greater occurrences of complaints in relation to prescriptions (Figure 4.3). Therefore, it is imperative that practitioners utilise moments of education with players to illustrate rationale with their prescriptions.

First and foremost, it is imperative to highlight the importance of building positive relationships with players, as this is the first step to any good working relationship (see *Chapter 11*). Pertaining to certain players having a negative attitude towards strength training, having a professional relationship, derived from respect, allows for greater compliance. Additionally, further education may be

100 Mike Beere et al.

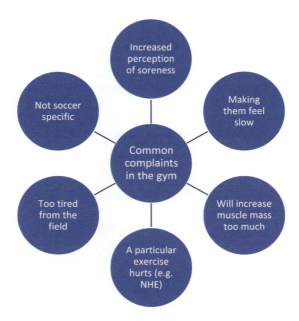

Figure 4.3 Common complaints from players, due to misconceptions of strength training in elite soccer.

Strategies to increase compliance	Reframing language (strength vs range of motion)
	Education (player, coach, staff)
	Microdosing across the week
	Exercise alternatives
	Exercise progressions/regressions
	Reduced complexity and volume
	Prescribing familiar exercises
	Relationship building

Figure 4.4 Strategies to increase compliance to strength training prescription.

necessary for support staff and coaching staff in relation to rationale of strength training variables and responses. Developing a professional relationship with players allows for greater understanding of player perspective and thought processes, potentially influenced by previous experience. During unwanted periods of low-compliance, practitioners may have to adjust training variables in order to develop trust. Practitioners may provide familiar exercises to player's previous exposures that illicit desired outcomes, amongst other strategies (Figure 4.4). Although alternative exercises to the practitioner's exercise menu may not be preferred, one should initially dedicate the outcome to improving compliance, with the long-term objective of providing appropriate stimulus.

Applying best practice or a performance teams' ideal prescription may not always be possible in a professional setting. However, with continued efforts to design programmes based off evidence-based principles, as well as keeping an open-mind to individual preferences and experiences, optimal compliance and performance enhancements can still be made. As performance departments continue to evolve and more research is done in the field of sports science, so too will the awareness of best practice strength prescriptions in elite soccer. It is the objective of this text to continue to educate and provide a resource of the current evidence-based principles to strength training, as well as provide strategies to apply in a real-world setting.

Conclusion

Strength is an integral piece of the performance programme for elite soccer teams. Understanding its role in performance, injury prevention and overall availability, is essential for any practitioner working at the elite level. Assessing strength and power will assist in profiling players and can influence prescription on and off the field. Knowledge of the key exercises used, as well as the benefits associated, will result in the most effective programme. Scheduling strength training during a week can vary greatly, depending on a variety of factors such as fixtures, player readiness, field load, and individual preference. Many barriers and cultural differences exist when it comes to strength training prescription. Knowing your cohort of players, their experiences, training age etc. will assist in the design process. Finally, effective, adaptable, and simple prescriptions are paramount to the overall effectiveness of programming.

References

1 Little, T. and A.G. Williams, *Measures of exercise intensity during soccer training drills with professional soccer players.* The Journal of Strength & Conditioning Research, 2007. **21**(2): p. 367–371.
2 Owen, A.L., et al., *Heart rate responses and technical comparison between small-vs. large-sided games in elite professional soccer.* The Journal of Strength & Conditioning Research, 2011. **25**(8): p. 2104–2110.
3 Barnes, C., et al., *The evolution of physical and technical performance parameters in the English Premier League.* International Journal of Sports Medicine, 2014. **35**(13): p. 1095–1100.
4 Bradley, P.S., et al., *Tier-specific evolution of match performance characteristics in the English Premier League: it's getting tougher at the top.* Journal of Sports Sciences, 2016. **34**(10): p. 980–987.
5 Chelly, M.S., et al., *Effects of a back squat training program on leg power, jump, and sprint performances in junior soccer players.* The Journal of Strength & Conditioning Research, 2009. **23**(8): p. 2241–2249.
6 Hoff, J. and J. Helgerud, *Endurance and strength training for soccer players.* Sports Medicine, 2004. **34**(3): p. 165–180.
7 Ronnestad, B.R., et al., *Short-term effects of strength and plyometric training on sprint and jump performance in professional soccer players.* The Journal of Strength & Conditioning Research, 2008. **22**(3): p. 773–780.

8 Cormie, P., M.R. McGuigan, and R.U. Newton, *Developing maximal neuromuscular power.* Sports Medicine, 2011. **41**(1): p. 17–38.
9 Suchomel, T., et al., *The importance of muscular strength: training considerations.* Sports Medicine, 2018. **48**(4): p. 765–785.
10 Wisløff, U., et al., *Strong Correlation of maximal squat strength with sprint performance and vertical jump height in elite soccer players.* British Journal of Sports Medicine, 2004. **38**(3): p. 285–288.
11 Morin, J.-B., et al., *A simple method for computing sprint acceleration kinetics from running velocity data: Replication study with improved design.* Journal of Biomechanics, 2019. **94**: p. 82–87.
12 Morin, J.-B., et al., *When jump height is not a good indicator of lower limb maximal power output: theoretical demonstration, experimental evidence and practical solutions.* Sports Medicine, 2019. **49**(7): p. 999–1006.
13 McGuigan, M.R., G.A. Wright, and S.J. Fleck, *Strength training for athletes: does it really help sports performance?* International Journal of Sports Physiology and Performance, 2012. **7**(1): p. 2–5.
14 Weldon, A., et al., *The strength and conditioning practices and perspectives of soccer coaches and players.* International Journal of Sports Science & Coaching, 2022. **0**(0): p. 17479541211072242.
15 Beere, M., I. Jeffreys, and N. Lewis, *Strength and conditioning provision and practices in elite male football.* Professional Strength & Conditioning, 2020. **58**: p. 21–40.
16 Meckel, Y., et al., *Seasonal variations in physical fitness and performance indices of elite soccer players.* Sports, 2018. **6**(1): p. 14.
17 Dellal, A., K. Chamari, and A. Owen, *How and when to use an injury prevention intervention in soccer.* Muscle Injuries in Sport Medicine, 2013: p. 241–273.
18 Hägglund, M., et al., *Injuries affect team performance negatively in professional football: an 11-year follow-up of the UEFA Champions League injury study.* British Journal of Sports Medicine, 2013. **47**(12): p. 738–742.
19 Ekstrand, J., *Keeping your top players on the pitch: the key to football medicine at a professional level.* 2013, BMJ Publishing Group Ltd and British Association of Sport and Exercise Medicine.
20 Turner, A.P., J.H. Barlow, and C. Heathcote-Elliott, *Long term health impact of playing professional football in the United Kingdom.* British Journal of Sports Medicine, 2000. **34**(5): p. 332–336.
21 Moreno-Pérez, V., et al., *Effects of home confinement due to COVID-19 pandemic on eccentric hamstring muscle strength in football players.* Scandinavian Journal of Medicine & Science in Sports, 2020. **30**(10): p. 2010–2012.
22 Fanchini, M., et al., *Exercise-based strategies to prevent muscle injury in elite footballers: a systematic review and best evidence synthesis.* Sports Medicine, 2020. **50**(9): p. 1653–1666.
23 O'Brien, J., W. Young, and C.F. Finch, *The delivery of injury prevention exercise programmes in professional youth soccer: Comparison to the FIFA 11+.* Journal of Science and Medicine in Sport, 2017. **20**(1): p. 26–31.
24 O'Brien, J. and C.F. Finch, *Injury prevention exercise programmes in professional youth soccer: understanding the perceptions of programme deliverers.* BMJ Open Sport & Exercise Medicine, 2016. **2**(1): p. e000075.
25 Mendonça, L.D.M., et al., *Sports injury prevention programmes from the sports physical therapist's perspective: an international expert Delphi approach.* Physical Therapy in Sport, 2022. **55**: p. 146–154.
26 Bittencourt, N.F., et al., *Complex systems approach for sports injuries: moving from risk factor identification to injury pattern recognition—narrative review and new concept.* British Journal of Sports Medicine, 2016. **50**(21): p. 1309–1314.

27 Parry, L. and B. Drust, *Is injury the major cause of elite soccer players being unavailable to train and play during the competitive season?* Physical Therapy in Sport, 2006. **7**(2): p. 58–64.
28 Bahr, R. and T. Krosshaug, *Understanding injury mechanisms: a key component of preventing injuries in sport.* British Journal of Sports Medicine, 2005. **39**(6): p. 324–329.
29 Buckthorpe, M., et al., *Recommendations for hamstring injury prevention in elite football: translating research into practice.* British Journal of Sports Medicine, 2019. **53**(7): p. 449–456.
30 Cronström, A., et al., *Modifiable factors associated with knee abduction during weight-bearing activities: a systematic review and meta-analysis.* Sports Medicine, 2016. **46**(11): p. 1647–1662.
31 Freckleton, G. and T. Pizzari, *Risk factors for hamstring muscle strain injury in sport: a systematic review and meta-analysis.* British Journal of Sports Medicine, 2012: p. bjsports-2011–090664.
32 McCall, A., et al., *Injury risk factors, screening tests and preventative strategies: a systematic review of the evidence that underpins the perceptions and practices of 44 football (soccer) teams from various premier leagues.* British Journal of Sports Medicine, 2015. **49**(9): p. 583–589.
33 McCall, A., et al., *Injury prevention strategies at the FIFA 2014 World Cup: perceptions and practices of the physicians from the 32 participating national teams.* British Journal of Sports Medicine, 2015. **49**(9): p. 603–608.
34 Thorpe, R.T., et al., *The tracking of morning fatigue status across in-season training weeks in elite soccer players.* International Journal of Sports Physiology and Performance, 2016. **11**(7): p. 947–952.
35 Bahr, R., K. Thorborg, and J. Ekstrand, *Evidence-based hamstring injury prevention is not adopted by the majority of Champions League or Norwegian Premier League football teams: the Nordic Hamstring survey.* British Journal of Sports Medicine, 2015. **49**(22): p. 1466–1471.
36 Lauersen, J.B., D.M. Bertelsen, and L.B. Andersen, *The effectiveness of exercise interventions to prevent sports injuries: a systematic review and meta-analysis of randomised controlled trials.* British Journal of Sports Medicine, 2014. **48**(11): p. 871–877.
37 Dellal, A., et al., *Comparison of physical and technical performance in European soccer match-play: FA Premier League and La Liga.* European Journal of Sport Science, 2011. **11**(1): p. 51–59.
38 Green, B., et al., *Recalibrating the risk of hamstring strain injury (HSI): A 2020 systematic review and meta-analysis of risk factors for index and recurrent hamstring strain injury in sport.* British Journal of Sports Medicine, 2020. **54**(18): p. 1081–1088.
39 Opar, D.A., M.D. Williams, and A.J. Shield, *Hamstring strain injuries.* Sports Medicine, 2012. **42**(3): p. 209–226.
40 Timmins, R.G., et al., *Short biceps femoris fascicles and eccentric knee flexor weakness increase the risk of hamstring injury in elite football (soccer): a prospective cohort study.* British Journal of Sports Medicine, 2016. **50**(24): p. 1524–1535.
41 Lloyd, R.S., et al., *Chronological age vs. biological maturation: implications for exercise programming in youth.* The Journal of Strength & Conditioning Research, 2014. **28**(5): p. 1454–1464.
42 Lievens, E., et al., *Muscle fibre typology as a novel risk factor for hamstring strain injuries in professional football (soccer): a prospective cohort study.* Sports Medicine, 2022. **52**(1): p. 177–185.
43 Coles, P.A., *An injury prevention pyramid for elite sports teams.* British Journal of Sports Medicine, 2018. **52**(15): p. 1008–1010.
44 Gabbett, T.J., *Debunking the myths about training load, injury and performance: empirical evidence, hot topics and recommendations for practitioners.* British Journal of Sports Medicine, 2020. **54**(1): p. 58–66.

45 West, S.W., et al., *More than a metric: how training load is used in elite sport for athlete management.* International Journal of Sports Medicine, 2021. **42**(04): p. 300–306.
46 Hulin, B.T. and T.J. Gabbett, *Indeed association does not equal prediction: the never-ending search for the perfect acute: chronic workload ratio.* 2019, BMJ Publishing Group Ltd and British Association of Sport and Exercise Medicine. p. 144–145.
47 Calder, A. and T. Gabbett, *Influence of tactical formation on average and peak demands of elite soccer match-play.* International Journal of Strength and Conditioning, 2022. **2**(1): p. 1–10.
48 Ekstrand, J., M. Hägglund, and M. Waldén, *Epidemiology of muscle injuries in professional football (soccer).* The American Journal of Sports Medicine, 2011. **39**(6): p. 1226–1232.
49 Ekstrand, J., et al., *Injury rates decreased in men's professional football: an 18-year prospective cohort study of almost 12 000 injuries sustained during 1.8 million hours of play.* British Journal of Sports Medicine, 2021. **55**(19): p. 1084–1091.
50 Jones, A., et al., *Epidemiology of injury in English professional football players: a cohort study.* Physical Therapy in Sport, 2019. **35**: p. 18–22.
51 Silvers-Granelli, H., et al., *Efficacy of the FIFA 11+ injury prevention program in the collegiate male soccer player.* The American Journal of Sports Medicine, 2015. **43**(11): p. 2628–2637.
52 Buchheit, M., C. Vassallo, and M. Waldron, *One box-to-box does not fit all-insights from running energetics.* Sport Performance & Science Reports, 2021. **1**(136): p. 1–11
53 Reiman, M.P. and D.S. Lorenz, *Integration of strength and conditioning principles into a rehabilitation program.* International Journal of Sports Physical Therapy, 2011. **6**(3): p. 241.
54 Opar, D.A., et al., *Eccentric hamstring strength and hamstring injury risk in Australian footballers.* Medicine and Science in Sports and Exercise, 2015. **47**(4): p. 857–865.
55 Thorborg, K., et al., *Hip adduction and abduction strength profiles in elite soccer players: implications for clinical evaluation of hip adductor muscle recovery after injury.* The American Journal of Sports Medicine, 2011. **39**(1): p. 121–126.
56 Van Wyngaarden, J.J., et al., *Quadriceps strength and kinesiophobia predict long-term function after ACL reconstruction: a cross-sectional pilot study.* Sports Health, 2021. **13**(3): p. 251–257.
57 Freckleton, G., J. Cook, and T. Pizzari, *The predictive validity of a single leg bridge test for hamstring injuries in Australian Rules Football Players.* British Journal of Sports Medicine, 2014. **48**(8): p. 713–717.
58 Toohey, L.A., et al., *The validity and reliability of the sphygmomanometer for hip strength assessment in Australian football players.* Physiotherapy Theory and Practice, 2018. **34**(2): p. 131–136.
59 Mendiguchia, J., et al., *Training-induced changes in anterior pelvic tilt: potential implications for hamstring strain injuries management.* Journal of Sports Sciences, 2021. **39**(7): p. 760–767.
60 Mendiguchia, J., et al., *Can we modify maximal speed running posture? Implications for performance and hamstring injury management.* International Journal of Sports Physiology and Performance, 2021. **1**(aop): p. 1–10.
61 Lahti, J., et al., *Multifactorial individualised programme for hamstring muscle injury risk reduction in professional football: protocol for a prospective cohort study.* BMJ Open Sport & Exercise Medicine, 2020. **6**(1): p. e000758.
62 Edouard, P., et al., *Sprinting: a potential vaccine for hamstring injury.* Sport Performance & Science Reports, 2019. **1**: p. 1–2.

63 Bourne, M.N., et al., *Impact of the Nordic hamstring and hip extension exercises on hamstring architecture and morphology: implications for injury prevention.* British Journal of Sports Medicine, 2016: p. bjsports-2016–096130.
64 Bourne, M.N., et al., *An evidence-based framework for strengthening exercises to prevent hamstring injury.* Sports Medicine, 2018. **48**(2): p. 251–267.
65 Hoff, J., *Training and testing physical capacities for elite soccer players.* Journal of Sports Science, 2005. **23**(6): p. 573–582.
66 Suchomel, T., et al., *The importance of Muscular Strength in athletic performance.* Sports Medicine, 2016. **46**(10): p. 1419–1449.
67 Abernethy, P., G. Wilson, and P. Logan, *Strength and power assessments issues, controversies and challenges.* Sports Medicine, 1995. **19**(6): p. 401–417.
68 Brady, C., et al., *Focus of attention for diagnostic testning of the force-velocity curve.* Strength and Conditioning Journal, 2017. **39**(1): p. 57–70.
69 Young, W., R. James, and I. Montogomery, *Is muscle power related to running speed with change of directions?* Journal of Sports Medicine and Physical Fitness, 2002. **42**(3): p. 282–288.
70 Paul, J., D and P. Nassis, Nassis, *Testing strength and power in soccer players: the application of conventional and traditional methods of assessment.* Journal of Strength and Conditioning Research, 2015. **29**(6): p. 1748–1758.
71 Hopkins, W., *Measures of reliability in sports medicine and science.* Sports Medicine, 2000. **30**(1): p. 1–15.
72 Hopkins, W., *How to interpret changes in athletic performance test.* Sportscience, 2004. **8**: p. 1–7.
73 Bishop, C., et al., *A novel approach for athlete profiling: the unilateral dynamic strength index.* Journal of Strength and Conditioning Research, 2018. **35**(4): p. 1023–1029.
74 Lopez-Valenciano, A., et al., *Epidemiology of injuries in professional football: a systematic review and meta-analysis.* British Journal of Sports Medicine, 2019. **54**(12): p. 1–9.
75 Pfirrmann, D., et al., *Analysis of injury incidences in male professional adult and elite youth soccer players: a systematic review.* Journal of Athletic Training, 2016. **51**(5): p. 410–424.
76 Vincens-Bordas, J., et al., *Eccentric hamstring strength is associated with age and duration of previous season hamstring injury in male soccer players.* International Journal of Sports Physcial Therapuy, 2020. **15**(2): p. 246–253.
77 Engebretsen, A.H., et al., *Intrinsic risk factors for groin injuries among male soccer players a prospective cohort study.* The American Journal of Sports Medicine, 2010. **38**(10): p. 2051–2057.
78 Perez, V.M., et al., *Adductor squeeze test and groin injuries in elite football players: a prospective study.* Physcial Therapy in Sports. 2019. **37**: p. 54–59.
79 Gülch, R., *Force-velocity relations in human skeletal muscle.* International Journal of Sports Medicine, 1994. **15**(S 1): p. S2-S10.
80 Suchomel, T.J., P. Comfort, and J.P. Lake, *Enhancing the force-velocity profile of athletes using weightlifting derivatives.* Strength & Conditioning Journal, 2017. **39**(1): p. 10–20.
81 Harris, N., J. Cronin, and J. Keogh, *Contraction force specificity and its relationship to functional performance.* Journal of Sports Sciences, 2007. **25**(2): p. 201–212.
82 Bisciotti, G.N., et al., *Return to sports after ACL reconstruction: a new functional test protocol.* Muscles, Ligaments and Tendons Journal, 2016. **6**(4): p. 499.
83 Stone, M., S. Plisk, and D. Collins, *Strength and conditioning: Training principles: evaluation of modes and methods of resistance training-a coaching perspective.* Sports Biomechanics, 2002. **1**(1): p. 79–103.

84 Baker, D., *The effects of an in-season of concurrent training on the maintenance of maximal strength and power in professional and college-aged rugby league football players.* Journal of Strength and Conditioning Research, 2001. **15**(2): p. 172–177.
85 Stone, M.H., et al., *The importance of isometric maximum strength and peak rate-of-force development in sprint cycling.* The Journal of Strength & Conditioning Research, 2004. **18**(4): p. 878–884.
86 Haff, G.G. and S. Nimphius, *Training principles for power.* Strength & Conditioning Journal, 2012. **34**(6): p. 2–12.
87 Haff, G.G., A. Whitley, and J.A. Potteiger, *A brief review: explosive exercises and sports performance.* Strength and Conditioning Journal, 2001. **23**(3): p. 13–25.
88 Lovell, D.I., R. Cuneo, and G.C. Gass, *The effect of strength training and short-term detraining on maximum force and the rate of force development of older men.* European Journal of Applied Physiology, 2010. **109**(3): p. 429–435.
89 Maffiuletti, N.A., et al., *Rate of force development: physiological and methodological considerations.* European Journal of Applied Physiology, 2016. **116**(6): p. 1091–1116.
90 Griffin, L., et al., *Motor unit firing variability and synchronization during short-term light-load training in older adults.* Experimental Brain Research, 2009. **197**(4): p. 337–345.
91 Harris, G.R., et al., *Short-term performance effects of high power, high force, or combined weight-training methods.* The Journal of Strength & Conditioning Research, 2000. **14**(1): p. 14–20.
92 Beere, M. and I. Jeffreys, *Physical testing and monitoring practices in elite male football overview testing and monitoring in elite male football.* Professional Strength & Conditioning, 2021. **62**: p. 29–42.
93 Leyva, W., et al., *Comparison of deadlift versus back squat postactivation potentiation on vertical jump.* Gavin Journal of Orthopedic Research and Therapy, 2016. **1**: p. 6–10.
94 Jones, T.W., et al., *Strength and conditioning and concurrent training practices in elite rugby union.* The Journal of Strength & Conditioning Research, 2016. **30**(12): p. 3354–3366.
95 Gee, T.I., et al., *Strength and conditioning practices in rowing.* The Journal of Strength & Conditioning Research, 2011. **25**(3): p. 668–682.
96 Ebben, W.P. and D.O. Blackard, *Strength and conditioning practices of National Football League strength and conditioning coaches.* The Journal of Strength & Conditioning Research, 2001. **15**(1): p. 48–58.
97 Ebben, W.P., R.M. Carroll, and C.J. Simenz, *Strength and conditioning practices of National Hockey League strength and conditioning coaches.* The Journal of Strength & Conditioning Research, 2004. **18**(4): p. 889–897.
98 Lindstedt, S.L., P. LaStayo, and T. Reich, *When active muscles lengthen: properties and consequences of eccentric contractions.* Physiology, 2001. **16**(6): p. 256–261.
99 Suchomel, T.J., et al., *Implementing eccentric resistance training—part 1: a brief review of existing methods.* Journal of Functional Morphology and Kinesiology, 2019. **4**(2): p. 38.
100 Prilutsky, B., *Eccentric muscle action in sport and exercise* in Biomechanics in Sport: Performance Enhancement and Injury Prevention. Oxford: Blackwell Science Ltd., 2000: p. 56–86.
101 LaStayo, P.C., et al., *Eccentric muscle contractions: their contribution to injury, prevention, rehabilitation, and sport.* Journal of Orthopaedic & Sports Physical Therapy, 2003. **33**(10): p. 557–571.
102 Duhig, S., et al., *Effect of high-speed running on hamstring strain injury risk.* British Journal of Sports Medicine, 2016. **50**(24): p. 1536–1540.

103 Anderson, L., et al., *Quantification of training load during one-, two-and three-game week schedules in professional soccer players from the English Premier League: implications for carbohydrate periodisation.* Journal of Sports Sciences, 2016. **34**(13): p. 1250–1259.
104 Anderson, L., et al., *Quantification of seasonal-long physical load in soccer players with different starting status from the English Premier League: Implications for maintaining squad physical fitness.* International journal of Sports Physiology and Performance, 2016. **11**(8): p. 1038–1046.
105 Akenhead, R. and G.P. Nassis, *Training load and player monitoring in high-level football: current practice and perceptions.* International Journal of Sports Physiology and Performance, 2016. **11**(5): p. 587–593.

5 Conditioning

Gary Walker, Mark Read, Darren Burgess, Ed Leng and Adam Centofanti

Importance of conditioning

Conditioning is a complex process that encompasses the strategic manipulation of training stress to produce a desired outcome. For elite soccer teams, the desired outcomes are to maximise overall squad availability, and to optimise player readiness by ensuring that each player has the physical capability to implement the required game tactics successfully [1]. A well-planned, progressive training programme with variation in frequency, duration, intensity, and type of activity should be implemented to aid these goals [2]. It is typical for elite soccer clubs to programme training load using a structured micro-cycle to prepare physically and tactically for match-day [3–5]. A micro-cycle period is often between three and fourteen days, with natural variation dependant on match turn around [5,6]. Planning a conditioning programme creates unique challenges for practitioners to achieve these desired goals whilst balancing the requirements of recovery, developing physical fitness, and adjusting the training load for freshness before each match [7].

Soccer has been described as intermittent, acyclical, variable, and unpredictable [8]. The physical demands vary between playing position and competition level, as well as changing longitudinally [9]. These factors are important considerations when planning conditioning programmes for elite teams as well as contextual factors such as coach philosophy, club culture, and age demographic of squad. Furthermore, the increasingly available data from sophisticated technology provide critical insights to aid programming.

Conditioning to maximise availability

Player availability is positively associated with team performance [10–13]. In contrast, injury or illness naturally impacts team selection and match success; and results in negative psychological effects and the longer-term quality of life for the player [14,15]. Injuries also affect sports teams financially through medical fees and insurance premiums [16]. Additionally, player conditioning levels are important modifiable risk factors and are part of the injury occurrence pathway [17]. It has been suggested that keeping players injury free and capable

DOI: 10.4324/9781003200420-5

of playing competitive games every three to four days, throughout their career is the primary purpose of conditioning [18]. Within a 10-month competitive season for club and international teams, players can now be exposed to up to 70 matches and 220 sessions per season [1,19]. Evidence showing the optimisation of modifiable factors is spearheaded by elements of conditioning and several reviews evaluate the training-injury relationship [20–23]. A consensus group broadly defines 'load' in a sport setting as 'the sport and non-sport burden (single or multiple physiological, psychological or mechanical stressors) as a stimulus that is applied to a human biological system (including subcellular elements, a single cell, tissues, one or multiple organ systems, or the individual)' [24]. It is concluded that if load is applied in a moderate and progressive manner, and rapid increases in load (relative to what the athlete is prepared for) are avoided, high loads and physically hard training may offer a protective effect against injuries. It is also advised that load must always be prescribed on an individual and flexible basis. There is variation in the timeframe of player response and adaptation to load, and therefore regular athlete monitoring is fundamental to ensure appropriate and therapeutic levels of external and internal loads *(see Chapter 6)*. It has become clear that increased robustness is an outcome of a successful conditioning programme that enhances the appropriate physical and physiological characteristics to match the demands imposed on the modern soccer player. Additionally, it is vital that a sound conditioning programme is complemented with a effective strength programme to further enhance physical robustness *(see Chapter 4)*. Furthermore, conditioning must also be a vehicle to maximise physical performance to increase chance of success.

Conditioning to optimise performance

As forementioned, the goal of conditioning is to optimise performance at a specific point in time – i.e. a match. Scientific research has become important to prescribe optimal training programmes that prevent both under and overtraining and increase the chance of achieving desired performance [25]. Measuring performance collectively and individually is vital to this process and even though soccer is the most popular sport world-wide, it is one of the least quantified in analysis of performance and the measurement of player contribution to success [26]. The task of objectively quantifying the impact of individual players actions during matches remains largely unexplored [27]. However, it is used in a variety of tasks including player acquisition and evaluation, fan engagement, media reporting and scouting. Soccer analytics is lacking a comprehensive approach to address performance-related questions due to the low-scoring and dynamic nature of the sport [28]. It is suggested that analysis methods that incorporate several facets of soccer, within a dynamic context, would appear to be superior and most appropriate to use [29]. Selecting valid performance metrics, especially at an individual player level, provides a significant challenge to researchers and practitioners alike *(see Chapter 7)* but the measurement of performance can support the identification of talent, opposition analysis to improve match preparedness and strategies for training intervention [29].

110 Gary Walker et al.

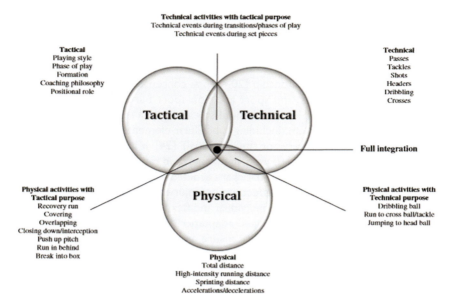

Figure 5.1 Venn diagram depicting a generalised integrated approach to quantifying and interpreting the physical match performance of soccer players (Adapted from Bradley and Ade [10]).

An integrated approach to measuring performance contextualises match demands by assimilating physical and tactical data effectively (Figure 5.1) [30].

The concept of metric integration is adopted by analytics organisations that provide performance feedback to clubs and media. These platforms quickly and accurately provide a large range of match performance data, allowing the simultaneous analysis of the physical efforts, movement patterns, and technical actions of players [31]. Examples include the Champion Data player ranking system in AFL [32] and InStat Index in soccer, recently used to analyse the association between running and match performance [33]. This automatic algorithm considers the contribution of the player to team success based on the significance of their actions, opponent level and the level of the championship they play in. For the full integration approach (Figure 5.1) to be effective, it is important for the clubs to consider its own performance quantification metrics specific to the playing style.

Type of conditioning

Teams should continually evolve their conditioning practice informed by advances in scientific evidence to enable players to develop elite levels of athleticism to support peak performance [34]. To design training strategies that maximise performance potential, practitioners must not only have a knowledge

Characteristic	ATP-PC energy system	Lactic acid system	Aerobic energy system
Intensity of activity	High intensity (95%+ max HR)	> High intensity (85%+ max HR) >Used for increases in intensity during long duration events when PC has not restored	>Resting >Sub maximal intensity (<85%+ max HR)
The duration that the energy systems are dominant during activity	Short duration (1 – 5 sec)	Intermediate duration (5 – 60 sec+)	Long duration (75 sec+)
Total% event duration	0 – 10sec	10 – 75 sec	75 sec+ It is the major contributor in events that are of more than 75 sec in total event duration
Fitness components	>Anaerobic: power and speed >Muscular strength (1-3sec) >Muscular power >Dynamic flexibility. >Agility	>Anaerobic: power and speed >Muscular power (when repeated efforts are made during activity. >Muscular strength (isometric >5sec). >Dynamic flexibility. >Local muscular endurance >Agility (only if fatiguing)	>Aerobic capacity/CV endurance >Local muscular endurance. >Static flexibility

Abbreviations – HR – heart rate; CV – cardiovascular; ATP-PC – adenosine triphosphate-phosphocreatine

Figure 5.2 Overview of the relationship between different physiological systems and the development of different fitness components. (Adapted from Morgans et al. [38]).

of the physical demands of the sport but also incorporate knowledge of the physiological requirements of elite soccer players [35]. The physiological capacities soccer players commonly have, which enable them to perform successfully, include a high level of aerobic and anaerobic conditioning, speed, agility, strength, and power [34,36]. These capacities are thoroughly investigated and discussed in previous research, and illustrated in Figure 5.2 [37,38]. However, it is important to emphasise the complexity of conditioning for the modern soccer player. Training programmes need to stress several energy systems, develop strength and range of movement, and all of which must be incorporated within a tactical and technical training schedule.

Aerobic capacity

A soccer player's aerobic capacity is dependent on three elements: maximal oxygen uptake (VO_{2MAX}), anaerobic threshold, and work economy [39]. This is a pivotal conditioning consideration as at least 90% of the energy demands of a soccer match are aerobic [37]. VO_{2MAX} is positively related to league position, and increasing VO_{2max} increases the distance covered during a match, linked to a corresponding 25% increase in ball involvements and 100% increase in number of sprints performed [40,41]. Extensive research has shown that appropriately planned training can improve aerobic capacity by affecting multiple factors, including the strength of the heart muscle, concentration of haemoglobin, capillary density, and activity of aerobic enzymes which can aid recovery between exhaustive power-demanding sprints and high-intensity bouts during matches [41]. Conditioning soccer players specifically to improve these capacities can use various methods including traditional running drills, specifically designed dribble tracks and small-sided games (SSGs) [39,42]. Additionally, SSG training can maintain cardiorespiratory fitness whilst eliciting a high level of enjoyment [43].

Where the body uses both aerobic and anaerobic systems to produce energy, the intensity of activity will determine which system is prominent. Components of anaerobic capacity have the biggest impact on the outcome of the match and are characterised by repeated short high-intensity activity [44]. To achieve a high capacity in these key elements, the anaerobic energy systems, including the ATP-PC and anaerobic glycolysis, need to be highly conditioned, affecting fitness components including speed, strength, power, and agility (Figure 5.2).

Speed

Sprinting is one of the most important activities in soccer, and although sprint volume (total distance accumulated >25.2 $km·h^{-2}$) only constitutes approximately 12% of the mean total match distance covered (position dependant), straight sprinting has been identified as the single most frequent locomotive action in goal situations performed by either the scoring or assisting player [45,46]. Therefore, improving sprint performance is critical. This can be achieved through specific sprint training coupled with strength and power training, but ultimately there is no substitute for running fast progressively and regularly. Exposure to maximal running speed is widely regarded as a method to improve physical performance and reduce the risk of injury, most prominently hamstring related [47,48].

Agility

Specific to a sporting context, agility is defined as a rapid whole-body movement with change of velocity or direction in response to a stimulus [49] and is influenced by many factors including speed, strength, power, co-ordination and running technique. Suggested to be one of the key performance indicators [50], players can carry out more than 1,200 changes in direction during the game [51]. The training of agility can be progressed through technical drills, pattern running, and then reactive agility training as part of both separated conditioning elements or integrated soccer work through SSGs. There is no 'one size fits all' approach to how elements of conditioning are developed, and the programme will be dictated by a multitude of factors principally led by the head coach (see Chapter 11). Overload of each element can be achieved through different methods in the previously mentioned forms of pure conditioning, position-specific or technical-tactical drills, intertwined with a carefully planned strength and power programme to complement and support these field loads.

Training approaches to conditioning

There is no one distinct way to develop players conditioning levels on the field. Over time, there have been a multitude of approaches utilised by professional soccer teams to optimise conditioning, with advantages and disadvantages to each of their approaches. Finding the balance between technical/tactical development, and physical conditioning during training, can be a difficult task if there is not a clear approach to what the team needs. Performance staff will often need to adapt to the coach's preferred style of conditioning, whether this be isolated conditioning and soccer drills, or a more integrated approach. Ultimately, it is part of the role of a performance team to identify strengths and weaknesses of the approach taken, and provide appropriate recommendations to achieve optimal conditioning, without compromising technical/tactical development. Being adaptable is an essential attribute for any practitioner undertaking this role of applying conditioning concepts to align with tactical objectives. The following approaches are some of the more common place training methodologies utilised in soccer across the globe (Figure 5.3):

- Isolated
- Hybrid
- Integrated

Isolated approach

The isolated approach to training in soccer usually involves separating soccer drills and physical drills with the objective of prioritising one of these objectives at a time (physical, technical, or tactical). This type of approach can be simpler in design, however, has the potential to compromise one of the objectives due to its isolated approach. Separate conditioning blocks, if managed appropriately, can lead itself to being a very effective modality to improving the team's physical condition. The same can be said for tactical drills whereby there is no restriction for the coach, enabling them to really emphasize specific elements, if necessary, without any physical objective. Although many drills will often overlap objectives by default of the sport, there does not tend to be much deliberate practice of concepts being integrated together. Whereas the focus leans more towards achieving one objective unrelated to the specific game model. With every approach, there is a spectrum as to what level of isolation or integration there may be. However, the isolated approach focuses on individual concepts without addressing the sub principles that lead into a particular concept. For example, a general possession grid designed to keep the ball without any specific principles being addressed prior to match play, followed by a 5-10 minute physical prescription.

Hybrid approach

The hybrid approach aims to incorporate both isolated objectives as well as integrated objectives. This approach can have a big fluctuation in terms of integration and isolation, however, tends to focus on being integrated with the supplementation of isolation. Having an integrated mindset towards training prescription and drill design enables the team/staff to still focus on game model principles. However, with the advantage of isolating concepts as they see fit to achieve global objectives. An example of a hybrid approach is high-speed running prescriptions at the end of a session. If the desired meterage is not attained during the session, or as part of the holistic plan towards physical development, extra controlled high-speed running is prescribed. This mixed-method approach if planned appropriately can be an excellent collaboration between game model development and physical development. It requires effective communication between performance and coaching staff to determine where/if isolated drills may be required for a training session. Depending on the desires of the coaching staff, conditioning can be incorporated into a technical drill to lift its intensity and allow for a conditioning prescription, in conjunction with game model development. For example, three-team possession grid focusing on the sub principle of reactive collective pressing after ball loss. Following each set of possession, players perform two linear runs before returning to the drill for the next set. Extended rest may be required to ensure intensity remains high; however, using the runs between repetitions increases the physical demand, whilst attaining some high-speed running that may not have been achieved.

Integrated approach

The integrated approach to training in soccer uses the game model as a basis to drive training drills, whilst also incorporating the physical element to each drill. This approach requires a lot of planning and excellent communication between technical and performance staff, to ensure each drill is meeting all objectives. Tactical periodisation has helped teams plan their technical/tactical drills across the week, to suit the physical objectives required for each day, ensuring physical adaptations occur. For this approach to be most successful, it is imperative that the performance staff have a clear understanding of the coach's game model, as well as technical skills required for specific drills. Utilising wearable technology, such as global positioning systems (GPS), to catalogue each drill is a great tool to gain thorough understanding of the physical output achieved in each drill. Where the integrated approach can fail is when neither the physical or technical/tactical objective is achieved during a particular drill, which is often the result of poor planning, or lack of understanding of a particular variable (physical, technical, and tactical). A common error in the integrated approach can be when the objective of hitting maximum velocity exposure in training is not met. If the incorrect drill is chosen to achieve this objective, the player may achieve neither the physical nor technical/tactical objectives. This can occur if there is poor implementation of the ball at the wrong time or distances not adequate to achieve desired speeds. The advantage of the integrated approach is the repeated practice of principles related to the team's game model, whilst also striving to achieve physical intensity during technical/tactical drills leading to more positive performance transfer in a match context. Drills as simple as a passing sequence in a warmup, will be based around sub principles related to the team's game model, which contribute to achieving the physical theme objectives for that day.

Conditioning 115

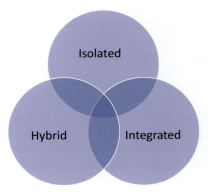

Figure 5.3 Training approach to conditioning.

The warm-up

The warm-up is an important time slot for practitioners to prepare their players, as well as developing physical attributes. There are several elements of the warm-up that practitioners need to consider when structuring the variables of exercises prescribed.

Elements of the warmup

The warm-up in soccer provides practitioners with an opportunity to

1   develop physical traits or characteristics,
2   set the tone for the session to follow,
3   implement aspects of injury prevention, and
4   introduce skill session themes.

Ideally, the practitioner is provided with the session details to follow so that the warm-up can be tailored to suit the themes of the skills session. For example, if the session is to involve SSGs, then it is best the warm-up includes aspects of agility and reaction time. Regardless of the specific themes of the skills session to follow, the warm-up represents an ideal period for the players to be exposed to fundamental movement patterns such as acceleration, deceleration, change of direction, and essential collision work.
   Sample:
   A typical warm-up for a SSG session might look like

- **0-10 minutes** – Muscle activation and individual prep – typically this may happen indoors and possibly involve dynamic resistance work (using bands) and basic injury prevention exercises (e.g. ankle mobility/proprioception);

- **10-15 minutes** – dynamic movement-based actions such as walking lunges, carioca, leg swings, run throughs etc. this section can involve basic ball passing/dribbling to apply specificity to the warm-up; and
- **15-20 minutes** – ballistic movements such as sharp accelerations/decelerations, plyometrics, change of direction (COD). This section ought to include the ball and include similar movements to those which will occur later in the session.

Ideally, warmups should not last more than 15-20 minutes, depending on the manager/head coach preference and the session to follow. It is crucial that the practitioner understands the preferences of both the manager and players and tailor the warmups accordingly. If, for example, a manager/head coach prefers shorter warmups without the use of the ball, then practitioners should look for other opportunities to develop physical traits, perhaps indoors prior to the warmup during 'activation' sessions.

Drill design

Practitioners will often make suggestions to soccer-specific drills to aid in the physical preparedness of players. Variables within soccer drills can be altered to create various physical adaptations. Utilising match data can help guide practitioners with feedback on the intensity of specific drills. Thus, practitioners can provide coaches with recommendations on how to alter drills to illicit desired physical adaptations. However, as aforementioned, coaches/managers may not always adhere to the recommendations, resulting in addition prescriptions by practitioners. Prescriptions can be with or without the ball, dependant on many variables, and implemented in different portions of the training session.

Peak match intensity and drill design

Although activity profiles have been well-documented throughout various levels of competition in soccer [52], various novel methods have been used to investigate the most-demanding passages of play. A rolling-duration method to determine peak intensities throughout match-play has been used to investigate a variety of sports (Figure 5.4) [53–55]. Specifically, when investigating professional soccer, identifying the most demanding passages of play can be used to assist coaches and practitioners in prescribing training intensities [56,57]. The most demanding passages of play vary dependent on several factors, including contextual elements (score line, tactics, formations etc) as well as position, physical qualities, and environmental factors. However, by constructing activity profiles categorised by position, period of play, and tactical formation, practitioners and coaches are better informed on the individual physical demands of match-play [56]. Furthermore, the outlined activity profiles can aid practitioners and coaches in prescribing and modifying training variables to elicit,

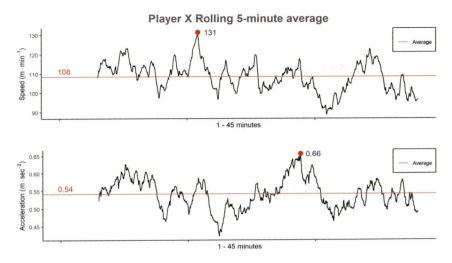

Figure 5.4 Extracted GPS data from a 1st half (45-minute period). A 5-minute rolling average applied to speed (m·min^{-1}) and acceleration (m·s^{-2}). The red dot indicates the peak intensity for a 5-minute period during match-play for the associated variables.

or even exceed, true "game-like" intensity. Thus, creating desired conditioning adaptations of the appropriate energy systems (as aforementioned; Figure 5.2).

Running only conditioning prescriptions

Performance practitioners should consider the following variables before incorporating running as a conditioning stimulus into a team's training programme:

1 **Timing** – time of week, month, and season
2 **Individual player training loads** – do all players require extra work or a select few
3 **Manager/player biases/preferences** – do the players and/or manager 'buy in' to extra conditioning with or without the ball?

Once the above points have been considered and extra conditioning is agreed to, where possible, performance staff should ensure the conditioning is specific to the players and, ideally the individual positional requirements of each player. For example, the 'outside' players (full-backs, wingers) ought to perform separate conditioning to the 'inside' players (central midfielders, central defenders). The work to rest ratios of each position should be established, preferably during the hardest parts of the game (peak match intensity), and the conditioning drills should be based on these requirements. The next decision to decide is whether to incorporate the ball into the prescribed conditioning work.

Conditioning without the ball

Conditioning without the ball offers several advantages, such as;

- set times/distances,
- competition between players, and
- specific – majority of individual running is without ball at feet, during match-play

If work without the ball is preferred, the conditioning should focus primarily on high intensity and/or sprint running. These sessions should be:

- **Specific** – both in terms of distance (i.e. replicate/overload match distances and number of efforts covered in specific positions) and work to rest ratios (i.e. replicate/overload the work and rest periods each position demands in the match)
- **Periodised** – these sessions need to be appropriately progressed and placed in the calendar so as not to negatively influence training or match outputs.

EXAMPLE

An example of a conditioning session, without the use of a soccer ball may look like the following.

- **Session Title** – High-Intensity Interval Training (HIIT) mid-season top up for central midfielder.
- **Parameters** –
  - *1:3 Work-to-rest ratio.* (to match game demands)
  - *Speed (approximately)* = 6–7 m·s^{-1}
  - *Total High-speed distance [HSR] (>5.5 m·s^{-1})* = 300 m
  - *Total Time* = 3 mins
- Details –
  - 2 × 60 m@8.5 s work and 24 s recovery
  - 2 × 50 m@7 s work and 21 s recovery
  - 2 × 40 m@6 s work and 18 s recovery

One of the advantages of this type of session is it can be manipulated to achieve various physiological demands. For example, the above session can be manipulated to be more aerobic in nature, such as the following.

- **Session Title** – HIIT pre-season aerobic top up for Central midfielder
- **Parameters** –
  - *1:1 work-to-rest ratio* (to match game demands)
  - *Speed (approximately)* = 5–6 m·s^{-1}
  - *Total High-speed distance [HSR] (>5.5 m·s^{-1})* = 450 m
  - *Total Time* = 3.5 minutess

- Details –
  - 2 × 60 m@11 s work and 11 s recovery
  - 2 × 50 m@9 s work and 9 s recovery
  - 2 × 40 m@7 s work and 7 s recovery

Conditioning with the ball

Some coaches insist on using the ball during conditioning sessions. This type of conditioning can be more specific to the game and more enjoyable to players. The above sessions can be altered to include the ball via:

- Adding passing/shooting after various distances (e.g. for the 60 m runs – sprint 30 m, pass into a target then sprint 30 m to return to start
- Adding skill execution (passing, juggling, etc.) during the recovery periods in between sprint bouts

EXAMPLE

Fullback extensive top up:

- 2 × 5 Overlap with cross + recovery run to defensive position (Figure 5.5). 60 s recovery between reps, 2 minutes recovery between sets.

The use of SSG for conditioning

Some coaches prefer to perform all conditioning with SSGs. This type of conditioning offers many advantages including the inclusion of tactics, skills and decision making during the conditioning process. However, this type of conditioning

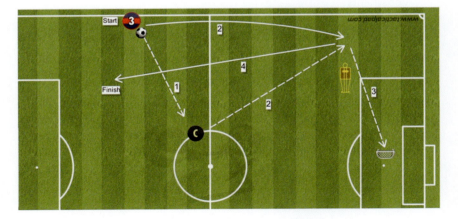

Figure 5.5 Extensive top-up conditioning: fullback position specific.

requires careful planning as often these games result in lower sprint/high speed numbers than players experience during matches. The following sections will cover the technical, tactical, and environmental constraints used to increase the physical demands of SSGs.

Constraints and drill design

Just as technical staff will use constraints in the design of drills to achieve technical and tactical objectives, applying constraints to drills can also aid in desired physical adaptation [58]. Rather than solely isolating soccer drills and conditioning drills, integration via the modification of constraints can lead to achieving physical objectives in conjunction with technical and tactical goals. Figure 5.6 highlights key constraints that can be modified to elicit desired physical objectives [42].

One of the most important physical components of training is the level of intensity, therefore the significance of using constraints to raise intensity is fundamental to the physical development of professional soccer players [46]. Understanding of peak match intensities can create a blueprint for drill design to ensure players are performing at peak match intensity for targeted variables (average speed and average acceleration) [55,57]. Using the peak match intensity data points can be a reference for drills to whether they result in true 'game-like' speeds. However, it may not always be appropriate to train at, or above, the peak match intensities. Specifically, the taper phase of the microcycle may contain drills that focus on more tactical/technical elements, requiring multiple stationary periods where coaches are instructing on tactical implications leading to the upcoming opponent. Therefore, comparing

Drill Constraints	
	Dimensions - small, medium, big
	Numbers - 1v1 -11v11 or uneven
	Task constraints (rules) - ball touches, zones, pressing rules, offside, scoring strategies
	Work : Rest - intensive or extensive prescription
	Equipment - balls available, big vs small goals vs no goals
	Opposition - Positional weighing. I.E. Defenders vs midfielders
	Support players - such as bumpers/neutrals

Figure 5.6 Examples of constraints within technical drills.

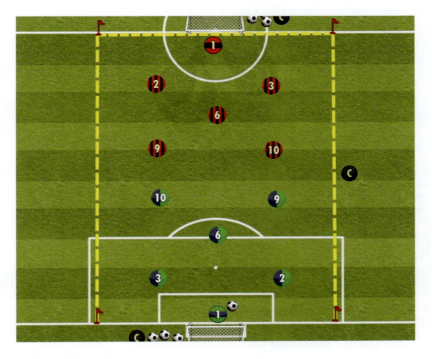

Figure 5.7 A 5v5 small-sided game example.

peak match intensities to drills is best suited for the physical acquisition days of the microcycle (Figures 5.4 and 5.7).

Additionally, the level of coach drive can also elicit different outcomes to the physical output. Specifically, coach encouragement has shown to increase the physical output of players compared to no coach driving intensity [59]. Therefore, there is great importance of the practitioner's collaboration with technical staff when it comes to drill design, as each constraint can have a tactical element attached that may or may not fit in with the club's/team's game model or philosophy of play. Understanding various elements of technical drills is essential in achieving desired physical objectives. The following questions can aid in the design of drills:

- What is the main conditioning objective? Aerobic, anaerobic?
- What physical variable are we looking to overload?
- Are we overloading a drill at peak match intensity or beyond?
- What type of training day is it? Intensive/extensive, etc.?
- What level are the players at physically? Is it appropriate for the cohort of players?
- What are the technical, tactical, and psychological implications of each drill?

Table 5.1 Example of constraints within a 5v5+Goalkeepers drill

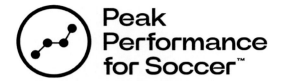

5v5 + Goalkeepers (GK)	
Constraints	
Dimensions	50 m × 35 m
Work: Rest	4 × 4 min: 90 s
Touches on ball	Two touches max
Offside	No offside
Defensive strategy	Must press the ball
Restarts	Always from GK – 3 s max
Support players	None
Equipment	Multiple balls on side of goal
Support staff	Serving balls to GK

Drill comments

Average acceleration greater than peak match intensity
Great aerobic and anaerobic conditioning stimulus (increased time above 85% HR max)
Increased technical demand with increased technical actions
High player enthusiasm and motivation

Common errors with drill design

Figure 5.8 highlights common errors that can occur with drill design in professional soccer. Without astute understanding of drill constraints and the affect they have on the drill being designed, the desired physiological adaptations may not be achieved. For example, if the SSG highlighted in Table 5.1 (5v5+GK) is played for 2 × 8 minutes instead of the recommended 4 × 4 minutes, players will be exposed to a different training stimulus. Although it still achieves the same total volume from a duration standpoint (16 minutes), the intensity of these games will likely be compromised and played under the desired intensity. Similarly, decreasing the dimensions of this drill from 50 m × 35 m to 35 m × 25 m will reduce the game speed and overall playing area per individual player. Coach intervention or the stop starting of a particular drill is commonplace in soccer, and often a very valuable and necessary process to ensure drill standards remain high, and learning takes place. However, it must be understood the potential negative affects this can have on the physical response of drills, particularly if the drill is designed to achieve a conditioning stimulus.

Common errors with drill design

- Timings - work:rest inappropriate to maintain intensity
- Stop/starting drill - too frequent stop starting of drill by techncial staff during games decreasing physical response
- Dimensions - inappropriate dimensions to achieve desired physical adaptation
- Rules - touch limit inapprorpiate to lift and maintain desired game speed
- Staffing - not enough avaiable staff to serve balls for quick restarts
- Equipment - insufficient balls to maintain game speed

Figure 5.8 Common errors with the drill design process.

Barriers to performance and conditioning

As aforementioned, the overall aim of a successful conditioning strategy is to maximise player availability within the squad, ensuring that each player has the physical capability to implement the required tactics within the game-model of the head coach, while optimising a players' readiness for each match to allow the player to demonstrate this capability. Therefore, to successfully manage the training requirements of a squad of players throughout a season, it is important to structure training appropriately using strategies to identify the individual needs of players, ensuring that those requirements are scientifically planned and delivered within the constraints of the annual fixture schedule [1]. It is therefore vital for the practitioner to consider several sources of objective and subjective information on a daily, weekly, and time-phase period, in order to design the ideal training programme given the considerable number of constraints that exist. These considerations are summarised in Figure 5.9, and include understanding your cohort of players, knowing how hard to train at specific times of the season, the head coach's mentality to fitness and conditioning, together with the environment that you are training in [1]. There is often no right or wrong answer to this and is particularly contextual, with successful outcomes combining objective data, experience, and intuition, blending both art and science to find a training 'sweet-spot' for each player.

Knowing your Cohort of Players

The main consideration for the practitioner when understanding the constraints and barriers to performance is fully understanding your players within a squad. Each player has a unique set of physical strengths and weaknesses, together with their individual characteristics, such as age, injury history, and player life cycle, which can impact upon their future risk and performance. For example, it is known that older players with previous injury are at increased

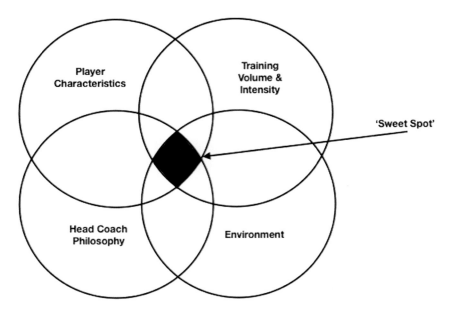

Figure 5.9 Identifying the constraints and barriers to performance within a professional soccer environment.

risk of sustaining a future injury [60,61]. Successful performance teams routinely perform a 'needs analysis' of each player from a holistic technical, tactical, physical and mental perspective using both objective assessment and subjective information to identify these strengths and weaknesses *(see Chapter 3)*. Importantly, this must be aligned with the game model of the head coach, identifying the positional role requirements for each player in all phases of the game (attack, defence, and transitional moments, both in and out of possession). By undertaking this process, each player can then be provided with a personal development plan by which the multi-disciplinary high-performance team can begin to more effectively plan and periodise training. For example, a needs analysis can be used to identify a mismatch between a young full-back with only moderate aerobic capability in a team in which the head coach wants him or her to perform continuous overlapping runs in attack. By combining objective data collection with subjective information, the performance practitioner may prescribe individual position-specific high-intensity aerobic training at the appropriate time to improve the players aerobic capability in performing match-specific actions, to aid their on-field performance.

The next major consideration is to understand each players' individual situation within a playing squad. For example, whether they are a starting player, substitute, non-starter, or injured or suspended which may provide additional conditioning opportunities. By adopting a holistic monitoring system, the performance practitioner can identify the acute training and match load that the player has experienced together with the chronic load over a particular period. Key questions to ask include the following:

- What was the players most recent match or training load?
- What has been their match/training load density in a particular period?
- How much time for training is there until the next match for each player?

The final barrier to performance at the individual level is identifying where each player is at on any given day and how they are responding to the imposed demands that have been placed upon them. This can be ascertained by performing daily and weekly objective and subjective monitoring assessments to determine each players' time-course of recovery *(see Chapter 6)*.

Knowing How Hard to Train

Elite soccer players are required to produce successful performances across many weeks and months throughout a season, and not just peak for a small number of competitions as in other sports. In team-based sports such as soccer, however, the end stage of the competitive season usually consists of the most important matches in both league and cup competitions. For this reason, practitioners are required to optimise the preparation and performance of players on a weekly basis, yet deliver them in the best condition to compete for the major prizes at the end of the season. In designing an appropriate training plan, it is important to consider the fitness-fatigue model, which proposes that different training stressors result in different physiological responses [62]. These stressors result in two after-effects, fitness and fatigue, and their interaction can positively or negatively influence performance. Understanding this model, together with each player's individual response to the training stimulus will further allow the practitioner to optimise player preparation and performance.

Head Coach's Philosophy

The head coach's philosophy to fitness and conditioning is a vitally important consideration when designing a team training programme. It is fundamental to understand the game model of the head coach, with a clear understanding of the physical requirements by position for each player within the team. This can be quantified using external load metrics to identify the total distance, high-speed and sprint running requirements during a match. Furthermore, this should be broken down into the specific movements that are required in offensive, defensive and transitional moments, that are performed both in and out of possession. This will provide the practitioner with a guide as to the most important physical actions and parameters to replicate and overload in training sessions. Following this, communication between the head coach, technical and conditioning staff is extremely important when subsequently planning training as there are several philosophical approaches to soccer conditioning.

Environment

The environmental situation can also act as a significant barrier to the performance of a training programme, notably the altitude and temperature that training is performed at. Several acute physiological changes are associated with exercise at altitude, particularly in athletes that are not acclimatised [63]. These changes have been demonstrated to impair aerobic performance and high-speed running in both youth, male, and female soccer players [64–66]. Furthermore, it is reported that in hot conditions, the performance of high-intensity running of players is reduced and that fatigue is associated with hyperthermia and dehydration [67]. The practitioner working in those environments should determine the amount of time that their squad of players will have to encounter the environmental conditions for, before devising an appropriate training and nutritional strategy for each situation.

Finding the Sweet-Spot

There is no perfect programme or 'one-size-fits-all' approach for designing conditioning plans for elite soccer players but the goal for the practitioner is to find the training sweet-spot for each player within the squad. It is likely that this blend of art and science will require the combination of objective and subjective information, together with experience and intuition; however, a number of guiding questions can assist in this process:

- How fit is fit enough?
- How do you know?
- Are the players physically capable of executing the game-model of the head coach (technical and tactical) for >90 minutes and for multiple matches per week?
- Are the players physically and mentally 'ready' for the next match?

Within this process, it is vital to be data-informed, collecting meaningful objective information about each player's training load (both acute and chronic), together with their response to the imposed demands *(see Chapters 6 and 7)*. With the increased utilisation of technology within elite soccer, monitoring each player's response may involve physiological, autonomic, biomechanical, and musculoskeletal objective markers, but it is important to maintain human interactions with players and to speak with them about how they feel within the training environment.

The 'holy grail' for the performance practitioner is to determine the optimal dose of training for each player to allow them to be available for matches, with capability to execute the game-model whilst being in an optimal state of readiness to perform successfully.

Practical application

One could be forgiven in thinking that the element of 'conditioning' for a team sport, such as soccer, is a relatively straight forward entity. Nevertheless, the topic is far more complex than we might first think and subsequently requires a much deeper understanding of the individual make-up of each team and furthermore the status of each player as we transition from day one of pre-season through to the final competitive game at the business end of the year.

Starting point

As aforementioned, once presented with a large majority of the variables which may dictate the base of a periodisation model, a backroom staff can begin to construct an effective strategy to prepare players from a technical, tactical, and physical standpoint. With enough detail, it becomes possible to plan and prepare not only for the immediate future but also for the longer term in the form of a mesocycle or macrocycle. Practitioners must pick a theoretical starting point to begin exploring the variety of conditioning practices available for soccer, and as a result, it would be only appropriate to begin at the start point of every season; the pre-season.

This specific time of the year lends itself to being possibly the best time to programme any form of fitness and conditioning. We are effectively not only dealing with a 'blank canvas' of readiness states across a group on return from an off-season break, but also this time of year can be portrayed as far less chaotic than the in-season period, where we must deal with multiple competitions and many more extraneous variables. Despite this, the ability to have all players at a similar 'readiness state' should not signify that we can comfortably lump all our athletes on an identical conditioning programme expecting identical results. Instead, we should look to prescribe workloads in a relative manner to allow our players to develop in the most optimal way for their individual physical make up, whilst avoiding any incidents of overreaching and subsequently overtraining *(see Chapter 8)*. With reasonable resources and staffing, it should be possible to group athletes into varying subunits to cater to their individual and positional needs. These subgroups could be dependent on a large series of factors such as age, training history, skill level, and, of course, conditioning status, normally quantified via a range of testing modalities on the return from the prescribed off-season. Through doing so, we avoid the 'one-size-fits-all' approach to conditioning, and instead incorporate a manageable level of individualisation within the wider context of preparing to meet the overarching team goals for the season to follow.

Once in suitable subgroups, most clubs will begin with a general preparatory phase, whereby players are re-introduced to the fundamental demands of the game carefully, and basic aerobic qualities will be developed to be able to cope with the demands of a more specific preparatory phase which will subsequently follow. The total length of such a phase is highly variable depending on the length of pre-season but could be anywhere between five days to three weeks. From this point forward, there are many ways to construct the remainder of a pre-season conditioning plan for a team, with some clubs opting for traditional large volumes of work in the initial stages of the mesocycle in order to 'push' physical fitness levels after a period of inactivity, whilst other approaches will work on more of a careful graduation of training load through the allocated pre-season period to prolong physical status throughout a 10–11-month season. Regardless of which, a large majority of teams will facilitate their conditioning philosophy through a linear periodisation model and will commonly transition from more of 'larger-volume-based' aerobic style blocks in the initial weeks, to more of a position-specific-based 'explosive' and 'realisation' phase immediately prior to the beginning of competition and at the end of pre-season.

One conditioning method which is becoming more popular, and one which would suit this 'big to small' linear transition model through pre-season, is the implementation of large-to-small-sided games. The transition from a quantity of large-sided games (LSGs) through to medium and then chronologically, small, offers a transition model of differing physical qualities, which could be treated as possibly the most 'specific' conditioning modality. An LSG format can be portrayed as a conditioning modality which brings about a similar rate of perceived exertion (RPE) as a medium or small format, however, will yield much greater total and higher speed running distances for every minute played, but at a lower heart rate. Essentially, a lower intensity yet volume producing aerobic workout. In contrast, from both a technical and physical standpoint, the smallest format of games (4v4–5v5 including GK's), can be observed to have a much greater occurrence of explosive and intense technical actions when contrasted to its larger counterparts. As such, there is a fair argument to suggest that by beginning pre-season with LSGs, when there is a greater requirement for a strong aerobic and volume foundational base, before then transitioning through and to a form of more 'intense' SSGs could be a protocol worth considering regardless of the standard of soccer.

Away from the extensive literature and data which has been completed surrounding this area of physical performance and conditioning, there are also some parallel thought processes which should be considered to help the understanding of why such a method may be useful for a pre-season period. As discussed earlier in this chapter, there is an ever growing need to prescribe work in a relative manner to our players, and through the early implementation of LSGs, we partially address this issue directly, even if only on a positional basis. Secondly, another consideration as to why to begin with LSGs in comparison to a SSG, is the reduction in shooting, which, when returning from a period of reduced activity (sometimes 4-6 weeks), could be advantageous as to not be faced with a 'spike' in acute load from a shooting perspective, and be faced with a form of repetitive overuse injury. The same can be said about plyometric exposure when the stimulus is downregulated for some time due to a similar period of inactivity.

Table 5.2 A sample template of constraints for a pre-season 'games-based' conditioning programme

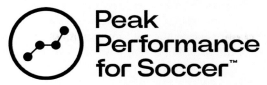

	Small-sided games – 4v4-5v5 (inc GK)	Medium-sided games – 6v6-8v8 (inc GK)	Large-sided games – 9v9-11v11 (inc GK)
Duration	90 s – 3 min	3–6 min	8–12 min
Repetition	4–8	3–6	2–4
Total volume	12–24 min	18–36 min	14–48 min
Frequency + volume	X1-2 per week (four total sessions)	X2 per week (four total sessions)	X2 per week (four total sessions)
Other	Coach encouragement, Competition format, limited touches (1–2)	Coach encouragement, Competition format	Coach encouragement, Match format

Finally, through beginning with a structured and planned 11v11 approach, we are essentially engineering in reverse from the first pre-season friendly match which commonly consists of players having to complete somewhere in the region of 45 minutes of match play. For that reason, by following a potential programme like that seen in Table 5.2, we could comfortably work towards a total volume of 30–40 minutes of 11v11 in smaller repetitions to best prepare for this first 'big' physical acute load of the season.

The second phase of pre-season essentially consists of players beginning to play friendly matches to gain match exposure. Many teams will progressively build their athletes through a process of 45 to 90 minutes of match load over a three to four game schedule. As a result, depending on the length of a given pre-season, in conjunction with a well-planned conditioning model, it is fair to assume that a large group of players within a squad will be at a relatively similar place from a fitness perspective. However, as a squad transitions from this 'match exposure' period into a competitive game schedule, the ability to prescribe specific practices to two to three subgroups and/or utilise an LSG to SSG protocol as aforementioned becomes far more challenging. Specifically, the selection of players moves from an all-inclusive fitness driven approach, to almost exclusively being led by results and performance. Consequently, this evokes a far less linear process of match exposure, and can result in two to three subgroups forming, into a large spectrum of fitness states across a team.

The 'Grey Zone'

A typical 'in-season' mesocycle seen across large parts of Europe can be a need for teams to compete every 72–96 hours, depending on the number of competitions exposed to [68]. The result of such a schedule is that 'acquisition/conditioning days' essentially being replaced by the game day itself. The main playing squad falls into a routine of the most important physiological stimulus now being that of the actual match [69]. What this means is that the playing group is effectively moved towards a 'High-Low' loading model, whereby they are either stimulated by a Match Day, or preparing for the upcoming fixture through a range of recovery modalities *(see Chapter 8)*. This is essentially a maintenance model and the only opportunities to implement any conditioning opportunities would be either when a player is suspended, a non-selected-player or in the later stages of competitions when perhaps there is a slightly less congested period of matches.

However, if we take the previous example, there is one stand out opportunity to implement 'conditioning' elements into a week, and that is of course with the players who are restricted match minutes, either due to non-selection or a lack of playing time (<30 mins). Unlike the 'High-Low' model which starting players may be exposed to, those athletes left on the fringe of a squad require a far more complex level of fitness application, and it is up to the physical performance coaches to best align all players *(see Chapter 10)*.

The Match Day 'Top Up'

Although one of the most important and hectic days of the week from a first team perspective, the match day itself provides many small pockets of opportunity ideal for the 'underloaded' athlete and should be seen as an opportunity missed if not utilised maximally. This theory holds even more weight during congested periods when the availability of a high training stimulus for the whole group is significantly reduced. Nevertheless, several practical and logistical considerations may modulate what specific activities can be performed directly after a match ends, and as such it is imperative that we touch upon these to highlight how best to approach the conditioning possibilities [70].

As in almost every sport, professional soccer fixtures are played either at home or at a venue away from the club's facilities, and in the case of the latter; it can be assumed that an extent of travel is required. In turn, it can be assumed that many away trips will be concluded by a return journey taking place immediately post game. This of course provides a challenge to the physical performance coach who must find the optimal way to deliver a training stimulus before re-joining the rest of the staff and players. Supplement this initial time constraint with the possibility of a restricted use of the playing surface or even detailed tactical debriefs, and the practitioner is left with a very small window of opportunity. To add even further context, guidelines from the English Premier League and several other leagues throughout Europe state that it is not permitted for players to train on the same pitch that the game was played on for any

Conditioning 131

more than 15 minutes after each game [71]. Therefore, we can safely assume that practitioners should be focusing their 'top-up' conditioning practices towards strategies that have a duration of between five and ten minutes.

This limiting time factor, in addition to the other uncontrollable restrictions, such as constraints on the usage of specific areas of the pitch and even confines of specific movement patterns by ground staff, essentially dictates that the Match Day Top Up needs to be short, effective, and most likely in a linear fashion. This may best suit different forms of high-speed running, repeated sprint, or even maximal speed exposure. Any other work generally includes a form of change of direction which may not be deemed 'acceptable' on an opposition or even home grounds playing surface.

Where and when practical, practitioners may find it useful to implement different conditioning strategies for each positional subgroup. Figure 5.10 presents one method which looks to address this through using a variety of distances and tempos.

Anecdotally, this type of work completed at around 70% effort, followed by periods of extended active or passive rest (typically up until the start of the next minute, for example, 8 s work; 52 s rest) allows for high quality of movement whilst also achieving large volumes of high-speed running, without the promotion of an injury risk. In addition, and although trivial, tempo runs also allow for the entire 'subgroup' of top up players to complete the same total duration of exercise vs all players completing an identical exercise prescription but perhaps a different number of reps. Furthermore, Table 5.3 outlines just some of the positional differences between such an approach and how it may be prescribed.

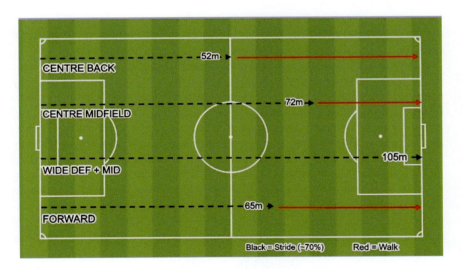

Figure 5.10 Position-specific high-speed-running protocol.

Table 5.3 Post-match top up – position-specific tempo-run prescription example

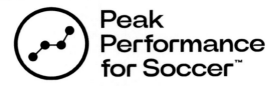

		Wide defender		
Shuttle distance	Duration	Rest	HSR yied per rep	Prescription
105 m	16 s	44 s	80–90 m	1 × 10 or 2 × 6
		Central defender		
Shuttle distance	Duration	Rest	HSR yied per rep	Prescription
52 m	8 s	52 s	35–40 m	1 × 10 or 2 × 6

Alternatives for volume

It could be acceptable to purely focus on 'off the ball' exercises to directly address any deficiencies in higher volume training loads for the non-playing subgroup; however, as with any type of physical preparation work, it is important to understand how and when is the best and most appropriate time to implement such methods. If we are to consider these conditioning exercises, it is imperative that we account for not only training quality and intensity but also player enjoyment and 'buy-in', especially with this group of players who may be at a different motivational state compared to those who are included and involved in regular match play.

An example 'off the ball' exercise modality which could be useful to implement for such a purpose would be in the form of aerobic blocks, which are essentially continuous bouts of running at a given submaximal intensity. A representation of such a modality was researched and illustrated that 'aerobic interval training' in the form of 4 × 4 minutes continuous running at 90%–95% maximal heart, performed twice per week and as an extension to regular training, significantly improved an array of physiological parameters in addition to in-game physical outputs after only eight weeks [72]. Furthermore, without the authors reporting how much extra work was summated using such practices, it could be speculated that somewhere in the region of an additional 1000–1200 m total running distance may be covered during each block of four minutes, which would significantly elevate the volume parameters accumulated for each training session. The same principles can be attributed to long distance tempo runs and even repeated sprint exercise modalities, which both have the capability to improve aerobic base whilst eliciting additional running demands. Nevertheless, all such modalities in general fail to meet the intermittent and varying speed characteristic of soccer, and as such it is fair to conclude that choices to implement these modes of training should be based only on practical necessity [73].

A final thought to consider on a topic already highlighted within this chapter is the use of SSGs. This type of conditioning modality tends to have an inability to meet the 'volume' demands from a distance and high-speed running perspective required for the non-playing subgroup. However, it could be feasible that through a careful manipulation of certain conditioning constraints, there may be a possibility to provide a stimulus which is more suited to replacing the demands missed via 'non-selection'. Specifically, a research study suggested that using a 200 m² playing area per outfield individual instead of a 100 m² alternative induces additional volume load-based metrics such as total running distance and distance spent at higher speed thresholds [74]. As such, this type of manipulation of constraints could be extremely advantageous for physical performance coaches in search for the perfect modality to apply to our 'non-starters'. Although such conditions would need to be carefully planned to not create working areas which are unrealistic for the players to perform in, whilst maintaining the required intensity and motivation.

Conditioning during congested periods

Table 5.4 portrays a potential method of how it may be possible to prescribe certain physical stimuli to a group of players even when faced with a congested fixture period. Understandably, the 'match day' itself will essentially be the most physically demanding exposure throughout the week and will accommodate two working days of a microcycle such as that highlighted. Thereafter, and depending on the working philosophy of a backroom staff, the day following a match and the subsequent one after as *'non acquisition days'*. On these specific days, players should be persuaded to do very little due to them being situated directly within a cycle of recovery. There may also be an opportunity to complete some form of off-feet physical work such as upper body strength and/or even where desired, it may also be feasible for athletes to perform some form of low intensity steady state aerobic work on one or two of these days if an athlete feels it may help reduce markers of fatigue or soreness.

Accordingly, if continuing to follow the schedule proposed in Table 5.4, we are essentially left with only two acquisition days of which could be utilised to integrate a form of physical development. After a thorough recovery period of 48-60 hours, players are required to re-group for MD-2 and train in preparation for the upcoming fixture. Subsequently, this is almost the only opportunity to implement any form of conditioning work into a session and the warm-up can play a significant role in offering an opportunity to implement such. On the assumption, 15 minutes will be attributed to the warm-up phase of a session; after an effective 'Raise', 'Activation' and period of Mobility work, practitioners are potentially left with somewhere in the range of five to seven minutes of duration to utilise for the development of physical capabilities.

In addition to the warm-up on MD-2 being a possible window of opportunity for implementation of physical work, there is also an argument to further

Table 5.4 A proposed schedule for conditioning and athletic development stimuli during a two-game week separated by four days*

	Match day	MD+1	MD−3	MD−2	MD−1	Match day
Conditioning stimulus	Match Exposure (100% Volume + Intensity)	Recovery + Regeneration (low level steady state aerobic work if desired)	Rest day	Small-medium-sided games (underloaded)		Match Exposure (100% Volume + Intensity)
Athletic development stimulus				Acceleration	Reactive/cognitive stimuli	
				Maximal speed exposure (for reduced minute players)	Priming + Potentiation activities	
				Movement quality	Movement quality	
				Running based plyometrics	Mobility	
				And/or		
				Change of direction		
				Deceleration		
				On pitch strength Qualities		

Dependent on match minutes.

increase the physical stimulus of such training sessions via the implementation of small-medium-sided games. Through doing so in perhaps an underloaded manner, with a greater number of teams (three teams for one pitch), a smaller playing area and perhaps no limitation on the number of touches, we might be able to provide an environment which induces a small quantity of aerobic conditioning, without causing excessive tiredness or fatigue for the upcoming match day.

Ultimately, the prescription of conditioning is very complex and much more difficult than what it may first seem to those entering the industry. As a practitioner, it is imperative that we continue to look for new ways to deal with the multiple subgroups which make up a squad of players; however, the fundamental takeaway should be that we must strive to provide as much individualism as possible, especially if we are to give our athletes the best possible environment to perform and remain robust and injury free.

Conclusion

The importance of conditioning in professional soccer cannot be understated, and is a prerequisite to high performance, injury prevention and increasing overall player availability. Maximising physical output from drills and warm-ups becomes important for the physical development of players and must be utilised as an opportunity to increase physical capacities, where appropriate. Drill constraints can be implemented to increase the physical demand of drills; however, it must be a collective decision with coaching staff as to the implication that these constraints can have on technical/tactical behaviours. Knowing your cohort of players, the environment, the head coach's philosophy on training, upcoming fixtures, and the training loads of past, present and future will heavily influence how conditioning is applied in your setting. Where possible, applying a more individualised approach to conditioning is considered advantageous. It is recommended that an evidence-based approach, combined with craft knowledge and an understanding of training culture be used to formulate best practice conditioning principles to the holistic programme.

References

1 Walker, G.J. and R. Hawkins, *Structuring a program in elite professional soccer.* Strength & Conditioning Journal, 2018. **40**(3): p. 72–82.
2 Jaspers, A., et al., *Relationships between training load indicators and training outcomes in professional soccer.* Sports medicine, 2017. **47**(3): p. 533–544.
3 Thorpe, R.T., et al., *Tracking morning fatigue status across in-season training weeks in elite soccer players.* International Journal of Sports Physiology and Performance, 2016. **11**(7): p. 947–952.
4 Los Arcos, A., A. Mendez-Villanueva, and R. Martínez-Santos, *In-season training periodization of professional soccer players.* Biology of sport, 2017. **34**(2): p. 149.
5 Malone, J.J., et al., *Seasonal training-load quantification in elite English premier league soccer players.* International journal of sports physiology and performance, 2015. **10**(4): p. 489–497.
6 Anderson, L., et al., *Quantification of training load during one-, two-and three-game week schedules in professional soccer players from the English Premier League: implications for carbohydrate periodisation.* Journal of sports sciences, 2016. **34**(13): p. 1250–1259.
7 Gastin, P.B., et al., *Influence of physical fitness, age, experience, and weekly training load on match performance in elite Australian football.* The Journal of Strength & Conditioning Research, 2013. **27**(5): p. 1272–1279.
8 Nicholas, C.W., F.E. Nuttall, and C. Williams, *The Loughborough Intermittent Shuttle Test: a field test that simulates the activity pattern of soccer.* Journal of sports sciences, 2000. **18**(2): p. 97–104.
9 Carling, C., et al., *The role of motion analysis in elite soccer.* Sports medicine, 2008. **38**(10): p. 839–862.
10 Arnason, A., et al., *Physical fitness, injuries, and team performance in soccer.* Medicine & Science in Sports & Exercise, 2004. **36**(2): p. 278–285.
11 Eirale, C., et al., *Low injury rate strongly correlates with team success in Qatari professional football.* British journal of sports medicine, 2013. **47**(12): p. 807–808.
12 Podlog, L., et al., *Time trends for injuries and illness, and their relation to performance in the National Basketball Association.* Journal of science and medicine in sport, 2015. **18**(3): p. 278–282.
13 Raysmith, B.P. and M.K. Drew, *Performance success or failure is influenced by weeks lost to injury and illness in elite Australian track and field athletes: a 5-year prospective study.* Journal of Science and Medicine in Sport, 2016. **19**(10): p. 778–783.

14 Hägglund, M., et al., *Injuries affect team performance negatively in professional football: an 11-year follow-up of the UEFA Champions League injury study.* British journal of sports medicine, 2013. **47**(12): p. 738–742.
15 King, T., et al., *Life after the game—Injury profile of past elite Australian Football players.* Journal of science and medicine in sport, 2013. **16**(4): p. 302–306.
16 Gallo, P.O., et al., *The epidemiology of injuries in a professional soccer team in Argentina.* International SportMed Journal, 2006. **7**(4): p. 255–265.
17 Windt, J. and T.J. Gabbett, *How do training and competition workloads relate to injury? The workload-injury aetiology model.* Br J Sports Med, 2017. **51**(5): p. 428–435.
18 Iaia, F.M. and R. Hawkins, *Fitness coaching in an elite soccer team: With special focus on individual-based approaches,* in Science and Football VIII. 2016, Routledge. p. 30–39.
19 Nassis, G.P., et al., *Elite football of 2030 will not be the same as that of 2020: Preparing players, coaches, and support staff for the evolution.* 2020, Wiley Online Library. p. 962–964.
20 Drew, M.K. and C.F. Finch, *The relationship between training load and injury, illness and soreness: a systematic and literature review.* Sports medicine, 2016. **46**(6): p. 861–883.
21 Eckard, T.G., et al., *The relationship between training load and injury in athletes: a systematic review.* Sports medicine, 2018. **48**(8): p. 1929–1961.
22 Jones, C.M., P.C. Griffiths, and S.D. Mellalieu, *Training load and fatigue marker associations with injury and illness: a systematic review of longitudinal studies.* Sports medicine, 2017. **47**(5): p. 943–974.
23 Gabbett, T.J., *Debunking the myths about training load, injury and performance: empirical evidence, hot topics and recommendations for practitioners.* British journal of sports medicine, 2020. **54**(1): p. 58–66.
24 Soligard, T., et al., *How much is too much?(Part 1) International Olympic Committee consensus statement on load in sport and risk of injury.* British journal of sports medicine, 2016. **50**(17): p. 1030–1041.
25 Borresen, J. and M.I. Lambert, *The quantification of training load, the training response and the effect on performance.* Sports medicine, 2009. **39**(9): p. 779–795.
26 Pelechrinis, K. and W. Winston, *Positional value in soccer: Expected league points added above replacement.* arXiv preprint arXiv:1807.07536, 2018.
27 Decroos, T., et al. *Actions speak louder than goals: Valuing player actions in soccer.* in *Proceedings of the 25th ACM SIGKDD international conference on knowledge discovery & data mining.* 2019.
28 Fernández, J., L. Bornn, and D. Cervone. *Decomposing the immeasurable sport: A deep learning expected possession value framework for soccer.* in *13th MIT Sloan Sports Analytics Conference.* 2019.
29 Ali, A., *Measuring soccer skill performance: a review.* Scandinavian journal of medicine & science in sports, 2011. **21**(2): p. 170–183.
30 P.S. and J.D. Ade, *Are current physical match performance metrics in elite soccer fit for purpose or is the adoption of an integrated approach needed?* International Journal of Sports Physiology and Performance, 2018. **13**(5): p. 656–664.
31 Dellal, A., et al., *Comparison of physical and technical performance in European soccer match-play: FA Premier League and La Liga.* European journal of sport science, 2011. **11**(1): p. 51–59.
32 Mooney, M., et al., *The relationship between physical capacity and match performance in elite Australian football: a mediation approach.* Journal of Science and Medicine in Sport, 2011. **14**(5): p. 447–52.
33 Modric, T., et al., *Analysis of the association between running performance and game performance indicators in professional soccer players.* International journal of environmental research and public health, 2019. **16**(20): p. 4032.
34 Orange, S. and A. Smith, *Evidence-based strength and conditioning in soccer.* The Health & Fitness Journal of Canada, 2016. **9**(2): p. 21–37.

35 Sporis, G., et al., *Fitness profiling in soccer: physical and physiologic characteristics of elite players.* The Journal of Strength & Conditioning Research, 2009. **23**(7): p. 1947–1953.
36 Turner, A.N. and P.F. Stewart, *Strength and conditioning for soccer players.* Strength & Conditioning Journal, 2014. **36**(4): p. 1–13.
37 Bangsbo, J., *Energy demands in competitive soccer.* Journal of sports sciences, 1994. **12**(sup1): p. S5–S12.
38 Morgans, R., et al., *Principles and practices of training for soccer.* Journal of Sport and Health Science, 2014. **3**(4): p. 251–257.
39 Hoff, J., et al., *Soccer specific aerobic endurance training.* British Journal of Sports Medicine, 2002. **36**(3): p. 218–21.
40 Wisloeff, U., J. Helgerud, and J. Hoff, *Strength and endurance of elite soccer players.* Medicine and science in sports and exercise, 1998. **30**(3): p. 462–467.
41 Helgerud, J., et al., *Strength and endurance in elite football players.* International journal of sports medicine, 2011. **32**(09): p. 677–682.
42 Hill-Haas, S.V., et al., *Physiology of small-sided games training in football.* Sports medicine, 2011. **41**(3): p. 199–220.
43 Los Arcos, A., et al., *Effects of small-sided games vs. interval training in aerobic fitness and physical enjoyment in young elite soccer players.* PloS one, 2015. **10**(9): p. e0137224.
44 Evangelos, B., et al., *Aerobic and anaerobic capacity of professional soccer players in annual macrocycle.* Journal of Physical Education and Sport, 2016. **16**(2): p. 527.
45 Rampinini, E., et al., *Variation in top level soccer match performance.* International journal of sports medicine, 2007. **28**(12): p. 1018–1024.
46 Faude, O., T. Koch, and T. Meyer, *Straight sprinting is the most frequent action in goal situations in professional football.* Journal of sports sciences, 2012. **30**(7): p. 625–631.
47 Djaoui, L., et al., *Maximal sprinting speed of elite soccer players during training and matches.* The Journal of Strength & Conditioning Research, 2017. **31**(6): p. 1509–1517.
48 Edouard, P., et al., *Sprinting: a potential vaccine for hamstring injury.* Sport Performance & Science Reports, 2019. **1**: p. 1–2.
49 Sheppard, J.M. and W.B. Young, *Agility literature review: Classifications, training and testing.* Journal of sports sciences, 2006. **24**(9): p. 919–932.
50 Svensson, M. and B. Drust, *Testing soccer players.* Journal of Sports Sciences, 2005. **23**(6): p. 601–18.
51 Mohr, M., P. Krustrup, and J. Bangsbo, *Match performance of high-standard soccer players with special reference to development of fatigue.* Journal of sports sciences, 2003. **21**(7): p. 519–528.
52 Cummins, C., et al., *Global positioning systems (GPS) and microtechnology sensors in team sports: a systematic review.* Sports Medicine, 2013. **43**(10): p. 1025–1042.
53 Delaney, J.A., et al., *Acceleration-Based Running Intensities of Professional Rugby League Match Play.* International Journal of Sports Physiology and Performance, 2016. **11**(6): p. 802–809.
54 Delaney, J.A., et al., *Establishing duration-specific running intensities from match-play analysis in rugby league.* International Journal of Sports Physiology and Performance, 2015. **10**(6): p. 725–31.
55 Calder, A.R., et al., *Physical demands of female collegiate lacrosse competition: whole-match and peak periods analysis.* Sport Sciences for Health, 2021. **17**(1): p. 103–109.
56 Calder, A. and T. Gabbett, *Influence of Tactical Formation on Average and Peak Demands of Elite Soccer Match-Play.* International Journal of Strength and Conditioning, 2022. **2**(1): p. 1–10.
57 Delaney, J.A., et al., *Modelling the decrement in running intensity within professional soccer players.* Science and Medicine in Football, 2017. **2**(2): p. 86–92.
58 Aguiar, M., et al., *A review on the effects of soccer small-sided games.* Journal of human kinetics, 2012. **33**: p. 103.
59 Rampinini, E., et al., *Factors influencing physiological responses to small-sided soccer games.* Journal of sports sciences, 2007. **25**(6): p. 659–666.

60 Opar, D.A., M.D. Williams, and A.J. Shield, *Hamstring strain injuries*. Sports medicine, 2012. **42**(3): p. 209–226.
61 Toohey, L.A., et al., *Is subsequent lower limb injury associated with previous injury? A systematic review and meta-analysis*. British journal of sports medicine, 2017. **51**(23): p. 1670–1678.
62 Banister, E.W. and T.W. Calvert, *Planning for future performance: implications for long term training*. Canadian Journal of Applied Sport Sciences. Journal Canadien Des Sciences Appliquees Au Sport, 1980. **5**(3): p. 170–176.
63 Wehrlin, J.P. and J. Hallén, *Linear decrease in $\dot V\hbox{O}_{2\max}$ and performance with increasing altitude in endurance athletes*. European Journal of Applied Physiology, 2006. **96**(4): p. 404–412.
64 Garvican-Lewis, L.A., et al., *Stage racing at altitude induces hemodilution despite an increase in hemoglobin mass*. Journal of Applied Physiology, 2014. **117**(5): p. 463–472.
65 Nassis, G.P., *Effect of altitude on football performance: analysis of the 2010 FIFA World Cup Data*. The Journal of Strength & Conditioning Research, 2013. **27**(3): p. 703–707.
66 Bohner, J.D., et al., *Moderate altitude affects high intensity running performance in a collegiate women's soccer game*. Journal of human kinetics, 2015. **47**: p. 147.
67 Mohr, M., et al., *Examination of fatigue development in elite soccer in a hot environment: a multi-experimental approach*. Scandinavian journal of medicine & science in sports, 2010. **20**: p. 125–132.
68 Morgans, R., et al., *An intensive Winter fixture schedule induces a transient fall in salivary IgA in English premier league soccer players*. Research in Sports Medicine, 2014. **22**(4): p. 346–354.
69 Thomas, K., et al., *Etiology and recovery of neuromuscular fatigue following simulated soccer match-play*. Medicine & Science in Sports & Exercise, 2017. **49**(5): p. 955–64.
70 Hills, S.P., et al., *Profiling the post-match top-up conditioning practices of professional soccer substitutes: An analysis of contextual influences*. The Journal of Strength & Conditioning Research, 2020. **34**(10): p. 2805–2814.
71 Anderson, L., et al., *Quantification of seasonal-long physical load in soccer players with different starting status from the English Premier League: Implications for maintaining squad physical fitness*. International journal of sports physiology and performance, 2016. **11**(8): p. 1038–1046.
72 Helgerud, J., et al., *Aerobic endurance training improves soccer performance*. Medicine and science in sports and exercise, 2001. **33**(11): p. 1925–1931.
73 Impellizzeri, F.M., et al., *Physiological and performance effects of generic versus specific aerobic training in soccer players*. International journal of sports medicine, 2006. **27**(06): p. 483–492.
74 Castillo, D., et al., *Influence of different small-sided game formats on physical and physiological demands and physical performance in young soccer players*. The Journal of Strength & Conditioning Research, 2021. **35**(8): p. 2287–2293.

6 Player monitoring and practical application

Andrea Riboli, Lewis MacMillan, Alex Calder and Lorcan Mason

Overview of monitoring

Within current professional sport, the monitoring of athletes has become a cornerstone of the daily training schedule. The monitoring systems implemented by the performance and medicine departments within clubs are dependent on its ability to reliability and accurately quantify the training dose and the individual response to the training dose of each player. This information, in turn, is then used to inform and assist the actions that are taken in terms of future planning of the training process to maximize player availability and performance through understanding the complex relationships between the training dose, performance outcomes, injury, and illness [1–6].

Specifically, soccer is vastly moving towards a higher physical and technical requirement. Moreover, players are faced with an even more congested schedule, especially for those competing in both national and international competitions. These factors lead to an even more complex and challenging training load management. For instance, teams playing in national championships, national cups, and international competitions (e.g. UEFA, CONCACAF, and AFC Champions Leagues) are faced with a very congested fixture schedule with often three matches per week. Additionally, also the transition periods (i.e. the off-season periods) are reduced for players competing with their national teams (i.e. in international tournaments such as World-, Europe-, Asian- and African-Cups). Therefore, coaches and sport scientists often have to be agile in their periodisation to account for match schedule; the competitive schedule negatively affects the training availability (e.g. due to a greater amount of recovery sessions for players who play the whole match), reducing the time for performance development and testing procedures.

The abovementioned complex scenario demands the need for coaches and practitioners to create a consistent analysis of information collected during practice (e.g. pre-training, post-training, on-field practice, and gym sessions). Meaning, that a detailed comprehension of the information collected daily during both training and matches should be integrated to inform performance and medical staffs about player readiness, performance development, and the rehabilitation process, when required. Therefore, in elite soccer, the performance and medical staff need to comply with objective and subjective information to maximize player's performance development, whilst minimizing the risk of injury.

Why we track and monitor

Approach to the problem

Tracking and monitoring players' well-being, training status, dose, and response can be accomplished a variety of ways [5, 7]. However, as practitioners, we must understand the rationale as well as the validity and reliability of the approaches. It is suggested that when attempting to answer questions within the performance departments, practitioners employ a systematic approach.

Figure 6.1 illustrates the appropriate steps, via a systematic approach, to defining procedures within a performance department. Developing and fine-tuning protocols via a systematic approach will help increase sustainability, organization, and effectiveness within a multi-disciplinary team [8]. When monitoring players, it is integral that all members of the performance and medical departments work cohesively in a systematic manner to effectively execute strategies and protocols.

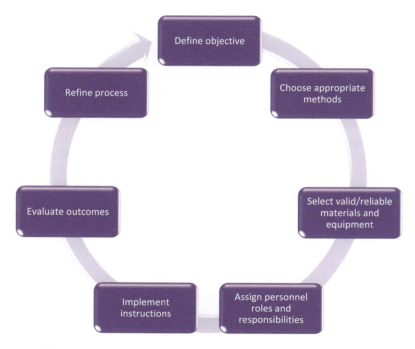

Figure 6.1 A systematic approach to solving problems and questions within a performance department of an elite soccer organization.

The training processes

The ultimate/continuous aim of the training process is to progressively develop the required qualities of the sport (soccer) in order to improve performance [2]. This is achieved via the balance between the application of an appropriate training dose and the time afforded to facilitate adequate recovery for sustained adaptations [9, 10].

In essence, for adaptations to occur, an overloading training dose must be applied to the individual and homeostasis must be disturbed resulting in reduced performance (fatigue) [11]. If appropriate recovery is afforded, adaptations occur which are protective against further fatigue arising from a similar training dose [12–14].

In essence, the training-recovery cycle can be partly explained based on three governing theories [15]:

1 Selye's general adaptation syndrome theory [11], which describes the body's response to a stressor/stimulus.
2 The stimulus-fatigue-recovery-adaptation theory [16–18], which proposes that the accumulation of fatigue is in proportion to the duration, volume, and/or intensity of the stressor/stimulus.
   a Furthermore, the frequency of subsequent stressors/stimuli is also crucial in order to optimize performance outcomes, with any subsequent training occurring during the supercompensation phase [14, 19–21], if the subsequent stressors/stimuli is applied too soon – the additional fatigue may accumulate which results in a prolonged return to homeostasis and reduced performance [19, 22, 23]. However, when the subsequent stressors/stimuli are applied at the appropriate time, during the supercompensation phase, performance can be enhanced [10].
3 The fitness-fatigue model [15, 24, 25], which advises that training doses which minimize fatigue accumulation while also maximizing adaptation will have the greatest transfer to performance outcomes.

However, to fully explain the training-recovery cycle, practitioners must also account for the multitude of additional internal psycho-physiological responses/adaptations that also occur during training which dilute the accuracy of quantifying the training response [26–28], resulting in the complex relationship between the training dose, performance outcomes, injury and illness [29, 30]. Therefore, a multi-dimensional monitoring approach to evaluate the individual response to the implied training stressor has become an essential part of informing the training process.

Subjective-objective/internal-external

A key component of any successful monitoring system is its ability to quantify the training load accurately and reliably. In soccer (along with many sports), training load can be categorized as either external or internal [31]. External training load refers to the physical work that players are exposed to via specific training prescriptions. The training prescriptions set by practitioners and coaches elicit a desired physiological response and adaptation, resembling the internal training load [32]. Internal training load often refers to the psychophysiological response that players/athletes experience in reaction to managing the requirements provoked by the external training load [31].

The collection of these measures form the foundations of a training process framework informing the monitoring process [27]. Ultimately, it is the athlete's internal load that determines the stress that governs the individual response to the implied external load training stressor [27]. Within the external/internal categories, measures can be collected subjectively or objectively (Table 6.1). Subjective measures refer to the myriad of internal factors that potentially reflect mental load, such as fatigue, effort, stress, motivation etc. [33]. Furthermore, subjective measures have shown to be a vital assessment for determining the relationship between injury and performance [34, 35].

Even though internal load measures are associated with adaptations, it is imperative that we understand and quantify the external loads that contribute to an athlete's internal response. Due to advancements in technology, the process of measuring external loads has become widespread across the sporting landscape [36] and is quantified depending on the context of the sport or mode of training [37].

The advantage of monitoring external loads is that it allows the practitioners to prescribe training more precisely in advance of the session being carried out

Table 6.1 Examples of external and internal measures, separated by subjective and objective categories

External	
Subjective	Objective

• Coaches interpretation
  • E.g. performance output/rating
	• Global Positioning System (GPS)
	• Video tracking
	• Force plate data
	• Gym monitoring equipment
	  • e.g. velocity-based training
	• Body weight markers
	• Biomechanical analysis

Internal	
Subjective	Objective

• Wellness questionnaires
• Rate of perceived exertion (RPE)
• Pain scales
	• Heart rate monitoring
	  • e.g. training data, and heart rate variability (HRV)
	• Blood markers
	  • e.g. creatine kinase

based on the valid and reliable variables collected during previous sessions and the athlete's prior response to the external load that was prescribed [38]. As mentioned, how external load is collected and prescribed is context-specific. However, in field-based team sports, the most commonly used technologies include both local and global positioning systems, along with accelerometers, inertial measurement units, and camera-based measurements [2].

Detailing each of these systems and their variables is beyond the scope of this section; however, they have been extensively researched within the literature [36, 39–43]. Nonetheless, it is not necessarily how (i.e. the technology used) the external load is quantified but rather the why (i.e. what is this tool used? Is it valid? or Is it reliable?), and that is to inform the training process in order to achieve the desired adaptations imposed by the external load prescribed [27]. As a result, these adaptations, either positive or negative, are what correspond to the internal load [26, 27].

In view of that, when monitoring athletes, it is recommended that measures of internal load are used as the primary means of determining the training outcomes (adaptations) [27]. This is since the internal load borne by an individual athlete corresponding to a specific external load will vary depending on the specific contextual factors, along with the nature of the sport [27, 44–47]. Hence, in a practical sense estimating one's internal load response prior to training or performance is at best, what all great practitioners have, an educated guess!

Nonetheless, internal load can be psychological/subjective or physiological/objective in nature [1, 27, 28] with the methods of assessment being context-specific [27] based on the nature of the sport and when used in combination reflects the type of fatigue experienced which will enhance a practitioners understanding of the internal load experienced to better inform the training process [26, 27]. However, it is important to note that when it comes to the level of evidence of objective and subjective measures, current research [48–50] demonstrates that there is little relationship between objective and subjective measures and suggests that subjective measures of internal load were more stable and responsive to training load.

Assessing fatigue

As aforementioned, the key to any monitoring system is to find the appropriate balance between an athlete's level of fatigue and their ability to perform [10, 15, 24–27], while also taking the numerous contextual factors that influence this equation [27]. Fatigue as a concept is extremely difficult to define due to its multifaceted origins [2] with numerous definitions proposed in the literature [6, 51]. Despite this ambiguity, there is mutual agreement that a central component of fatigue is the failure to produce or maintain the required force or power output for a given task that was previously attainable resulting from both central and peripheral factors [51], including activation of the motor command, propagation of the action potential through the descending motor pathway, myofilament excitation-contraction coupling, and the status of the intracellular milieu [52], which can persist for days at a time if not addressed [53].

However, despite this agreement, there is a failure to acknowledge the mental component of fatigue which must be considered [51, 53] due to the suggestion that when fatigue is reported as a symptom by an individual, it can only be evaluated by self-reporting and categorized as a trait characteristic or state variable [53]. Despite this, physiology remains the central focus of the numerous models proposed to define fatigue [51, 53, 54], all of which fail to account for the perception of effort required to maintain the required force or power output for a given task (i.e. the definition of fatigue) [55]. To address this omission of perception of effort two main concepts have been developed: the Psychobiological Model of Fatigue (PBM) [55] and Integrative Governor Theory (IGT) [56] which are defined below; however, it must be noted that there is some criticisms of these concepts [57]. Nevertheless, quantifying an athlete's fatigue status and its time-course remains a central component of any monitoring system [56, 58]; however, it must be noted that there is no current gold-standard of measurement and misconceptions are still prevalent within the literature [27]. To account for the ambiguities of the definition, of fatigue, the term 'Readiness' has been utilized in athletic populations [1, 59] and has been defined as a state 'where an athlete has no impairment of physical performance, no mental fatigue or excessive psychological distress' [3].

Understanding the physical demands of soccer

The quantification of physical demands has become crucial for leading the performance development towards an evidence-based practice. Coaches and practitioners can collect and track a variety of information about the individual- and team-based training loads during both training and matches. In practice, daily training load management is manipulated accordingly with the demands imposed on each player across the day-to-day training routine. To quantify the locomotor demands, semi-automated video-based tracking technologies and global-positioning system (GPS) are frequently utilized [60, 61]. Understanding of the interplay of an athlete's internal and external training loads is imperative when attempting to monitor fatigue and optimize performance. The information gained by GPS may allow for better analysis and planning of training loads [61, 62]. However, subsequent match-play data may provide a greater understanding of the specific demands during official matches (see Chapter 7).

Locomotor demand can be defined as the work completed by the players, measured independently of their internal characteristics and physiological responses [37, 38]. In top-class soccer, semi-automated video-based tracking technologies, GPS and inertial sensors such as accelerometers, magnetometers, and gyroscopes allow us to measure the total distance, the distance covered at different running speed and the distance covered accelerating/decelerating [38]. Tracking technologies, such as GPS and semi-automated video-based tracking technologies, allow us to determine the locomotor demands imposed on each player during daily routine (see Chapter 7). However, to better understand the complexity of individual physiological responses to training [27], we must not forget the importance of the physiological measurements (i.e. internal load) [27] and the individual cardiorespiratory and metabolic capacities [63–65] that are still lacking using tracking technologies.

Validity and reliability of tracking technologies

The validity of an instrument reflects the ability to accurately measure what the device intends to measure [66, 67]. The reliability refers to the reproducibility of a value on repeat occasions [66, 68]. Despite validity and reliability, it was also demonstrated that such differences using different tracking technologies could still exist [69]. Therefore, practitioners should be aware that these differences may affect the between-systems interchangeability [69]. In real-life soccer-specific context, GPS and semi-automated video-based tracking technologies are often utilized during training and match, respectively; this may affect data comparison. To overlap these differences, an accurate between-systems comparison should be performed for providing specific calibration equations as previously proposed for both integrating different tracking technologies [69] and using match demands as a reference for small-sided games [70].

Monitoring strategies

The use of force plate testing

The force plates are a useful tool in screening, profiling, monitoring and rehabilitating elite athletes, especially across competitions and leagues with irregular and congested competitive schedule [71]. The counter movement jump (CMJ) is the most detailed test with an easy setup up and great athlete compliance. Additionally, several research projects stated the validity and reliability of CMJ [72, 73]. In sports with congested fixture schedules, CMJ has been reported as the test upon which other results could be compared [71]. When deeper analysis is required, single leg jumps (SLJ) assessment is strongly recommended. SLJ and/or SL-CMJ are useful to assess bilateral asymmetry and as an important benchmark during rehabilitation process (see Chapter 9). The squat jump (SJ) creates the opportunity to test neuromuscular power during concentric phase, testing the rate of force and power development without the effect of eccentric and elastic activation as a boost for neuromuscular effort. The drop jump (DJ) provides information about amortization and the individual ability to jump after a landing phase; however, the DJ has been reported as less reliable and it requires a greater familiarization process [73].

Through force plates testing procedures, stakeholders should manage the training process regarding the individual neuromuscular capacity determined towards the medium to long term training periodisation. A battery of different tests such as bilateral and single leg CMJ, SJ, etc. should be administered regularly (e.g. monthly or weekly) to assess progress on prescribed goals determining possible potential injuries or negative deviations. The results obtained throughout the season should be compared with the individual's previous data to determine possible positive or negative effects by individual standard deviation, coefficient of variation and smallest worthwhile change [74, 75]. As such, more information collected during in-season and off-season period provide a more valid and reliable benchmark to assess individual positive and negative changes in neuromuscular training status.

Several variables can be utilized to determine different neuromuscular aspects. The jump height is somewhat representative of generic athletic ability and relatively easy to administer, given the simplified motivation for athletes. The reactive strength index modified is a more robust indicator of jump performance inclusive of jump height and contraction time considering both concentric and eccentric phases. The Eccentric Utilization Ratio (EUR) between CMJ and SJ heights is highly recommended to determine the effect of training on muscle-contraction force excluding pre-activation during eccentric pre-jump phase [76]. EUR results can be a useful tool to discriminate neuromuscular, power, and strength requirements, therefore informing the training prescriptions. The rate of force development (RFD) demonstrates the effectiveness of the neuromuscular power during both concentric and eccentric phases. In the context of rehabilitation processes, between-limbs differences, landing analysis and CMJ depth during both bilateral and SL-CMJ and/or SJ tests should be utilized to determine the effectiveness of return to play process. Consequently, helping the performance and medical staff to review objective data together to create collaborative, deliberate plans, thus ensuring coherence across training prescription for both health and performance purposes. In conclusion, a strong neuromuscular testing battery (i.e. a composite score of several neuromuscular tests) should help practitioners to collect information for players' profiling across the season. However, due to the very congested environment in elite sport, CMJ with reactive strength index (RSI) modified (i.e. jump height and contraction time) and/or rate of force development analysis may be a useful and a less-consuming tool to create a consistent neuromuscular assessment across the season. Single leg analysis and other tests (e.g. SJ, DJ, etc.) may help further analysis and can be utilized in some key-periods during the season or when particular deeper analysis is required in some players.

The rate of perceived exertion

The physiological demand, also referred as 'internal load', can be defined as the summation of the physiological stimulation/stress imposed during training activities [38]. This can vary accordingly with the locomotor demands imposed (e.g. total load, sets, and repetitions) and with the type of training performed (e.g. strength or endurance exercise) as well as environmental factors. The heart rate (HR) is one of the best objective ways to quantify aerobic training intensity [77, 78]. Monitoring players' HR during training can lead to an indirect measure of energy expenditure and reflect the rate of the maximum oxygen uptake [79]. However, HR could fail to describe the individual subjective perception of exercise efforts [37].

The rate of perceived exertion (RPE) can help the understanding of stress each athlete perceived in his/her bodies during exercise, with the assumption that an athlete might be able to adjust their training intensity using their own perceptions of effort [80, 81]. Therefore, the RPE is a rating of the overall difficulty perception of the exercise bout obtained ~30 minutes after the completion of the training session [82].

It was demonstrated that the RPE correlated to the average HR and acute changes in HR during steady-state exercise [81], high-intensity interval cycling [83] and soccer-specific drills [79]. In soccer, it was demonstrated *large* to *very large* correlations (i.e. ranging from 0.50 to 0.85) between HR responses and RPE-based approach; similarly, the HR-RPE relationship showed *very large* to *nearly perfect* association (i.e. ranging from 0.75 to 0.90) in endurance athletes [84]. A subsequent review [80] reported *large* to *very large* correlations between RPE and HR, blood lactate, $\%VO_{2max}$, VO_2 and ventilation rate [80]. Therefore, the RPE is extensively used during practice to inform about individual perceived and physiological responses to exercise at different playing levels [37].

The overall quantification of training load using RPE can be described also through the session-RPE (sRPE). The sRPE is calculated by multiplying RPE (1–10 scale) by the duration of the exercise or activity (in minutes) [82]. The pattern of the differences between sRPE and the summated HR zone score during aerobic exercise was very consistent [85, 86]. Therefore, RPE was proposed as a valid and reliable measure of exercise intensity [80, 85, 87]. Practitioners may consider RPE as a valid tool to report and calculate training load during aerobic exercise [87]. Additionally, differential-RPE (dRPE) can be supplemented, alongside traditional RPE methods, to detect isolated individual differences in perceived efforts [88].

However, RPE and sRPE cannot replace the HR-based methods due to the complex interaction of many factors that contribute to the personal perception of physical effort, including hormone concentrations, substrate concentrations, personality traits, ventilation rate, neurotransmitter levels, environmental conditions or psychological states [80, 89]. The RPE-based methods can be considered as a supplemental tool to detect the perception of effort during aerobic exercise in conjunction with individual physiological responses (i.e. HR indexes). Amalgamating the various subjective information (i.e. HR and RPE) may accurately describe actual physiological and perceived training loads and their interaction to describe possibly the acute and/or chronic adaptations [37]. Conversely, if HR monitors are not available, the RPE method may give an accurate supplemental assessment of aerobic training load [37, 80, 87].

Self-report measures of wellbeing

One method of assessing readiness is through the use of athlete self-reported measures (ASRMs) [1, 49, 59, 90–92] due to their sensitivity and consistency in reflecting changes in training load [49, 59]. Athlete self-report measures often comprise brief, single-item checklists derived from validated questionnaires to assess possible symptoms of overtraining, fatigue and/or other problems [93]. Self-report measures, such as wellness surveys are intended to be completed daily [94]. Single item refers to the single-question measurement of an aspect of wellbeing, such as rating general fatigue on a Likert scale, as opposed to a multi-item measure in which several questions may be used to quantify fatigue. The most used measures have been muscle soreness, fatigue, sleep quality, stress, and mood [95]. Other variables such as motivation to training, sleep quantity, time of sleep, mental fatigue, energy and perceived recovery has been previously reported [94]. In practice, the performance and medical staff could use a summed wellness score and/or an average wellness score to inform the decision-making process. However, there seems to be no clear consensus about the preferential use of a summarize and/or an averaged wellness score.

Practitioners are often faced with the high-performance management that usually seems interested in exploring the relationship between pretraining wellness and subsequent load output (i.e. the same day) [96–98] and/or the relationship between training load and subsequent wellness (i.e. next day) [99, 100]. The overall results, from previous research, showed mainly *trivial* to *moderate* associations between single-item self-report measures and the measurements of workload [94, 99]. Specifically, muscle soreness showed *trivial* to *large* positive and negative associations [94, 96, 101]; fatigue showed no correlations or small to *very large* negative and positive associations [94, 100, 102]; sleep quality showed no correlations or *trivial* to *very large* negative and positive associations [27, 100, 103]; stress showed no correlation or *small* to *large* positive and negative associations [78, 96, 99]. Therefore, the main findings showed a paucity of significant associations between self-report measures and training load. Where associations were found, the directions of the relationship were negative (i.e. a higher training load, large wellness decrease). However, despite the interest to determine possible relationships with training loads, such an association may not be expected to be especially useful. A possible dissociation between the expected wellbeing-score and the locomotor/physiological demands may highlight symptoms of fatigue providing helpful information in clinical assessment and actual training prescriptions.

Self-report measures may help practitioners to improve certain aspects, such as communication with athletes and within stakeholders (e.g. coaches, practitioners, and other support staff). The wellness score may be used to modulate the daily training load management and to individualize exercise prescriptions for avoiding possible injuries and/or other problems. In elite soccer, players should avoid the likelihood of missing training sessions and increase the possibility for team selection. A consistent self-report measurement may help practitioners prescribe individual exercise programmes before and after each training session, with the overall goal to avoid time-lost from on-field practice and increasing odds of match-roster selection. Practitioners should not forget that the self-report measures are influenced by several psychological and social factors [93]. The nature of the self-reported information reflects a complex 'readiness', not just a training response. For this reason, stakeholders should create appropriate relationships within each player, allowing high individual involvement for accurate self-measure data collection.

Table 6.2 Example of a wellness questionnaire (ASRM*)

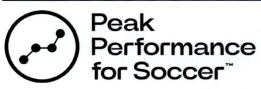

	Scale
Sleep quantity	_____ PM to _____ AM
Sleep quality	/5
Mood	/5
Stress	/5
Readiness to train	/5
Fatigue	/5
Soreness	/5

*ASRM: athlete self-reported measure

The use of self-reported measures may add new insights to the more objective locomotor and physiological measurements. The inconsistent findings about the relationship between training load and self-report measures, reinforce the use of wellbeing information to strengthen their use as supplemental tools in the clinical decision-making process. In practice, the performance and medical staff may consider wellbeing information such as muscle soreness, fatigue, sleep quality, stress, etc. for practical and clinical decisions (Table 6.2). This information should be added to the objective locomotor and physiological demands for creating an overall training load description using both the objective measures (i.e. GPS, HR, etc.) and the perceived wellbeing of each player.

Physical performance analysis

Understanding the activities of match-play is crucial for soccer-specific training prescriptions [70, 104–106]. The activities recorded during the matches are used to plan the training workload and as a reference for soccer-specific drills (e.g., small-sided games), technical-tactical drills and/or individual positional exercises [70, 107, 108]. The intermittent nature of soccer is characterized by high-intensity interspersed with low-intensity running activities [109, 110]. Therefore, the understanding of the locomotor and physiological demands during both training and matches may inform practitioners about the daily training load management. Several studies highlighted that professional soccer players should be trained based on the match physical demands for a successful performance and injury prevention [111–113]. The training prescription may provide a progressive adaptation up to official match demands contextualizing soccer-specific and/or general exercises across both the average and the maximal competition demands [70, 106, 108].

Although the most common time-motion analysis has been focused on the 90-min [114], 15-min [115] and 5-min [111] match demands, the attention has been raised on the most demanding passages of match-play also known as peak match intensities. [116–119]. During the training process, the relative whole-match running distances fail to fully account for the worst-case scenario that occurs during official matches [120] and it may be responsible for underpreparing players for the peak match intensity [117, 119, 121]. This may negatively affect performance capacity [106, 112, 122, 123] and possibly increase the occurrence of injuries [124, 125]. The use of a rolling average method, where distance is divided in set intervals from every time point sampled, could be a more appropriate method when quantifying the running intensity periods in team sports [106, 120, 126]. This approach may help practitioners to plan the locomotor activities during soccer-specific drills (e.g. small- or large-sided games) in accordance with the peak match intensities [107, 127, 128]. For example, a previous study suggested that if the players covered a specific intensity during the match, these players might to be trained for similar demands [111]. For this purpose, coaches may design their training drills (e.g., modifying area per player in small-sided games) to elicit average [70, 108] and/or peak demands [129]. For instance, a recent study reported professional players may cover ~200 m (being ~61 m at high-speed running and ~30 m sprinting) in 1 minute [122]. Additionally, the one-minute periods have been recently described across formation, ball in play and ball possession to help practitioner for contextualizing the maximal technical-tactical match demands during practice [130]. This study showed an increase in maximal relative distances as the time-dependent period decreases across different metrics within each playing position [130]. For high-speed, sprint and acceleration/deceleration distances, the 1-min$_{peak}$ showed fourfold higher locomotor requirements than whole match (90 min). Interestingly, although the authors reported no between-formation differences in total distance and the distance in different speed thresholds, the 1-min$_{peak}$ for Acc/Dec appears the lowest in 4-4-2 on average but the highest in 4-3-3 for forwards, central and wide midfielders [130]. Moreover, the intermittent nature of soccer is also characterized by game interruptions (i.e. when the ball is out of play,) [110, 131]. During official matches, an average of ~54 to ~57 min ball-in-play (BiP) time across the whole match time was observed in Italian Serie A, French Ligue 1, German Bundesliga, FIFA World Cup and UEFA Euro tournaments [110, 130, 131]. The official match-play demands which include ball out-of-play time may underestimate the highest intensity of competitions not preparing the player for the actual maximum match demands [132, 133]. Therefore, practitioners should also consider the time with/without ball-in-play for individual match analysis. The BiP cycles seem to be more appropriate for designing training sessions [132, 133]. Recently, the peak match intensity during BiP for total distance, high-speed running, accelerating/decelerating and high-metabolic load distance were suggested to gain maximal physical-performance development [133]. Interestingly, in Italian Serie A soccer players, the BiP$_{peak}$ was found lower than 1-min$_{peak}$ for high-speed running, sprint and acceleration/deceleration [130]. This was due to the distance covered for tactical organization when the ball was out-of-play after very high-intensity actions (i.e. counterattacks) [112].

Nevertheless, it should be noted that these peak locomotor demands may occur only once throughout a match so this approach does not reflect the overall physical demands (especially when it comes to the volume completed at, or close to such peak demands) [123, 134]. In Australian football and rugby league, the greatest volume of activity during official matches was at ~60% of the 1-min$_{peak}$ demands [104]. Therefore, a detailed description of the match intensity rather than only 1-min$_{peak}$ may be useful for exercise prescriptions during daily routine [104]. The distribution of the match activities during official soccer matches with regard to 1-min$_{peak}$ was recently showed for the first time in Italian Serie A [123]. Interestingly, the most locomotor activities occurred at an intensity higher than the average 90-min match demand (>90-min$_{avg}$). In details, with the exception of the *small* difference for acceleration, the relative distance >90-min$_{avg}$ was *largely* to *very largely* higher than the 90-min$_{avg}$ for each metric. The time spent and the distance covered at different percentages than 1-min$_{peak}$ were calculated for different high-speed and acceleration/deceleration metrics. The time spent and the distance covered at different percentages of 1-min$_{peak}$ should be used as reference for the durations, repetitions and/or sets that should be utilized during practice to recreate or to overload such sport-specific metrics [123]. As a mere example, ~6 min at intensity higher than 80% of the 1-min$_{peak}$ for the distance > 20 km·h^{-1} could be used as a minimal reference to plan at least 6 repetitions of 1-min using soccer-specific positional drills [123]. Moreover, the overall training intensity and its distribution across different percentages that 1-min$_{peak}$ should inform practitioners for training load management [123, 130]. Therefore, coaches and sport scientist should manipulate small-sided games, technical-tactical drills and/or positional exercise to replicate and/or overload the 90-min average match demands [70, 108, 119] and the most demanding passages of match play (e.g. 1-min$_{Peak}$) [130]. However, all the intermediate intensities between average and peak match demands should be considered for the overall training intensity [123]. This information may guide the prescription of training intensity for both the overall training session demands and for each drill prescriptions.

Heart rate responses

The assessment of HR derived measurements including resting HR (RHR), exercising HR (HRex), HR variability (HRV), and HR recovery (HRR) has also received some attention within the literature [59, 135] due to their ability to be utilized as surrogate markers of an individual's autonomic nervous system (ANS) and cardiovascular fitness [136] in a time-efficient, inexpensive, and non-invasive manner [135–139]. However, despite the relative ease of data collection, HR measures remain cautiously implemented [135, 136] as ambiguity exists in the interpretation of the data collected [136, 140] due to contradictory results [138, 140], inconsistent methods [141], and misinterpretation of the data reported within the literature [136]. Also, as the majority of the research has been conducted in endurance sports [135] the interpretation of the results remains speculative due to the inherent complex nature of team sport [37, 136]. Furthermore, despite the use of HRex & HRR to infer changes in fitness from standardized protocols [59, 135, 136], morning resting HRV is currently the only viable option to guide the training process [135, 142, 143] in a non-invasive and non-fatiguing manner, although it is important to state the lack of sensitivity of HR measures to perturbations of other internal load measures as HRV is solely a marker of cardiac ANS function and cannot infer any additional information [144]. Despite this ambiguity, Schneider et al. [135] has provided an excellent overview of currently utilized HR measures and their context for interpretation in practice.

Tracking/Monitoring injury risk

Unfortunately, training loads can be easily mismanaged and can become a major cause of soft tissue injuries [145]. When the load demanded exceeds that which the body can tolerate, 'overtraining syndrome', characterized by 'too much, too fast', can lead to an increased occurrence of soft tissue injury and fatigue in the athlete, so that rest and rehabilitation is required [145, 146]. Conversely, during rehabilitation, athletes may be underloaded and consequently either unable to re-entre training with the correct fitness or requiring longer recovery to be 'fit to train'. This can be seriously problematic as underloading can lead to a cyclical

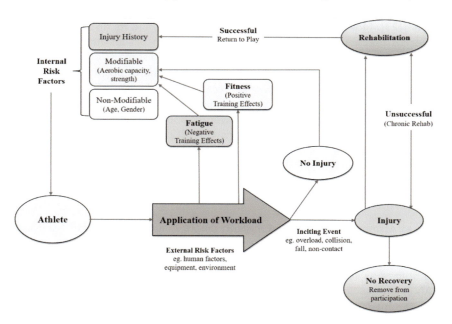

Figure 6.2 An investigation of the athlete workload injury cycle, its effects, and modification of risk factors (Adapted from Windt and Gabbett [145]).

pattern known as 'chronic rehabilitation' [147]. Often, in striving to achieve 'marginal gains', the athlete workload balance is not successfully maintained, perhaps seen in the higher rate of injury in football compared to other contact sports [148]. Therefore, daily athlete monitoring has become a necessity to reduce injury occurrence and has led to a recent massive expansion in sport scientist employment in this field in elite level football [149].

The balance of loading is highly individualized due to the influence of many confounding variables (reflecting both internal and external stressors) (Figure 6.2). During adolescence, young athletes enter a critical stage of rapid physical and psychological maturity. This period is incredibly important for an individual's future career as well as their current situation. Unfortunately, little research has been conducted on workloads, performance and injury in adolescence and early adulthood – especially in team sports [148]. However, the relationship between training load and injury has been reported in a variety of adult team sports [150, 151] and has been inferred to be the same in adolescent populations [148]. Yet, due to the lack of research in adolescent populations, it is unclear.

Training load and injury risk

Injury risk and training load have a paradoxical relationship. While higher training loads have often been associated with causing injury, it is also observed that higher training loads can also be associated with protection against injury [152–154]. The introduction of new models on sport injury risk has tried to clarify this. Is has been suggested that instead of 'high' training loads being problematic, it is training load errors that cause increased risk [155]. Furthermore, it was proposed that underloading and overloading were the cause of decreased fitness, performance, and increased injury risk. This suggests that there is an 'optimum' load for an individual and that training load-related injuries are, in fact, 'preventable injuries'. Hence, it has become the responsibility of the performance and medical staff in soccer clubs to prevent these injury occurrences by correctly adding load in a safe way, specific to the player.

Underloading occurs when an athlete does not have a training regime sufficient to maintain or improve the training status across the season and/or to meet the demands of competition, which leads to increased risk of injury. This most commonly occurs during a period of training tapering, rest, or rehabilitation. Moreover, Selye's general adaptation syndrome suggests that training stimuli below 'optimum' are insufficient to produce the athletic adaptation necessary for increased performance in sport [156].

Overloading is likely to occur when training regimes exceeds the 'normal' range. The associated risk of injury can last up to a month (28 days) and is known as the 'injury delay period' [157, 169]. Figure 6.3 represents an example of the 'injury delay period'. Often this occurs during pre-season training during the prescribed 'shock weeks' [28].

Soccer clubs may be hindered in using empirical evidence to evaluate training loads for several reasons, e.g., lack of resources, time, and buy in from coaching

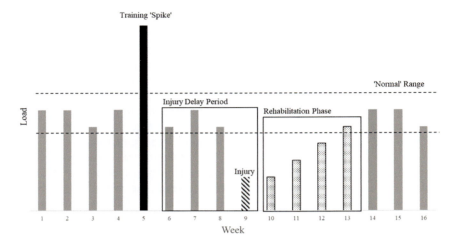

Figure 6.3 Injury delay period. Showing weekly loads and the occurrence of a 'spike' (Week 5) causing a 'delayed injury' (Week 9) and return to training protocol (Adapted from Charlton and Drew [169]).

staff [149]. Knowledge of the athlete is necessary to understanding their loading needs. However, this knowledge must be used in conjunction with empirical data to support and provide evidence for any prescribed course of action. Recently, there has been an increasing emphasis on monitoring athletes through training load management [154].

Training stress balance

Originally, Banister and colleagues designed a 'Training Stress Balance' (TSB) model to describe the training-performance relationship and to describe the athlete's response to a specific training stimulus [158, 159]. Akin to the dose-response relationship reported in pharmacology, Banister's model has the primary goal of reducing injury risk whilst maximizing performance so that optimum athletic performance can be assessed between negative (fatigue) and positive (fitness) aspects of training [160].

The Acute:Chronic Workload Ratio

Adapting the ideas from the TSB design, Gabbett and colleagues created the Acute:Chronic Workload ratio (ACWR) model [157]. This model compares the acute load (fatigue) to a chronic load (fitness) to create a ratio. Typically, acute load is the accumulated load of 1-week and is compared to a 4-week rolling average chronic load [157]. After the initial construction of the ACWR, researchers have investigated multiple approaches to identifying injury risk within their cohort, including mathematically coupling, exponentially weighting, and altering the acute/chronic time periods [161–163]. Regardless of the mathematical alterations to the ACWR, the result provides a ratio which, research shows, corresponds well with injury risk [161, 164].

A ratio between 0.8 and 1.3 was dubbed the 'sweet spot' in which athletes had the lowest risk of injury occurrence [147]. Loads greater than 1.3 (overloading) and loads less than 0.8 (underloading) were associated with higher rates of injury (Figure 6.4). Thus, a quantifiable way of keeping athletes at a reduced risk of injury from loading errors was created. This has significant practical use for the practitioner, allowing timely viewing of current athlete outputs and, accordingly, weekly load alteration to prevent sustained under or over loading.

However, due to the time and cost involved with athlete monitoring, there seems to be little application of ACWR in soccer academies. This is also apparent in research into ACWR, having almost exclusively been conducted in adult populations, with only one paper specifically focused on academy soccer [148]. It is also known that age plays a significant factor in an athlete's ability to cope with workload [165]; therefore, there is a suggestion that youths may have a different 'sweet spot' ratio compared to adult populations.

Conversely, recent research has disputed the accuracy and practicality of the ACWR to determine injury risk within sport [166]. Specifically, it has been found that the use of ACWR using a 4-week average caused spurious mathematical coupling increasing the likelihood of false positives of athletes being flagged as a risk of injury [167]. Additionally, a literature review suggests it was an ambiguous metric that is not consistent or have a unidirectional relationship with injury risk [166]. In essence, it is important for practitioners to note that the injury risk is multifactorial, something the ACWR does not take into consideration. The ACWR is purely a ratio between two numbers, the chronic, and the acute load of an individual. For example, we have two athletes to consider: Athlete A with a chronic load of 25 m and athlete B with 300 m of sprint distance (25.2 km). In their acute week, athlete, A is exposed to 50 m across seven sessions and

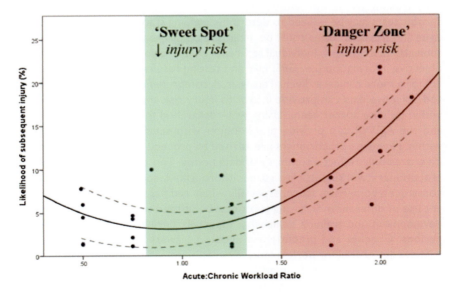

Figure 6.4 The sweet spot. Shows reduction in injury risk when the A:C workload ratio is between 0.8 and 1.3 (Adapted from Blanch and Gabbett [147]).

athlete B to 600 m in one session. Both athletes will have a weekly ACWR of 200% and both suggested to be exposed to high risk of injury in the proceeding 3-week period according to the previous research in ACWR. Here we can see that reliance on purely the ACWR inappropriate management of load can easily occur. As previously suggested [166], there is far more context that we need to understand than one arbitrary ACWR. Rather than using the ACWR as a 'gospel' for injury likelihood, it should be used within the practitioner's wheelhouse of tools to understand load management of athletes. It is vital that practitioners considering internal risk factors as well as the load itself when understanding injury risk. Furthermore, modifiable risk factors such as aerobic capacity, athletes chronic loads, and strength capacity have all been found to reduce the risk of load-related injury risks and deal with fluctuations in load greater than when they are at high levels [168].

Conclusion

During an elite soccer training routine in a high-performance environment, coaches and sport scientists must manipulate training load within a very congested competitive schedule. When international competitions are played, the time for training is reduced and the time available should be used to maximize the training stimulus. In this highly stressful environment, performance and health management should be a process in which different stakeholders have to be involved (i.e. coaches, sport scientists, physicians, physiotherapists, and players). Practitioners could manage simple tests such as CMJ several times over the season (e.g. weekly and/or monthly bases); additionally, other supplemental tests (i.e. single-leg tests, SJ, or DJ) could be scheduled in some key-periods across the season. This may help to assess individual variations in neuromuscular training status and acute/chronic readiness. Similarly, several submaximal aerobic tests may be utilized to determine training status across the season. Fatigue and wellness scales could be proposed on daily bases for a more individual subjective assessment. Individual self-report information may be integrated with objective information (i.e. GPS, HR, and testing results) and used by practitioners for a more clinical individual analysis. A comprehensive analysis of subjective and objective data can provide insight to injury risk and performance readiness within an elite soccer team. Using well-researched methods, such as the TSB and the ACWR can provide practitioners with specific parameters to work within. However, practitioners are advised to proceed with caution as composite scores only reflect a summary of data points. Therefore, it is suggested that practitioners working in elite soccer thoroughly inspect raw data points that construct a composite score, especially when 'red flags' are resulted. A consistent use of different monitoring tools may be utilized to maximize performance development and training availability, especially during very congested fixture periods. Coaches and practitioners should be aware that individual objective analyses are crucial for performance development and to possibly avoid injuries in high-performance environments.

References

1 Halson, S.L., *Monitoring training load to understand fatigue in athletes.* Sports Medicine, 2014. **44**(S2): p. S139–147.
2 Coutts, A., S. Crowcroft, and T. Kempton, *Developing athlete monitoring systems: Theoretical basis and practical applications*, in Sport, recovery, and performance: Interdisciplinary insights. 2017, Routledge: London. p. 19–32.
3 Ryan, S., et al., *Training monitoring in professional Australian football: Theoretical basis and recommendations for coaches and scientists.* Science and Medicine in Football, 2019. **4**(1): p. 52–58.
4 West, S.W., et al., *More than a metric: How training load is used in elite sport for athlete management.* International Journal of Sports Medicine, 2021. **42**(4): p. 300–306.
5 Thornton, H.R., et al., *Developing athlete monitoring systems in team sports: Data analysis and visualization.* International Journal of Sports Physiology and Performance, 2019. **14**(6): p. 698–705.
6 French, D.N. and L. Torres Ronda, *National strength & conditioning association's essential of sport science.* 2021, Champaign, IL: Human Kinetics.
7 Bourdon, P.C., et al., *Monitoring athlete training loads: Consensus statement.* International Journal of Sports Physiology and Performance, 2017. **12**(s2): p. S2–161-S2–170.
8 Schalock, R.L., M. Verdugo, and T. Lee, *A systematic approach to an organization's sustainability.* Evaluation and Program Planning, 2016. **56**: p. 56–63.
9 Matveev, L.P. and A.P. Zdornyj, *Fundamentals of sports training.* 1981, Moscow: Progress Publishers.
10 Halson, S.L. and A.E. Jeukendrup, *Does overtraining exist? An analysis of overreaching and overtraining research.* Sports Medicine, 2004. **34**(14): p. 967–981.
11 Selye, H., *The stress of life.* 1956: McGraw-Hill.
12 Bompa, T.O., *Theory and methodology of training.* 1983, Dubuque, IA: Kendall/Hunt, p. 91–97.
13 Harre, D., *Principles of sports training: Introduction to the theory and methods of training.* 1982: Imported Publication.
14 Kukushkin, G., *The system of physical education in the USSR.* 1983, Moscow: Raduga Publishers.
15 Stone, M.H., M. Stone, and W.A. Sands, *Principles and practice of resistance training.* 2007, Champaign: Human Kinetics.
16 Verkhoshansky, Y., *Principles of planning speed/strength training program in track athletes.* 1979, Moscow: Legaya Athleticka. **8**: p. 8–10.
17 Verkhoshansky, Y., *Fundamentals of special strength-training in sport.* 1986: Sportivny Press.
18 Verkhoshansky, Y. and M.C. Siff, *Supertraining.* 6 ed. 2009, Rome: Verkhoshansky SSTM. 592.
19 Fry, R.W., A.R. Morton, and D. Keast, *Periodisation of training stress--a review.* Canadian Journal of Sport Sciences, 1992. **17**(3): p. 234–240.
20 Kuipers, H. and H.A. Keizer, *Overtraining in elite athletes. Review and directions for the future.* Sports Medicine, 1988. **6**(2): p. 79–92.
21 Viru, A., *The mechanism of training effects: a hypothesis.* International Journal of Sports Medicine, 1984. **5**(5): p. 219–27.
22 Rowbottom, D., D. Keast, and A. Morton, *Monitoring and preventing of overreaching and overtraining in endurance athletes.* Overtraining Sport, 1998: p. 47–66.
23 Snyder, A.C., et al., *Overtraining following intensified training with normal muscle glycogen.* Medicine & Science in Sports & Exercise, 1995. **27**(7): p. 1063–1070.
24 Chiu, L.Z. and J.L. Barnes, *The fitness-fatigue model revisited: Implications for planning short-and long-term training.* Strength & Conditioning Journal, 2003. **25**(6): p. 42–51.
25 Plisk, S.S. and M.H. Stone, *Periodization strategies.* Strength & Conditioning Journal, 2003. **25**(6): p. 19–37.

26. Kalkhoven, J.T., et al., *Training load and injury: Causal pathways and future directions.* Sports Medicine, 2021. **51**(6): p. 1137–1150.
27. Impellizzeri, F.M., S.M. Marcora, and A.J. Coutts, *Internal and external training load: 15 Years on.* International Journal of Sports Physiology and Performance, 2019. **14**(2): p. 270–273.
28. Drew, M.K. and C.F. Finch, *The relationship between training load and injury, illness and soreness: A systematic and literature review.* Sports Medicine, 2016. **46**(6): p. 861–883.
29. Schwellnus, M., et al., *How much is too much?(Part 2) International olympic committee consensus statement on load in sport and risk of illness.* British Journal of Sports Medicine, 2016. **50**(17): p. 1043–1052.
30. Soligard, T., et al., *How much is too much?(Part 1) International olympic committee consensus statement on load in sport and risk of injury.* British Journal of Sports Medicine, 2016. **50**(17): p. 1030–1041.
31. Impellizzeri, F.M., E. Rampinini, and S.M. Marcora, *Physiological assessment of aerobic training in soccer.* Journal of Sports Sciences, 2005. **23**(6): p. 583–592.
32. Riboli, A., et al., *Can small-sided games assess the training-induced aerobic adaptations in elite football players?* The Journal of Sports Medicine and Physical Fitness, 2021. Online ahead of print.
33. Coyne, J.O., et al., *The current state of subjective training load monitoring—a practical perspective and call to action.* Sports Medicine-Open, 2018. **4**(1): p. 1–10.
34. Rogalski, B., et al., *Training and game loads and injury risk in elite Australian footballers.* Journal of Science and Medicine in Sport, 2013. **16**(6): p. 499–503.
35. Brink, M.S., et al., *Monitoring stress and recovery: New insights for the prevention of injuries and illnesses in elite youth soccer players.* British Journal of Sports Medicine, 2010. **44**(11): p. 809–815.
36. Crang, Z.L., et al., *The validity and reliability of wearable microtechnology for intermittent team sports: A systematic review.* Sports Medicine, 2021. **51**(3): p. 549–565.
37. Bourdon, P.C., et al., *Monitoring athlete training loads: Consensus statement.* International Journal of Sports Physiology and Performance, 2017. **12**(Suppl 2): p. S2161–S2170.
38. Cardinale, M. and M.C. Varley, *Wearable training-monitoring technology: Applications, challenges, and opportunities.* International Journal of Sports Physiology and Performance, 2017. **12**(Suppl 2): p. S255–S262.
39. Coutts, A.J. and R. Duffield, *Validity and reliability of GPS devices for measuring movement demands of team sports.* Journal of Science and Medicine in Sport, 2010. **13**(1): p. 133–135.
40. Malone, J.J., et al., *Unpacking the black box: Applications and considerations for using GPS devices in sport.* International Journal of Sports Physiology and Performance, 2017. **12**(s2): p. S2–18–S2–26.
41. Lacome, M., B. Simpson, and M. Buchheit, *Monitoring training status with player-tracking technology. Still on the road to Rome. Part 2.* Aspetar Journal, 2018. **7**: p. 64–66.
42. Lacome, M., B. Simpson, and M. Buchheit, *2018 Monitoring training status with player-tracking technology. Still on the road to Rome. Part 1.* Aspetar Journal, 2018. **7**: p. 55–63.
43. Cormack, S. and A.J. Coutts, *Training load model*, in *National strength & conditioning association's essential of sport science*, D.N. French and L. Torres Ronda, Editors. 2021, Champaign, IL: Human Kinetics.p. 13–26.
44. Vellers, H.L., S.R. Kleeberger, and J.T. Lightfoot, *Inter-individual variation in adaptations to endurance and resistance exercise training: Genetic approaches towards understanding a complex phenotype.* Mammalian Genome, 2018. **29**(1–2): p. 48–62.
45. Smith, D.J., *A framework for understanding the training process leading to elite performance.* Sports Medicine, 2003. **33**(15): p. 1103–1126.
46. Bouchard, C., T. Rankinen, and J.A. Timmons, *Genomics and genetics in the biology of adaptation to exercise.* Comprehensive Physiology, 2011. **1**(3): p. 1603–1648.

47 Mann, T.N., R.P. Lamberts, and M.I. Lambert, *High responders and low responders: Factors associated with individual variation in response to standardized training.* Sports Medicine, 2014. **44**(8): p. 1113–1124.
48 Jeffries, A.C., et al., *Athlete-reported outcome measures for monitoring training responses: A systematic review of risk of bias and measurement property quality according to the COSMIN guidelines.* International Journal of Sports Physiology and Performance, 2020. **15**(9): p. 1–13.
49 Saw, A.E., et al., *Athlete self-report measures in research and practice: Considerations for the discerning reader and fastidious practitioner.* International Journal of Sports Physiology and Performance, 2017. **12**(Suppl 2): p. S2127–S2135.
50 Saw, A.E., L.C. Main, and P.B. Gastin, *Monitoring the athlete training response: Subjective self-reported measures trump commonly used objective measures: A systematic review.* British Journal of Sports Medicine, 2016. **50**(5): p. 281–291.
51 Taylor, J.L., et al., *Neural contributions to muscle fatigue: From the brain to the muscle and back again.* Medicine and Science in Sports and Exercise, 2016. **48**(11): p. 2294.
52 Enoka, R.M. and J. Duchateau, *Muscle fatigue: What, why and how it influences muscle function.* The Journal of Physiology, 2008. **586**(1): p. 11–23.
53 Enoka, R.M. and J. Duchateau, *Translating fatigue to human performance.* Medicine & Science in Sports & Exercise, 2016. **48**(11): p. 2228–2238.
54 Abbiss, C.R. and P.B. Laursen, *Models to explain fatigue during prolonged endurance cycling.* Sports Medicine, 2005. **35**(10): p. 865–898.
55 Marcora, S.M., *Do we really need a central governor to explain brain regulation of exercise performance?* European Journal of Applied Physiology, 2008. **104**(5): p. 929–931.
56 St Clair Gibson, A., J. Swart, and R. Tucker, *The interaction of psychological and physiological homeostatic drives and role of general control principles in the regulation of physiological systems, exercise and the fatigue process – The integrative governor theory.* European Journal of Sport Science, 2018. **18**(1): p. 25–36.
57 Strojnik, V. and P.V. Komi, *Fatigue after submaximal intensive stretch-shortening cycle exercise.* Medicine & Science in Sports & Exercise, 2000. **32**(7): p. 1314–1319.
58 Rowell, A.E., et al., *Identification of sensitive measures of recovery after external load from football match play.* International Journal of Sports Physiology and Performance, 2017. **12**(7): p. 969–976.
59 Thorpe, R.T., et al., *Monitoring fatigue status in elite team-sport athletes: Implications for practice.* International Journal of Sports Physiology and Performance, 2017. **12**(Suppl 2): p. S227–S234.
60 Almulla, J., A. Takiddin, and M. Househ, *The use of technology in tracking soccer players' health performance: A scoping review.* BMC Medical Informatics and Decision Making, 2020. **20**(1): p. 1–10.
61 Ravé, G., et al., *How to use global positioning systems (GPS) data to monitor training load in the 'real world' of elite soccer.* Frontiers in Physiology, 2020. **11**: p. 944.
62 Kupperman, N. and J. Hertel, *Global positioning system–derived workload metrics and injury risk in team-based field sports: A systematic review.* Journal of Athletic Training, 2020. **55**(9): p. 931–943.
63 Riboli, A., et al., *Comparison between continuous and discontinuous incremental treadmill test to assess velocity at VO2max.* Journal of Sports Medicine and Physical Fitness, **57**(9): p. 1119–1125.
64 Riboli, A., et al., *Testing protocol affects the velocity at VO2max in semi-professional soccer players.* Research in Sports Medicine, 2021. **30**(2): p. 1–11.
65 Riboli, A., et al., *Training status affects between-protocols differences in the assessment of maximal aerobic velocity* European Journal of Applied Physiology, 2021. **121**(11): p. 3083–3093. Epub ahead of print.
66 Scott, M.T., T.J. Scott, and V.G. Kelly, *The validity and reliability of global positioning systems in team sport: A brief review.* Journal of Strength and Conditioning Research, 2016. **30**(5): p. 1470–1490.

67 McDermott, V., *Validity and reliability*. Encyclopedia of communication theory. Littlejohn, S. W., & Foss, K. A. (Eds.), 2009, Thousand Oaks, CA: Sage Publication, Inc.
68 Hopkins, W.G., *Measures of reliability in sports medicine and science*. Sports Medicine, 2000. **30**(1): p. 1–15.
69 Buchheit, M., et al., *Integrating different tracking systems in football: Multiple camera semi-automatic system, local position measurement and GPS technologies*. Journal of Sports Sciences, 2014. **32**(20): p. 1844–1857.
70 Riboli, A., et al., *Area per player in small-sided games to replicate the external load and estimated physiological match demands in elite soccer players*. PLoS One, 2020. **15**(9): p. e0229194.
71 Schuster, J., D. Bove, and D. Little, *Jumping towards best-practice: Recommendations for effective use of force plate testing in the NBA*. Sport Performance & Science Reports, 2020. **97 vl**. p. 1–7.
72 Paul, D.J. and G.P. Nassis, *Testing strength and power in soccer players: The application of conventional and traditional methods of assessment*. Journal of Strength and Conditioning Research, 2015. **29**(6): p. 1748–1758.
73 Schuster, J., D. Bove, and D. Little, *Jumping towards best-practice: Recommendations for effective use of force plate testing in the NBA*. Sport Performance & Science Reports, 2019. **97**(v1).
74 Lohse, K.R., et al., *Systematic review of the use of 'magnitude-based inference' in sports science and medicine*. PLoS One, 2020. **15**(6): p. e0235318.
75 Impellizzeri, F.M., T. Meyer, and S. Wagenpfeil, *Statistical considerations (or recommendations) for publishing in science and medicine in football*. Science and Medicine in Football, 2019. **3**: p. 1–2.
76 McGuigan, M.R., et al., *Eccentric utilization ratio: Effect of sport and phase of training*. The Journal of Strength & Conditioning Research, 2006. **20**(4): p. 992–995.
77 Achten, J. and A.E. Jeukendrup, *Heart rate monitoring: Applications and limitations*. Sports Medicine, 2003. **33**(7): p. 517–538.
78 Gilman, M.B., *The use of heart rate to monitor the intensity of endurance training*. Sports Medicine, 1996. **21**(2): p. 73–79.
79 Esposito, F., et al., *Validity of heart rate as an indicator of aerobic demand during soccer activities in amateur soccer players*. European Journal of Applied Physiology, 2004. **93**(1–2): p. 167–172.
80 Borresen, J. and M.I. Lambert, *The quantification of training load, the training response and the effect on performance*. Medicine, 2009. **39**(9): p. 779–795.
81 Robinson, D.M., et al., *Training intensity of elite male distance runners*. Medicine & Science in Sports & Exercise, 1991. **23**(9): p. 1078–1082.
82 Foster, C., et al., *Athletic performance in relation to training load*. Wisconsin Medical Journal, 1996. **95**(6): p. 370–374.
83 Green, J.M., et al., *RPE association with lactate and heart rate during high-intensity interval cycling*. Medicine & Science in Sports & Exercise, 2006. **38**(1): p. 167–172.
84 Foster, C., *Monitoring training in athletes with reference to overtraining syndrome*. Medicine & Science in Sports & Exercise, 1998. **30**(7): p. 1164–1168.
85 Foster, C., et al., *A new approach to monitoring exercise training*. Journal of Strength and Conditioning Research, 2001. **15**(1): p. 109–115.
86 Edwards, S., *The heart rate monitor book*. 1993: Fleet feet Press.
87 Impellizzeri, F.M., et al., *Use of RPE-based training load in soccer*. Medicine & Science in Sports & Exercise, 2004. **36**(6): p. 1042–1047.
88 McLaren, S.J., et al., *The sensitivity of differential ratings of perceived exertion as measures of internal load*. International Journal of Sports Physiology and Performance, 2016. **11**(3): p. 404–406.
89 Williams, J.G. and R.G. Eston, *Determination of the intensity dimension in vigorous exercise programmes with particular reference to the use of the rating of perceived exertion*. Medicine, 1989. **8**(3): p. 177–189.
90 Akenhead, R. and G.P. Nassis, *Training load and player monitoring in high-level football: Current practice and perceptions*. International Journal of Sports Physiology and Performance, 2016. **11**(5): p. 587–593.

91 Taylor, K., et al., *Fatigue monitoring in high performance sport: A survey of current trends.* Journal of Strength and Conditioning Research, 2012. **20**(1): p. 12–23.
92 Weston, M., *Training load monitoring in elite English soccer: A comparison of practices and perceptions between coaches and practitioners.* Science and Medicine in Football, 2018. **2**(3): p. 216–224.
93 Saw, A.E., L.C. Main, and P.B. Gastin, *Monitoring athletes through self-report: Factors influencing implementation.* Journal of Sports Science & Medicine, 2015. **14**(1): p. 137.
94 Duignan, C., et al., *Single-item self-report measures of team-sport athlete wellbeing and their relationship with training load: A systematic review.* Journal of Athletic Training, 2020. **55**(9): p. 944–953.
95 Otero-Esquina, C., et al., *Is strength-training frequency a key factor to develop performance adaptations in young elite soccer players?* European Journal of Sport Science, 2017. **17**(10): p. 1241–1251.
96 Clemente, F.M., et al., *Seasonal player wellness and its longitudinal association with internal training load: Study in elite volleyball.* Journal of Sports Medicine and Physical Fitness, 2019. **59**(3): p. 345–351.
97 Sampson, J.A., et al., *Subjective wellness, acute: Chronic workloads, and injury risk in college football.* Journal of Strength and Conditioning Research, 2019. **33**(12): p. 3367–3373.
98 Wellman, A.D., et al., *Perceived wellness associated with practice and competition in national collegiate athletic association division i football players.* Journal of Strength and Conditioning Research, 2019. **33**(1): p. 112–124.
99 Fessi, M.S., et al., *Changes of the psychophysical state and feeling of wellness of professional soccer players during pre-season and in-season periods.* Research in Sports Medicine, 2016. **24**(4): p. 375–386.
100 Rabbani, A., et al., *Monitoring collegiate soccer players during a congested match schedule: Heart rate variability versus subjective wellness measures.* Physiology & Behavior, 2018. **194**: p. 527–531.
101 Buchheit, M., et al., *Monitoring fitness, fatigue and running performance during a pre-season training camp in elite football players.* Journal of Science and Medicine in Sport, 2013. **16**(6): p. 550–555.
102 Mara, J.K., et al., *Periodization and physical performance in elite female soccer players.* International Journal of Sports Physiology and Performance, 2015. **10**(5): p. 664–669.
103 Haller, N., et al., *Circulating, cell-free dna for monitoring player load in professional football.* International Journal of Sports Physiology and Performance, 2019. **14**(6): p. 718–726.
104 Johnston, R.D., et al., *The distribution of match activities relative to the maximal mean intensities in professional rugby league and australian football.* Journal of Strength and Conditioning Research, 2020. **Epub ahead of print**.
105 Martin-Garcia, A., et al., *Quantification of a professional football team's external load using a microcycle structure.* Journal of Strength and Conditioning Research, 2018. **32**(12): p. 3511–3518.
106 Riboli, A., et al., *Effect of formation, ball in play and ball possession on peak demands in elite soccer.* Biology of Sport, 2021. **38**(2): p. 195–205.
107 Lacome, M., et al., *Small-sided games in elite soccer: Does one size fit all?* International Journal of Sports Physiology and Performance, 2018. **13**(5): p. 568–576.
108 Riboli, A., et al., *Training elite youth soccer players: Area per player in small-sided games to replivcate the match demands.* Biology of Sport, 2022. **39**(3): p. 579–598.
109 Lago-Peñas, C., E. Rey, and J. Lago-Ballesteros, *The influence of effective playing time on physical demands of elite soccer players.* The Open Sports Sciences Journal, 2012. **5**: p. 188–192.
110 Siegle, M. and M. Lames, *Game interruptions in elite soccer.* Journal of Sports Sciences, 2012. **30**(7): p. 619–624.
111 Bradley, P.S. and T.D. Noakes, *Match running performance fluctuations in elite soccer: Indicative of fatigue, pacing or situational influences?* Journal of Sports Sciences, 2013. **31**(15): p. 1627–1638.

112 Oliva-Lozano, J.M., et al., *Worst case scenario match analysis and contextual variables in professional soccer players: A longitudinal study.* Biology of Sport, 2020. **37**(4): p. 429–436.
113 Gomez-Carmona, C.D., et al., *Accelerometry as a method for external workload monitoring in invasion team sports. A systematic review.* PLoS One, 2020. **15**(8): p. e0236643.
114 Di Salvo, V., et al., *Performance characteristics according to playing position in elite soccer.* International Journal of Sports Medicine, 2007. **28**(3): p. 222–227.
115 Bradley, P.S., et al., *High-intensity activity profiles of elite soccer players at different performance levels.* Journal of Strength and Conditioning Research, 2010. **24**(9): p. 2343–2351.
116 Casamichana, D., et al., *The most demanding passages of play in football competition: A comparison between halves.* Biology of Sport, 2019. **36**(3): p. 233–240.
117 Cunningham, D.J., et al., *Assessing worst case scenarios in movement demands derived from global positioning systems during international rugby union matches: Rolling averages versus fixed length epochs.* PLoS One, 2018. **13**(4): p. e0195197.
118 Ferraday, K., et al., *A comparison of rolling averages versus discrete time epochs for assessing the worst-case scenario locomotor demands of professional soccer match-play.* Journal of Science and Medicine in Sport, 2020. **23**(8): p. 764–769.
119 Calder, A. and T. Gabbett, *Influence of tactical formation on average and peak demands of elite soccer match-play.* International Journal of Strength and Conditioning, 2022. **2**(1): p. 1–10.
120 Varley, M.C., G.P. Elias, and R.J. Aughey, *Current match-analysis techniques' underestimation of intense periods of high-velocity running.* International Journal of Sports Physiology and Performance, 2012. **7**(2): p. 183–185.
121 Delaney, J.A., et al., *Peak running intensity of international rugby: Implications for training prescription.* International Journal of Sports Physiology and Performance, 2017. **12**(8): p. 1039–1045.
122 Oliva-Lozano, J.M., et al., *Differences in worst-case scenarios calculated by fixed length and rolling average methods in professional soccer match-play.* Biology of Sport, 2021. **38**(3): p. 325–331.
123 Riboli, A., F. Esposito, and G. Coratella, *The distribution of match activities relative to the maximal intensities in elite soccer players: Implications for practice.* Research in Sports Medicine, 2021: **30**(5): p. 1–12.
124 Van den Tillaar, R., J.A. Solheim, and J. Bencke, *Comparison of hamstring muscle activation during high-speed running and various hamstring strengthening exercises.* International Journal of Sports Physical Therapy, 2017. **12**(5): p. 718–727.
125 Beato, M., B. Drust, and A.D. Iacono, *Implementing high-speed running and sprinting training in professional soccer.* International Journal of Sports Medicine, 2021. **42**(4): p. 295–299.
126 Young, D., et al., *The match-play activity cycles in elite U17, U21 and senior hurling competitive games.*, Sport Sciences for Health, 2019. 15(2): p. 351–359.
127 Martin-Garcia, A., et al., *Positional demands for various-sided games with goalkeepers according to the most demanding passages of match play in football.* Biology of Sport, 2019. **36**(2): p. 171–180.
128 Wass, J., et al., *A comparison of the match demands using ball-in-play vs. whole match data in elite male youth soccer players.* Science and Medicine in Football, 2019. **9**(6): p. 2–6.
129 Riboli, A., F. Esposito, and G. Coratella, *Small-sided games in elite football: Practical solutions to replicate the 4-min match-derived maximal intensities.* Journal of Strength and Conditioning Research, Ahead of print.
130 Riboli, A., et al., *Effect of formation, ball in play and ball possession on peak demands in elite soccer.* Biology of Sport, 2021. **38**: p. 195–205.
131 Lagos-Penas, C., E. Rey, and J. Lago-Ballesteros, *The influence of effective playing time on physical demands of elite soccer players.* Open Sports Sciences Journal, 2012. **5**: p. 188–192.

132 Young, D., et al., *The match-play activity cycles in elite U17, U21 and senior hurling competitive games*. Sport Sciences for Health, 2019. **15**: p. 351–359.
133 Wass, J., et al., *A comparison of match demands using ball-in-play vs. whole match data in elite male youth soccer players*. Science and Medicine in Football, 2020. **4**(2): p. 142–147.
134 Johnston, R.D., et al., *The distribution of match activities relative to the maximal mean intensities in professional rugby league and australian football*. Journal of Strength and Conditioning Research, 2020. **36**(5): p. 1360–1366.
135 Schneider, C., et al., *Heart rate monitoring in team sports-a conceptual framework for contextualizing heart rate measures for training and recovery prescription*. Frontiers in Physiology, 2018. **9**:p. 639.
136 Buchheit, M., *Monitoring training status with HR measures: Do all roads lead to Rome?* Frontiers in Physiology, 2014. **5**: p. 73.
137 Aubert, A.E., B. Seps, and F. Beckers, *Heart rate variability in athletes*. Sports Medicine, 2003. **33**(12): p. 889–919.
138 Alexandre, D., et al., *Heart rate monitoring in soccer: Interest and limits during competitive match play and training, practical application*. Journal of Strength and Conditioning Research, 2012. **26**(10): p. 2890–2906.
139 Michael, S., K.S. Graham, and G.M.O. Davis, *Cardiac autonomic responses during exercise and post-exercise recovery using heart rate variability and systolic time intervals-a review*. Frontiers in Physiology, 2017. **8**(301): p. 301.
140 Bellenger, C.R., et al., *Monitoring athletic training status through autonomic heart rate regulation: A systematic review and meta-analysis*. Medicine, 2016. **46**(10): p. 1461–1486.
141 Plews, D.J., et al., *Monitoring training with heart rate-variability: How much compliance is needed for valid assessment?* International Journal of Sports Physiology and Performance, 2014. **9**(5): p. 783–790.
142 Kiviniemi, A.M., et al., *Daily exercise prescription on the basis of HR variability among men and women*. Medicine & Science in Sports & Exercise, 2010. **42**(7): p. 1355–1363.
143 Stanley, J., J.M. Peake, and M. Buchheit, *Cardiac parasympathetic reactivation following exercise: Implications for training prescription*. Sports Medicine, 2013. **43**(12): p. 1259–1277.
144 Force, T., *Heart rate variability: Standards of measurement, physiological interpretation and clinical use. Task force of the european society of cardiology and the north american society of pacing and electrophysiology*. Circulation, 1996. **93**(5): p. 1043–1065.
145 Windt, J. and T.J. Gabbett, *The workload—injury aetiology model*. 2016: BMJ Publishing Group Ltd and British Association of Sport and Exercise Medicine.
146 Kenttä, G. and P. Hassmén, *Overtraining and recovery*. Sports Medicine, 1998. **26**(1): p. 1–16.
147 Blanch, P. and T.J. Gabbett, *Has the athlete trained enough to return to play safely? The acute: Chronic workload ratio permits clinicians to quantify a player's risk of subsequent injury*. British Journal of Sports Medicine, 2016. **50**(8): p. 471–475.
148 Bowen, L., et al., *Accumulated workloads and the acute: Chronic workload ratio relate to injury risk in elite youth football players*. British Journal of Sports Medicine, 2016: **51**(5): p. 452–459.
149 McCall, A., et al., *Injury risk factors, screening tests and preventative strategies: A systematic review of the evidence that underpins the perceptions and practices of 44 football (soccer) teams from various premier leagues*. British Journal of Sports Medicine, 2015. **49**(9): p. 583–589.
150 Gabbett, T.J. and D.G. Jenkins, *Relationship between training load and injury in professional rugby league players*. Journal of Science and Medicine in Sport, 2011. **14**(3): p. 204–209.
151 Gabbett, T.J., *Debunking the myths about training load, injury and performance: Empirical evidence, hot topics and recommendations for practitioners*. British Journal of Sports Medicine, 2020. **54**(1): p. 58–66.

152 Hulin, B.T., et al., *Low chronic workload and the acute: Chronic workload ratio are more predictive of injury than between-match recovery time: A two-season prospective cohort study in elite rugby league players.* British Journal of Sports Medicine, 2016. **50**(16): p. 1008–1012.
153 Malone, S., et al., *High chronic training loads and exposure to bouts of maximal velocity running reduce injury risk in elite Gaelic football.* Journal of Science and Medicine in Sport, 2017. **20**(3): p. 250–254.
154 Gabbett, T.J., *The training-injury prevention paradox: Should athletes be training smarter and harder?* British Journal of Sports Medicine, 2016. **50**(5): p. 273–280.
155 Orchard, J.W., et al., *Cricket fast bowling workload patterns as risk factors for tendon, muscle, bone and joint injuries.* British Journal of Sports Medicine, 2015. **49**(16): p. 1064–1068.
156 Selye, H., *The general adaptation syndrome and the diseases of adaptation.* The Journal of Clinical Endocrinology, 1946. **6**(2): p. 117–230.
157 Hulin, B.T., et al., *Spikes in acute workload are associated with increased injury risk in elite cricket fast bowlers.* British Journal of Sports Medicine, 2013. **48**(8): p. 708–712.
158 Calvert, T.W., et al., *A systems model of the effects of training on physical performance.* IEEE Transactions on Systems, Man, and Cybernetics, 1976. **2**: p. 94–102.
159 Morton, R.H., J.R. Fitz-Clarke, and E.W. Banister, *Modeling human performance in running.* Journal of Applied Physiology, 1990. **69**(3): p. 1171–1177.
160 Morton, R., *Modelling training and overtraining.* Journal of Sports Sciences, 1997. **15**(3): p. 335–340.
161 Griffin, A., et al., *The association between the acute: Chronic workload ratio and injury and its application in team sports: A systematic review.* Sports Medicine, 2020. **50**(3): p. 561–580.
162 Murray, N.B., et al., *Calculating acute: Chronic workload ratios using exponentially weighted moving averages provides a more sensitive indicator of injury likelihood than rolling averages.* British Journal of Sports Medicine, 2016. **51**(9): p. 749–754.
163 Windt, J. and T.J. Gabbett, *Is it all for naught? What does mathematical coupling mean for acute: Chronic workload ratios?* 2019: BMJ Publishing Group Ltd and British Association of Sport and Exercise Medicine. p. 988–990.
164 Blanch, P. and T.J. Gabbett, *Has the athlete trained enough to return to play safely? The acute: Chronic workload ratio permits clinicians to quantify a player's risk of subsequent injury.* British Journal of Sports Medicine, 2015. **50**(8): p. 471–475.
165 Gabbett, T.J. and R. Whiteley, *Two training-load paradoxes: Can we work harder and smarter, can physical preparation and medical be teammates?* International Journal of Sports Physiology and Performance, 2017. **12**(Suppl. 2): p. 50–54.
166 Impellizzeri, F.M., et al., *Acute: Chronic workload ratio: Conceptual issues and fundamental pitfalls.* International Journal of Sports Physiology and Performance, 2020. **15**(6): p. 907–913.
167 Lolli, L., et al., *Mathematical coupling causes spurious correlation within the conventional acute-to-chronic workload ratio calculations.* British Journal of Sports Medicine, 2019. **53**(15): p. 921–922.
168 Andrade, R., et al., *Is the acute: Chronic workload ratio (acwr) associated with risk of time-loss injury in professional team sports? a systematic review of methodology, variables and injury risk in practical situations.* Sports Medicine, 2020. **50**(9): p. 1613–1635.
169 Charlton P, Drew MK. *Can We Think About Training Loads Differently?.* Canberra, Australia: Australian Institute of Sport, 2015.

7 Wearable technology

Joshua Rice, Damian Kovacevic, Alex Calder and Joel Carter

Wearable technology overview

In order to accurately assess and analyse the impact of both training and matches across the entirety of a macrocycle, the variables within training and match load must be thoroughly observed. Over the past 15–20 years, new technology has been developed in the form of sport specific global positioning system (GPS), designed with the aim of performing such tasks. The introduction of these GPS devices, in the 2000s, dramatically increased the provision of data available to practitioners regarding players' training and match activity. Commonly described as 'sports bras' by the onlooking public, these vests/performance garments in fact house the technology, allowing practitioners to monitor and track players performance. The performance garment, supplied by the GPS manufacturer, is designed to stabilise the device between the player's shoulder blades to minimise the amount of noise associated with various movement patterns. Each GPS device is designed to acquire performance variables such as distance the player has run, the intensity/speed of the run, the speed, the number of sprints, accelerations and decelerations which have occurred along with integrating with heart rate (HR) collection devices. These data points are often collated together to form what is widely known in the scientific literature as objective training load (TL) [1, 2].

Training load, by definition, is an input variable that is manipulated to elicit a desired training response [3]. In addition, it has also been well-researched that individuals respond to this same training load and physical exercise in different ways [4]. As such, successful training programmes require the systematic manipulation of key training load variables related to the duration, frequency and intensity of the training stimulus [5]. In order to achieve optimal physiological adaptation, training sessions need to be programmed and adjusted to meet the requirements of individual athletes [6]. To achieve the required training load and training adaptations, the use of wearable technology such as GPS and HR is commonplace within the elite soccer environment [7]. Although not imperative due to some practitioners operating within clubs with lesser budgets (see Chapter 1), where available, the use of GPS is extremely advantageous in guiding the prescription and monitoring of the overall training load/response. GPS

DOI: 10.4324/9781003200420-7

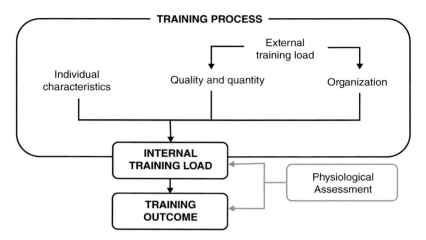

Figure 7.1 The training outcome is the consequence of the internal training load determined by (1) individual characteristics, such as genetic factors and previous training experience, and (2) the quality, quantity and organisation of the external training load (Extracted from Impellizzeri et al. [3]).

examines the external load, in conjunction with HR monitors that measure the internal response to such load (Figure 7.1).

The external aspect of training load refers to the specific training prescribed by coaches and practitioners, such as the number of sets/reps of a drill. The internal training load refers to the physiological stress that is imposed on the player (see Chapter 6 for more detail). As such, it is this stress (internal load) imposed on the athlete that stimulates the training-induced adaptations produced from the exercise [8, 9]. It has been noted that practitioners' most frequent methods to monitor these changes were the aforementioned GPS and HR monitors [10].

Validity and reliability

Player-tracking technology is an ever-evolving process which is continually developing due to advancements in microprocessors, software, and hardware. As a result, researchers continue to conduct validity and reliability studies as each device is updated from suppliers [11–13]. However, due to the time publications take to be processed and published, GPS devices are utilised within soccer before essential information on precision of measurement is available.

The use of methods to quantify elite soccer training has helped understand and quantify the following: external training load in the context of periodisation across the training week [14, 15]; a link between high-speed running (HSR) and injury risk [16]; and dose–response relations between internal load and fitness changes [17–19] (Figure 7.2). It appears the improvement in understanding

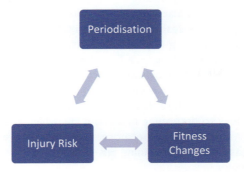

Figure 7.2 Factors that can be quantified by wearable technology in elite soccer.

surrounding training load has allowed for increased performance and decreased injury risk of soccer players [20, 21]. Quantifying the external and internal loads objectively and subjectively provides the practitioner with crucial information on the individual response to each soccer training session, indicating the need for individualised training programmes to be developed [22]. In response to both the volume and periodisation of these training strategies, the body adapts on a cellular and tissue level. As such, monitoring external loads provides an objective measure to provide the consequential internal load, in turn, predicting adaptation.

Unlike many linear-based sports, such as running and cycling, soccer's multi-directional nature reduces the likelihood that players receive individual specific training loads if not monitored closely [23]. As a result, GPS-and HR-based technologies have been widely implemented to attempt to quantify the training and match load accurately [24–26]. Elite soccer teams have extensively used GPS tracking devices to provide objective measures of external TL. Therefore, the importance of the GPS devices to be both reliable and valid is clear for practitioners working within soccer [11, 12, 25, 27–29].

Heart rate monitoring

Prior to the use of GPS, the primary technology used to quantify training was via the use of HR monitors. HR monitors have been commonplace in soccer for the past 20 years [30]. The development of this technology, concurrently to GPS, has allowed for the external and internal load stressed upon the body as a result of training to be monitored. The internal response to a given external stimulus can be influenced by factors such as genetic background and previous training experience [22]. These responses have allowed for an understanding and discrimination between different training drills based on pitch dimensions [31] and technical/tactical conditions [32, 33] implemented in training. Team HR systems are predominantly employed to monitor both the total cardiovascular exertion in the session and the responses to individual drills during the training bout.

To monitor the internal response of training, HR monitors are used to quantify the cardiovascular strain placed on an individual in a response to a given external TL [34]. Despite its widespread use in sport, there are several limitations associated with HR monitoring in sports such as soccer [35]. It has been suggested that graded exercise testing (GXT) is the gold standard for measuring an individual's maximum HR [36]. However, practicality has been used to question whether GXT is appropriate, or even feasible, in team-settings, and alongside budgetary constraints. Therefore, there is yet to be a consensus as to the gold standard methodology to determine maximum HR which is used to create HR zones for training monitoring. Furthermore, practitioners are currently reliant on proxy field measures in determining HR variables, due to the ease of use, and overall practicality.

The evaluation of training impulse (TRIMP) has been applied by practitioners for decades [37, 38]. TRIMP is a composite score, attempting to integrate multiple components, which allows practitioners to periodise training loads using one variable. Originally identified as the product of mean HR (intensity) and time-exercising (duration), TRIMP has been used to help identify TL in intermittent team sports [39]. However, the limitations of TRIMP have challenged researchers to investigate how zones can be applied to HR data, in order to better understand the demands of high-intensity exercise training [38]. One of the original HR zone summations illustrated the zones as: zone 1: 50%–60%, zone 2: 60%–70%, zone 3: 70%–80%, zone 4: 80%–90%, and zone 5: 90%–100% of maximal HR [40]. Researchers and practitioners have since tried to examine the most valid approach to identifying HR data and TL. A variety of calculations have been applied to determine HR zones, such as incorporating the ventilatory threshold and respiratory-compensation points [41]. However, the practicality of obtaining these markers is questioned, calling for a feasible way of identifying valid and reliable HR zones. Incorporating the RPE-scale (see *Chapter 6*) with the above-listed HR zones, also known as the RPE-method, has shown to be a valid and reliable measure of exercise intensity [38]. Furthermore, the application of use for this method in elite soccer is considered an accurate indicator of global internal TL [42]. However, in order to establish valid HR zones, practitioners must collect each player's individual maximum HR. In elite soccer, there are many different approaches in establishing maximum HRs in the team setting. It has been suggested that field-based testing, such as the 30-15 intermittent test or YoYo test (or derivatives of), may be beneficial in collecting maximum HRs [43–45].

Global Positioning System

Soccer teams have extensively used GPS tracking devices to provide objective measures of external training loads [46, 47]. Therefore, the importance of the GPS devices to be both reliable and valid is clear for practitioners working within elite soccer. For example, poor validity in GPS devices have been previously observed when measuring high-velocity decelerations (>5 $m·s^{-2}$) [25]. Therefore, considerations should be made when making decisions based upon certain information to ensure accuracy. One method to ensure that information is both reliable and valid is to quantify the error surrounding each specific metric for players.

These GPS devices rely on space navigation that provides the location and movement of individuals through a radio signal-based calculation between the satellite and the GPS receiver [48]. When the GPS receiver is connected to the satellite, an accurate location can be seen, allowing for velocity-based calculations to be derived [49]. However, to quantify the frequency and magnitude of multidirectional-based movements in all three dimensions (anterior-posterior, mediolateral and longitudinal) GPS systems are required to have triaxial accelerometers [50]. With the capability to monitor a wide variety of variables, many studies have attempted to understand the movement patterns employed during both match and training activities [51]. Variables including total distance, distances measured at various intensities, and whole-body load have been shown to correlate significantly with other load-based measures such as RPE [52].

As aforementioned, there have been numerous improvements in GPS over recent times [53]. In general, the measurement precision has improved with the increased sampling rate. While factors such as processors and the position of the device of the body remain extremely important an improvement in sampling rate is still of benefit to the quality of the GPS data. For instance, it has been illustrated that 10 Hz devices were found to be superior to 15 Hz devices, as the 15 Hz device used interpolated data which was not 'true' GPS sampling [53, 54]. However, to this date, both 10 Hz and 15 Hz are shown to be incapable of reliably measuring movements above 20 km·h [53, 54]. Additionally, most metrics have been considered reliable to interpret (within 5%, depending on the manufacturer); however, it is suggested that practitioners proceed with caution when analysing acceleration and deceleration movements [55]. Although average acceleration presented reliable data, when recording *efforts of acceleration and deceleration*, reliability decreased as the intensity increased. Thus, there is a requirement to conduct further testing using true higher-sampling GPS devices for further clarification.

Finally, when collecting GPS data for both practice and research, it is important that practitioners adhere to recommended guidelines for collection, processing, and reporting [56]. For example, all devices must be calibrated and worn in tight fitting garments provided by the manufacturer and athletes should be encouraged to use the same GPS devices across all sessions to ensure there are no issues with inter-unit reliability [51].

Using the data

Practitioners use GPS technology to quantify and monitor the player's locomotion, including distance, speed, and change of direction–based actions during training and matches. While there is widespread use of these devices, there is still much confusion around the most appropriate metrics to use and how to effectively report and generate the information to provide effective feedback to both coaches and players. Most manufacturers offer a long list of metrics that can be obtained via GPS devices; however, the question of interpretation must be asked when determining the validity/reliability of those metrics. Of the long list of metrics, many can be divided into bands (or thresholds) to better assess intensity of specific outputs. Specifically, when investigating velocity-based metrics, many practitioners are interpreting intensity by applying thresholds based on the individual (relative) or uniform across the cohort (absolute). Although less frequent, a variety of acceleration and deceleration thresholds have been identified in previous literature [57].

Additional wearable technology, such as HR monitors, allow practitioners to quantify individual players' responses from allocated training prescriptions. Like GPS technology, HR monitors have developed over the past few decades, allowing for more accurate depiction of HR data. Wearable HR monitors are used in training sessions and match-play to examine the internal response. Similar to GPS metrics, a myriad of data points is available for interpretation, including some composite scores (dependant on manufacturer). Additionally, HR monitors can also be applied to monitor HR variability, potentially indicative of fatigue or overtraining [35].

Speed and acceleration metrics

Depending on the GPS manufacturer, practitioners often have the ability to develop their own analysis by altering individual thresholds within a variety of popular metrics. A common quandary for performance practitioners in the choice between applying relative or absolute thresholds for measuring velocity thresholds, when detailing external loads. Whilst each approach has its rationale, they do have benefits and limitations associated. Determining an approach between absolute and relative thresholds allow practitioners to carefully dissect locomotive behaviour from training and games, allowing a greater opportunity to develop appropriate training prescriptions.

Relative thresholds

Relative thresholds are determined by the player's capacities to produce certain physical outputs. Although not specifically quantified, some of the earliest relative thresholds, in elite soccer, were established as early as the 1980s [58]. The first noted relative thresholds for velocity were determined, via a walking-sprinting continuum, as the following [58]:

- Standing: no locomotor movement
- Walking: forwards, sideways and backwards strolling locomotor movement
- Jogging: non-purposeful, slow running where the individual did not have a specific goal for his movements, such as to recover on defence
- Running: combined striding and sprinting; running with purpose and effort
- Utility: combined backwards running, sideways shuffling, and jumping

Due to the vagueness at determining when soccer players move from jogging to running, or commencing high-intensity efforts, it was suggested that there is a large potential for error if relative thresholds were not used [59]. Given the need for individuality, defining the onset of the second ventilatory threshold (VT_2) has been recommended in differentiating when one is working in moderate or high intensity zones [60, 61]. With that notion, relative positional English Premier League match profiles where established using ventilatory thresholds (VT_1 and VT_2), peak oxygen uptake (VO_{2peak}), and maximum aerobic speed (MAS) [62]. Furthermore, utilising additional individual measurements of fitness capacities, obtained via testing protocols (see Chapter 3), has shown to be advantageous in developing relative thresholds in elite soccer [63]. Researchers have investigated the use of MAS, Anaerobic Speed Reserve (ASR), and maximum velocity achieved in training (V_{MAX}), for establishing relative individual thresholds in elite soccer [63]. It was noted that although significant measurement bias was found between relative thresholds and absolute (arbitrary) thresholds, they are both beneficial in interpreting distance covered in specific speed zones. However, it was also stated that relative and absolute thresholds should not be used interchangeably. Overall, the consensus is that applying individualised thresholds provides additional and practically significant information [62].

Absolute thresholds

Absolute (or arbitrary) thresholds are typically fixed values that have been derived from research in the field to quantify general physical outputs for a variety of velocity and acceleration metrics. Some of the first arbitrary thresholds for the walking-sprinting continuum were established in the mid-1990s [64, 65]. However, since the introduction of wearable technology, researchers have had the ability to interpret and establish absolute thresholds with greater ease of use. Utilising some of the first accessible GPS devices (1 Hz), researchers were able to establish some specific velocity thresholds, categorised by sport [66]. Recently, the verbiage of the running parameters has changed to the commonly used HSR and sprinting. The threshold for HSR has either been a specified range, or a minimum threshold. Specifically, researchers have specified HSR, in soccer, to be accumulated distance between 19.8 and 25.1 km·h [63, 67, 68]. Whereas various research has identified all accumulated distance above 19.8 km·h is considered HSR [69, 70]. While both approaches are deemed valid, it is imperative that practitioners are concise when analysing and comparing HSR parameters. On the contrary, sprinting distance has been consistently identified as accumulated distances above 25.2 km·h [46, 63, 70, 71].

When investigating acceleration thresholds, efforts that are considered accelerations or decelerations are commonly arbitrarily defined as $+3/-3 m·s^{-2}$, respectively [46]. However, some research has defined multiple categories within acceleration bandwidths. Some of the bandwidths are simply labelled as low, moderate, or high, with thresholds of 1–2 $m·s^{-2}$ (low), 2–3 $m·s^{-2}$ (moderate), and >3 $m·s^{-2}$ (high) [70]. While the need for accurate acceleration measurements has been heavily stressed [72, 73], the quantification process for accelerations comes with limitations. Often, the speed is not known from which acceleration and deceleration measurements begin [46, 74]. However, when examining exposures at higher thresholds (>3.0m·s^{-2}), soccer players have shown to produce 26.5–34.9 acceleration exposures throughout a 90-minute match, dependant on position [75]. The majority, roughly 48%, of high acceleration outputs are when players are at a starting velocity of 0–1.0 m·s^{-1}, and have resulted in around 70 s between bouts [75–77]. Another limitation when examining acceleration outputs is the sensitivity associated with the thresholds and data-processing. It has been noted that most differences illustrated between manufacturers was the acceleration and deceleration metrics [78]. Furthermore, as the intensity of acceleration and deceleration increased (greater thresholds), the reliability decreased [78]. Thus, making the recommendation that practitioners approach with caution when attempting to make comparisons, especially between manufacturers.

Overall, in a large analysis involving 82 professional soccer clubs, some of the top-ranked variables for analysis included total distance, HSR (distance covered >5.50 m·s^{-1} [or 19.8 km·h]), sprint distance (distance covered >7.0 m·s^{-1} [or 25.2 km·h]), and acceleration variables [57]. Therefore, it is strongly suggested that practitioners employ a systematic process in the data collection process and monitor valid/reliable speed and acceleration-based metrics (Table 7.1.)

Table 7.1 Examples of absolute and relative speed and acceleration-based thresholds

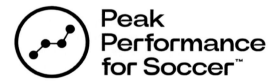

Absolute thresholds				
Metric:	Total distance	HSR	Sprint	Acc/Dec
Calculation	All distance covered	Distance covered >5.50 m·s^{-1} (or 19.8 km·h)	Distance covered >7.0 m·s^{-1} (or 25.2 km·h)	Exposures above or below 3.0 m·s^{-2} (±3.0 m·s^{-2})
Relative thresholds				
Metric:	Total distance	HSR	Sprint	Acc/Dec
Calculation	All distance covered	Distance covered >100% MAS	Distance covered >70% of V$_{MAX}$	Exposures above or below 3.0 m·s^{-2} (±3.0 m·s^{-2})

Acc/Dec = Total acceleration and deceleration exposures.

Other metrics

Arbitrary metrics

Once practitioners have established what GPS metrics the manufacturer offers, it is imperative that the validity and reliability are assessed. More importantly, practitioners must evaluate how they can use the metrics in a manipulatable manner to positively affect training. Specifically, GPS manufacturers often provide arbitrary metrics with their system in an attempt to simplify data analysis for users. Although often considered valid and reliable [79, 80], some of the composite metrics that manufacturers make available should be approached with caution. Practitioners should have a true understanding of the calculations within the composite metrics, such as Dynamic Stress Load (DLS) and Player-Load (PL), before attempting to analyse and alter training variables [81]. For example, if a player results in a statistically larger output in DLS/PL compared to the team average, how will the practitioner explain that outlier to the coaching staff. Whereas, simplified metrics, based on measurable units (i.e. distance-related), can be easier to determine and explain outliers.

Average acceleration

Due to the limitations, such as poor reliability, associated with acceleration-threshold measures, researchers have introduced a novel metric to investigate player locomotion [82]. Investigating acceleration and deceleration as a cumulative metric (Average acceleration, AvgAcc) allows for representation of total multi-directional load, thus considered appropriate for the game of soccer [23]. GPS manufacturers often allow the user to export raw data; therefore, extracting raw acceleration and converting all data points to positive obtains the validated AvgAcc metric [82]. Although AvgAcc doesn't reflect the high-energetic demands that acceleration thresholds illustrate, AvgAcc does offer an overall depiction of drill intensity. AvgAcc has been investigated in professional soccer as a reflection of some of the most demanding passages of play [83, 84]. This metric can help aid practitioners and coaches in establishing intensities of small-sided activities that may not result in high-acceleration exposures (>3.0 m·s^{-2}), due to size constraints [84].

Metabolic power

Although less popular, compared to the aforementioned metrics, metabolic power (P$_{MET}$) can be collected and examined via wearable technology [85]. P$_{MET}$ is representative of locomotive metrics, including speed, acceleration and deceleration. The notion of P$_{MET}$ is to quantify the concept of 'high intensity' via the energy cost of an individual, using W·kg^{-1} [86]. However, since the inception of analysing P$_{MET}$ in elite soccer, researchers have identified a myriad of limitations with the method [87]. P$_{MET}$ has often largely underestimated the actual metabolic demands of soccer-specific drills [87, 88]. Furthermore, the high-intensity thresholds (>20 W·kg^{-1}) for P$_{MET}$ also showed very large typical error and a very low intraclass correlation coefficient [87]. Thus, practitioners are encouraged to use caution with P$_{MET}$ metrics until further examination of validity is available in the literature.

Heart rate measures

While the use of wearable HR monitors in elite soccer is common practice, there still surrounds questions in relation to the use and interpretation of HR data. HR measures can reflect players' adaptation and training/fatigue status. However, in order to specifically identify adaptations, zones (or thresholds) are established to better categorise intensity. Additionally, when interpreting fatigue/training status, heart rate variability (HRV) measures are often recommended.

Heart rate thresholds/zones

As aforementioned, some of the original heart-rate threshold summations illustrated are as follows: zone 1: 50%–60%, zone 2: 60%–70%, zone 3:70%–80%, zone 4: 80%–90%, and zone 5: 90%–100% of maximal HR [40]. As suggested over the past few decades, merely recording HR data points is not sufficient in analysing effort from training sessions [39]. TRIMP has been established in the early 1990s to better allow practitioners to investigate HR responses in sport-related activities [39]. TRIMP is specified from training time and HR data points (within span) during activity. The original equation is as follows;

TRIMP = duration of training (min) × (HR$_{ex}$ − HR$_{rest}$)/ (HR$_{max}$ − HR$_{rest}$)

HR$_{ex}$ = Mean heart rate during exercise
HR$_{rest}$ = Heart rate at rest
HR$_{max}$ = Maximum heart rate

Although the initial TRIMP metric (listed above) seems simple in nature, this method comes with limitations. Due to mean (HR$_{ex}$) being used for calculation, there may be under-or-over estimations when analysing intermittent based activities, such as soccer drills [89]. Researchers have since established novel methods to account for intermittent locomotion. A modified version of the above-mentioned TRIMP, known as TRIMP$_{MOD}$, was introduced with associated HR zones and exponentially weighted factors [90] (Table 7.2).

Although various zones and methods can be applied when interpreting HR responses, it is imperative that practitioners monitor HR data in conjunction with other collection data. The importance of aligning HR data with other internal metrics (e.g. RPE), as well as external loads (GPS), has been noted extensively [3, 42, 91, 92]. A thorough analysis of HR and other data points is integral for both training and match-play [93–95].

Table 7.2 Heart rate zones, corresponding weight factors and training descriptors

Zone	% Maximal heart rate	Weighting	Training type
5	93–100	5.16	Maximal training
4	86–92	3.61	OBLA training
3	79–85	2.54	Steady-state training
2	72–78	1.71	Lactate-threshold training
1	65–71	1.25	Moderate activity

Source: Modified from Stagno et al. [90].

Heart rate variability

HRV refers to the amount of fluctuations in the average HR [96]. HRV has been considered a useful method to monitor the sympathetic and parasympathetic function of the autonomic nervous system (ANS) [96, 97]. Decreases in HRV, when recovering, have been associated with fitter individuals, potentially predictive of exercise performance [98, 99]. However, post-exercise HRV is influenced by a variety of factors, creating questions around the practicality [100]. Monitoring resting HRV can be done frequently, or across set chronic periods. Either approach has been proposed to be sensitive in interpreting both positive and negative adaptations [100]. In relation to elite soccer, resting HRV has been suggested to be the most valuable physiological marker to monitor fatigue [101]. With the validation and accessibility of smartphone applications to measure HRV, practitioners should consider methods to establish resting HRV within their environment [102]. However, understandably, more data collection requires more manpower and data analysis, and, therefore, may not be applicable in all settings.

Practical application of wearable technology in elite soccer

Arguably, the most valuable use of monitoring external training load via wearable technologies is when such monitoring modulates subsequent training prescription [57, 103, 104]. For this practice to be maximised efficiently, the data that is collected, analysed, interpreted, and reported on must be clear and simple, robust yet concise, powerful (i.e. relevant and actionable), and delivered in a highly organised, consistent, and timely manner (Figure 7.3) [105].

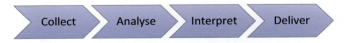

Figure 7.3 The process for practitioners in elite soccer examining physiology related data.

Delivering the data

It is recommended practitioners endeavour to report exclusively on the most important and useful metrics specific to their own, individually unique high-performance programme, and metrics that will ultimately have an actual impact on the programme [105]. Through being highly judicious with which metrics to include and/or exclude, subsequent analysis and delivery of said reports may have a more profound influence on the programme, an impact which has been shown to contribute towards:

- The planning of subsequent training prescription, be it monitoring training loads to increase player fitness (including return-to-play rehabilitation and reconditioning), or conversely, tapering loads to manage fatigue and/or mitigate future injury risk;
- The assessment of individual player intensity and output within training, relative to the competitive match play demands;
- Guidance during team selection; and ultimately;
- Helping increase on-field physical performance [106].

Reporting

The process of reporting is highly dependent on the coaching department's needs and expectations. Specifically, practitioners should cater the visual content of the reports to ensure the accurate message is being delivered to the coaches. As aforementioned, it is of high importance that practitioners firstly examine and interpret the data for its validity and reliability prior to delivery (Figure 7.3) [107]. For example, if the coaching and performance departments are wanting to compare the current training session to its average, in relation to match day (i.e. MD-3, MD-2, and MD-1), then the report should reflect the current average with the associated average (Figure 7.4).

Categorising wearable data by playing position can help aid coaches in overall feedback from the session. Specifically, positionally categorised data sets can help highlight positional characteristics, and determine whether certain drills were more demanding for certain positions. For example, if coaches had planned a 'patterns to goal' drill, mimicking offensive transitions up the wide areas of the field, full-backs and wingers may produce higher intense markers (e.g. HSR), compared to centre-backs and central midfielders. Additionally, coaches may want to identify where specific loads were accumulated. For instance, displaying a breakdown of drills from the training session will help indicate intensities as well as overall volume allocation.

Goalkeeper reports

Whilst often overlooked due to their lack of running actions compared to field-players, goalkeepers exhibit a variety of physical actions during match-play [108]. Goalkeepers frequent mostly around their penalty area (~44% of total match-play), yet still manage to demonstrate various explosive movements

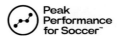

Date: 31-Mar   To Game: MD-2
Total Time: 70 mins   Duration: 1:01   N:19

OUTSIDE BACKS		DISTANCE	HSR (>5.5m·s⁻¹)	ACC/DEC	Sprint (>7.0m·s⁻¹)	RPE	Max Speed (m·s⁻¹)	%Max Speed
LB	Player 1	4539	138	37	47	3	7.8	84%
RB	Player 2	3867	125	26	46	4	8.2	87%
LB	Player 3	3739	111	28	19	5	7.7	82%
RB	Player 4	3134	75	11	10	4	7.2	85%
RB	Player 5	3210	17	23	0	6	6.3	70%
RB	Player 6	3402	8	17	0	5	5.8	65%
	Average	3649	79	24	30	5	7.2	79%
CENTRE BACKS								
CB	Player 7	2860	384	28	56	6	7.6	88%
CB	Player 8	2921	18	25	0	4	6.9	77%
CB	Player 9	2980	14	10	5	4	7.1	81%
	Average	2920	139	21	30	5	7.2	82%
MIDFIELDERS								
DMF	Player 10	3651	133	10	0	3	6.9	79%
ATT	Player 11	4219	78	19	0	4	6.8	79%
DMF	Player 12	3365	33	11	3	5	7.1	81%
CM	Player 13	3883	24	14	0	5	6.4	76%
	Average	3780	67	14	3	4	6.8	79%
ATTACKERS								
WG	Player 14	4103	342	28	102	4	8.3	87%
CF	Player 15	3605	267	24	32	5	7.9	84%
ST	Player 16	3595	238	25	18	6	7.7	81%
WG	Player 17	3465	204	20	38	4	7.6	82%
CF	Player 18	3354	196	19	4	4	7.2	78%
WG	Player 19	3943	160	19	8	4	7.4	85%
	Average	3678	234	23	34	5	7.7	83%
	Team Average	3628	118	22	7	4.0	7.2	81%
	MD-2 Average	4147	195	25	27	5.0	7.6	84%

Figure 7.4 An example of a daily GPS report for a MD-2. HSR = Total distance accumulated above 5.5 m·s⁻¹. ACC/DEC = Total exposures above or below 3.0 m·s⁻². Sprint = Total distance accumulated above 7.0 m·s⁻¹.

at different angles [109]. Therefore, with the development of technology, it seems appropriate for practitioners to attempt to quantify load and report to the goalkeeper coach. Although explosive movements, such as collisions in Rugby League, have been quantifiable via GPS units, goalkeeper-related metrics are still scarce [70, 110]. Due to the explosive, multi-directional outputs of

178 *Joshua Rice et al.*

goalkeepers during match-play, it seems appropriate to monitor the amount of high accelerations/deceleration exposures (>3.0 m·s^{-2}) [111]. Furthermore, research has indicated that goalkeepers often yield more acceleration/deceleration efforts in certain training days compared to match-play [112]. Additionally, some GPS manufacturers offer the measurement of jump intensities; however, it is important that practitioners understand the validity and reliability of accelerometer-based tracking [81].

Longitudinal reports

Practitioners are encouraged to provide objective feedback to coaches in regard to the training week or build-up to games. Regardless of the microcycle build-up preference, dictated by coaching or club (see *Chapter 11*), all stakeholders of the technical department should be provided with a weekly report

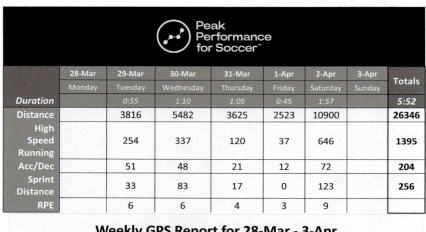

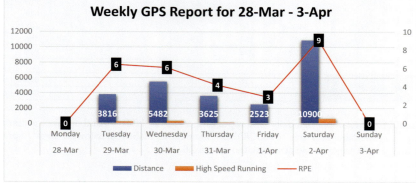

Figure 7.5 An example of a weekly report. HSR = Total distance accumulated above 5.5 m·s^{-1}. ACC/DEC = Total exposures above or below 3.0 m·s^{-2}. Sprint = Total distance accumulated above 7.0 m·s^{-1}.

for feedback on whether the resulted outputs reflect the proposed training plan (Figure 7.5). These weekly reports often display daily comparisons to match-play data. Specifically, research has used percentage of match-data to determine and highlight differences within the acquisition days of the training week (e.g. MD-4 and MD-3) [113].

Reflecting weekly percentage changes for players, across a variety of valid metrics, can aid practitioners in training prescriptions/recommendations to help mitigate the risk of injury. When a player is exposed to =>15% increase in training load from the preceding week, research has indicated that the risk if injury is significantly greater [114]. Additionally, research in elite soccer showed that comparisons to season averages, using four-week blocks, have been purposeful in determining injury risk [115]. Furthermore, illustrations of microcycles can aid practitioners on selecting appropriate days for scheduling additional training stimulus and/or recovery modalities (see *Chapter 8*) [116]. Therefore, it is highly recommended that practitioners develop a reporting system to indicate weekly change as well as seasonal comparisons.

Displaying change

Illustrating worthwhile change on one sheet of paper (physical data daily report, such as Figure 7.4) can be a challenging task for practitioners. Practitioners often conform to using percentage change, smallest worthwhile change (SWC) and/or other statistical methods. It is incredibly important that practitioners are thorough with the comparison process, ensuring the correct message is perceived by the coaching staff. For example, while a percentage change may be appropriate for determining differences in total distance, more sensitive metrics may result in exacerbated comparisons. Using Figure 7.4 in this example, the reported session is only 12.5% ((3628/4147)-1) lower than the averaged MD-2 for total distance covered (team average). However, when examining the sprint distance covered (team average), the same approach yields a percentage difference of 74% ((7/27)-1) less than the MD-2 average. As discussed previously, GPS-related metrics have varied typical errors associated. Having knowledge of validity/reliability of GPS-related metrics allows for practitioners to appropriately account for typical errors of measurement during the comparison process. Therefore, it is integral that practitioners thoroughly investigate the various comparison approaches and allow themselves the best chance to illustrate significant differences in metrics used in the daily report.

Note: It is recommended practitioners define SWC as $0.2 \times$ the between-player standard deviation, until new evidence is shown [117].

Primary barriers of delivery

Researchers identified, in English professional soccer, that stakeholders within the coaching process wanted to see measures reflecting 'high-intensity actions' (82%), and 'work rate/intensity' (74%), and 'comparing physical outputs to what players do in a match' (59%) [106]. For practitioners, within the same research, were primarily sought after observing 'individual player workload' (77%) [106]. 'Too much information and poor communication' have been identified as primary barriers of use for coaches when attempting to read and review GPS reports [106]. Coaches are typically more interested in the qualitative inferences of the report – specifically, the final outcomes, recommendations, and injury implications of the dataset – than the minutia involved in the statistical analysis that was applied to the quantitative data. With that in mind, reports should utilise appropriate user-friendly language when delivering qualitative inferences, supported by attractive visual aids to present the associated data. Of these visual aids, graphical representation of data is typically both attractive and informative (Figure 7.4).

Applying the findings in practice

In elite soccer, a popular use of GPS-guided training prescription involves progressively programming portions of match demands throughout the course of a training week. This method of training prescription allows for players to be better prepared physiologically (i.e. high fitness levels and more resilient tissue) for the demands of the match. Through a specific, periodised training programme, coping with the physical demands of match play – including its peak periods – should be less confronting for players, physically, (theoretically) less injurious, and ultimately, result in increased physical performance.

For example, categorised by individual positions, the average ~90-minute match day output of each GPS metric could be extrapolated by 120%–150%, with the aim to incrementally accumulate this output (or *training benchmark*) throughout the course of a training week. For instance, if wingers typically accrue ~1,000 m of HSR in ~90 minutes of match-play, then those wingers would attempt to incrementally accumulate ~1,200 to ~1,500 m of HSR throughout the course of a training week (excluding the match itself). In this example, the majority of this weekly benchmark would typically be accrued on the heaviest training session(s) of the week (i.e. 3 and 4 days until match day, or MD-3 and -4, respectively) [118–120].

It should be noted, higher HSR output within MD-3 and -4 sessions has been shown to have a positive influence of subsequent match-day performance [121]. This is most likely due to the distant proximity these sessions hold from match day. With 3 and 4 days until match day, compared to heavy output 1 day out from match day, players are afforded the time to adequately recover from the fatiguing training stimulus, and subsequently, express their physical capacities in competition more purely.

It should be acknowledged that these percentages (i.e. 120%–150%) are highly arbitrary. Each set of training benchmarks should be specific to the individually unique high-performance programme being implemented at the club (see *Chapter 11*). Some clubs may need a wider bandwidth for their benchmarks (i.e., 80%–150%), whilst others may need lower absolute benchmarks (i.e. 80%–120% at academy level), whereas some may need different benchmarks for each individual performance metric (i.e. ~120% for HSR distance vs >200% for high-intensity acceleration efforts vs no percentage-based benchmark for more highly sensitive metrics like sprint distance). Some clubs may preserve static benchmarks (i.e. benchmarks representing the *peak* physical output from past seasons), while others may utilise dynamic benchmarks (i.e. benchmarks represent a rolling average of match day demands, updated after each competitive round is played throughout the season). In that sense, there is infinite nuance that must be accounted for when applying this method of guided prescription. For example, modifications to training benchmarks are dependent on those who played for >90 minutes, substitutes, unused substitutes, as well as adjusting benchmarks during periods of high accumulative acute fatigue and soreness. Other content considered are some non-modifiable factors such as periods of congested fixtures, travel schedules, and the historical load of specific players.

Utilising live data

Nowadays, some of the more developed wearable manufacturers offer live tracking, for practitioners to make accurate decisions during training. Live feedback of physical outputs helps illustrate to practitioners the current intensity of drills, potential fatigue patterns, speed exposures, and overall goal setting. Specifically, if multiple bouts of a soccer-specific drill were prescribed for the session, and the coaches and/or practitioners notice a physical decrement, the live feedback can help quantify the severity of that decline. For example, at the conclusion of the second set (out of four), of an 8v8 drill, coaches may suspect a physically lower output during that set. Practitioners could then inspect the live feedback system and notice the average $m \cdot min^{-1}$ dropped by ~X% from first set to second set. Therefore, given the myriad of factors within the training session, practitioners could make some instantaneous recommendations, such as more rest between sets, to increase the likelihood of obtaining the desired physical outputs. However, it must be noted that some live wearable feedback systems will have associated standard errors of measurement [55]. Therefore, to increase the likelihood of accuracy of information, practitioners must be intentional with satellite placement as well as understanding which metrics may have greater errors of measurement. Additionally, practitioners may opt to use live feedback during match-play. Whilst the information is important, it is highly unlikely that any decisions made on game-day will be based on the GPS and/or HR information. Furthermore, it is more likely that the equipment needed to collect live data will merely be seen as a distraction on game day, creating greater potential for a negative environment.

Methodological considerations

The processes, systems, methods, etc. delineated in this chapter are just one effective way to analyse, deliver, and utilise external training load monitoring in elite soccer. If the principles of exercise physiology are adhered to, there are many different, yet still highly effective ways to utilise wearable technology.

This chapter did not discuss several recurrent situations pertinent to external training load monitoring in elite soccer, including:

- GPS- and HR-guided reconditioning of an injured athlete during their return to play rehabilitation (see Chapter 9)
- monitoring training loads during weeks of congesting fixtures (see Chapters 6 and 10)
- strategies to effectively manage deloads (see Chapters 8 and 10)
- dealing with missing data (i.e. National team duties, indoor stadiums, GPS- and/or HR-dropout, etc.), including equations that interchange player output between systems (optical vs GPS) with reduced error [122].

Furthermore, the mentioned methods in this chapter pertained to the delivery of wearable reports to technical coaches exclusively. Although there is always some overlap between departments within soccer clubs, this sub-chapter did not pertain to the delivery of reports to say, the medical department. For example, the medical department may often request elaborated versions of a report to aid in the return-to-play process.

Conclusion

When establishing protocols for usage of wearable technology in elite soccer environments, practitioners must first assess the validity and reliability of each device. Furthermore, practitioners should evaluate the validity and reliability of desirable metrics for collection. While manufacturers offer a variety of arbitrary metrics within their system, it is advised that practitioners only use data points that are valid and actionable in training. There are a variety of ways to illustrate a training report based on the wearable data collected. However, it is recommended that practitioners keep the reports as simple as possible (1-page) and can highlight any substantial differences, if necessary.

References

1. Jaspers, A., et al., *Relationships between training load indicators and training outcomes in professional soccer.* Sports Medicine, 2017. **47**(3): p. 533–544.
2. Casamichana, D., et al., *Relationship between indicators of training load in soccer players.* The Journal of Strength & Conditioning Research, 2013. **27**(2): p. 369–374.
3. Impellizzeri, F.M., E. Rampinini, and S.M. Marcora, *Physiological assessment of aerobic training in soccer.* Journal of Sports Sciences, 2005. **23**(6): p. 583–592.
4. Impellizzeri, F.M., S.M. Marcora, and A.J. Coutts, *Internal and external training load: 15 years on.* International Journal of Sports Physiology and Performance, 2019. **14**(2): p. 270–273.
5. Bosquet, L., et al., *Effects of tapering on performance: A meta-analysis.* Medicine & Science in Sports & Exercise, 2007. **39**(8): p. 1358–1365.
6. Bompa, T.O. and G. Haff, *Periodization: Theory and Methodology of Training.* 5 ed. 2009, Champaign: Human Kinetics. 411.

7. Almulla, J., A. Takiddin, and M. Househ, *The use of technology in tracking soccer players' health performance: A scoping review*. BMC Medical Informatics and Decision Making, 2020. **20**(1): p. 1–10.
8. Mujika, I. and S. Padilla, *Detraining: Loss of training-induced physiological and performance adaptations. Part I*. Sports Medicine, 2000. **30**(2): p. 79–87.
9. Laughlin, M.H., C.L. Oltman, and D.K. Bowles, *Exercise training-induced adaptations in the coronary circulation*. Medicine & Science in Sports & Exercise, 1998. **30**(3): p. 352–360.
10. McLaren, S.J., et al., *The relationships between internal and external measures of training load and intensity in team sports: A meta-analysis*. Sports Medicine, 2018. **48**(3): p. 641–658.
11. Huggins, R.A., et al., *The validity and reliability of global positioning system units for measuring distance and velocity during linear and team sport simulated movements*. The Journal of Strength & Conditioning Research, 2020. **34**(11): p. 3070–3077.
12. Pino-Ortega, J., et al., *Comparison of the validity and reliability of local positioning systems against other tracking technologies in team sport: A systematic review*. Proceedings of the Institution of Mechanical Engineers, Part P: Journal of Sports Engineering and Technology, 2021. **236**(2): p. 73–82.
13. Scott, M.T., T.J. Scott, and V.G. Kelly, *The validity and reliability of global positioning systems in team sport: A brief review*. The Journal of Strength & Conditioning Research, 2016. **30**(5): p. 1470–1490.
14. Malone, J.J., et al., *Seasonal training-load quantification in elite English premier league soccer players*. International Journal of Sports Physiology and Performance, 2015. **10**(4): p. 489–497.
15. Thorpe, R.T., et al., *The tracking of morning fatigue status across in-season training weeks in elite soccer players*. International Journal of Sports Physiology and Performance, 2016. **11**(7): p. 947–952.
16. Malone, S., et al., *High-speed running and sprinting as an injury risk factor in soccer: Can well-developed physical qualities reduce the risk?* Journal of Science and Medicine in Sport, 2018. **21**(3): p. 257–262.
17. Castagna, C., et al., *Effect of training intensity distribution on aerobic fitness variables in elite soccer players: A case study*. The Journal of Strength & Conditioning Research, 2011. **25**(1): p. 66–71.
18. Akubat, I., *Training load monitoring in soccer: The dose-response relationships with fitness, recovery and fatigue*. 2012, University of Hull.
19. Akubat, I., et al., *Methods of monitoring the training and match load and their relationship to changes in fitness in professional youth soccer players*. Journal of Sports Sciences, 2012. **30**(14): p. 1473–1480.
20. Thornton, H.R., et al., *Developing athlete monitoring systems in team sports: Data analysis and visualization*. International Journal of Sports Physiology and Performance, 2019. **14**(6): p. 698–705.
21. Gabbett, T.J., *The training-injury prevention paradox: Should athletes be training smarter and harder?* British Journal of Sports Medicine, 2016. **50**(1): p. 273–280.
22. Bouchard, C. and T. Rankinen, *Individual differences in response to regular physical activity*. Medicine and Science in Sports and Exercise, 2001. **33**(6; SUPP): p. S446–S451.
23. Taylor, J.B., et al., *Activity demands during multi-directional team sports: A systematic review*. Sports Medicine, 2017. **47**(12): p. 2533–2551.
24. Jennings, D., et al., *The validity and reliability of GPS units for measuring distance in team sport specific running patterns*. International Journal of Sports Physiology and Performance, 2010. **5**(3): p. 328–341.
25. Varley, M.C., I.H. Fairweather, and R.J. Aughey, *Validity and reliability of GPS for measuring instantaneous velocity during acceleration, deceleration, and constant motion*. Journal of Sports Sciences, 2012. **30**(2): p. 121–127.

26 Vickery, W.M., et al., *Accuracy and reliability of GPS devices for measurement of sports-specific movement patterns related to cricket, tennis, and field-based team sports.* The Journal of Strength & Conditioning Research, 2014. **28**(6): p. 1697–1705.
27 Aughey, R.J., *Applications of GPS technologies to field sports.* International Journal of Sports Physiology and Performance, 2011. **6**(3): p. 295–310.
28 Gray, A.J., et al., *Validity and reliability of GPS for measuring distance travelled in field-based team sports.* Journal of Sports Sciences, 2010. **28**(12): p. 1319–1325.
29 Hoppe, M.W., et al., *Validity and reliability of GPS and LPS for measuring distances covered and sprint mechanical properties in team sports.* PloS one, 2018. **13**(2): p. e0192708.
30 Ali, A. and M. Farrally, *Recording soccer players' heart rates during matches.* Journal of Sports Sciences, 1991. **9**(2): p. 183–189.
31 Kelly, D.M. and B. Drust, *The effect of pitch dimensions on heart rate responses and technical demands of small-sided soccer games in elite players.* Journal of Science and Medicine in Sport, 2009. **12**(4): p. 475–479.
32 Casamichana, D., et al., *Effect of number of touches and exercise duration on the kinematic profile and heart rate response during small-sided games in soccer.* Journal of Human Kinetics, 2014. **41**(1): p. 113–123.
33 Owen, A.L., et al., *Heart rate responses and technical comparison between small-vs. large-sided games in elite professional soccer.* The Journal of Strength & Conditioning Research, 2011. **25**(8): p. 2104–2110.
34 Drust, B., G. Atkinson, and T. Reilly, *Future perspectives in the evaluation of the physiological demands of soccer.* Sports Medicine, 2007. **37**(9): p. 783–805.
35 Achten, J. and A.E. Jeukendrup, *Heart rate monitoring.* Sports Medicine, 2003. **33**(7): p. 517–538.
36 Shookster, D., et al., *Accuracy of commonly used age-predicted maximal heart rate equations.* International Journal of Exercise Science, 2020. **13**(7): p. 1242–1250.
37 Banister, E.W., et al., *A systems model of training for athletic performance.* Australian Journal of Sports Medicine, 1975. **7**(3): p. 57–61.
38 Foster, C., et al., *A new approach to monitoring exercise training.* The Journal of Strength & Conditioning Research, 2001. **15**(1): p. 109–115.
39 Banister, E.W., *Modeling elite athletic performance.* Physiological Testing of Elite Athletes, 1991. **347**: p. 403–422.
40 Edwards, S., *Heart rate monitoring book.* 1993, Fleet Feet Press.
41 Alejandro, L., et al., *versus Vuelta a España: Which is harder.* Medicine & Science in Sports & Exercise, 2003. **35**(5): p. 872–878.
42 Impellizzeri, F.M., et al., *Use of RPE-based training load in soccer.* Medicine & Science in Sports & Exercise, 2004. **36**(6): p. 1042–1047.
43 Dellal, A., B. Drust, and C. Lago-Penas, *Variation of activity demands in small-sided soccer games.* International Journal of Sports Medicine, 2012. **33**(05): p. 370–375.
44 Krustrup, P., et al., *The yo-yo intermittent recovery test: Physiological response, reliability, and validity.* Medicine & Science in Sports & Exercise, 2003. **35**(4): p. 697–705.
45 Buchheit, M., et al., *Cardiorespiratory and cardiac autonomic responses to 30-15 intermittent fitness test in team sport players.* The Journal of Strength & Conditioning Research, 2009. **23**(1): p. 93–100.
46 Ravé, G., et al., *How to use Global Positioning Systems (GPS) data to monitor training load in the 'Real World' of elite soccer.* Frontiers in Physiology, 2020. **11**: p. 944.
47 Kupperman, N. and J. Hertel, *Global positioning system–derived workload metrics and injury risk in team-based field sports: A systematic review.* Journal of Athletic Training, 2020. **55**(9): p. 931–943.
48 Tamazin, M., et al., *GNSSs, signals, and receivers* in R. B. Rustamov, & A. M. Hashimov (Eds.), Multifunctional Operation and Application of GPS, 2018. London: IntechOpen. p. 119–139.

49 Larsson, P., *Global positioning system and sport-specific testing.* Sports Medicine, 2003. **33**(15): p. 1093–1101.
50 Krasnoff, J.B., et al., *Interunit and intraunit reliability of the RT3 triaxial accelerometer.* Journal of Physical Activity and Health, 2008. **5**(4): p. 527–538.
51 Johnston, R.J., et al., *Validity and interunit reliability of 10 Hz and 15 Hz GPS units for assessing athlete movement demands.* The Journal of Strength & Conditioning Research, 2014. **28**(6): p. 1649–1655.
52 Scanlan, A.T., et al., *The relationships between internal and external training load models during basketball training.* The Journal of Strength & Conditioning Research, 2014. **28**(9): p. 2397–2405.
53 Scott, M.T.U., T.J. Scott, and V.G. Kelly, *The validity and reliability of global positioning systems in team sport: A brief review.* Journal of Strength and Conditioning Research, 2016. **30**(5): p. 1470–1490.
54 Calder, A.R., *Physical profiling in lacrosse: A brief review.* Sport Sciences for Health, 2018. **14**(3): p. 475–483.
55 Thornton, H.R., et al., *Inter-unit reliability and effect of data processing methods of global positioning systems.* International Journal of Sports Physiology and Performance, 2018. **14**(4): p. 432–438.
56 Malone, J.J., et al., *Unpacking the black box: Applications and considerations for using GPS devices in sport.* International Journal of Sports Physiology and Performance, 2017. **12**(s2): p. S2–18–S2–26.
57 Akenhead, R. and G.P. Nassis, *Training load and player monitoring in high-level football: Current practice and perceptions.* International Journal of Sports Physiology and Performance, 2016. **11**(5): p. 587–593.
58 Mayhew, S. and H. Wenger, *Time-motion analysis of professional soccer.* Journal of Human Movement Studies, 1985. **11**(1): p. 49–52.
59 Abt, G. and R. Lovell, *The use of individualized speed and intensity thresholds for determining the distance run at high-intensity in professional soccer.* Journal of Sports Sciences, 2009. **27**(9): p. 893–898.
60 Beaver, W.L., K. Wasserman, and B.J. Whipp, *A new method for detecting anaerobic threshold by gas exchange.* Journal of Applied Physiology, 1986. **60**(6): p. 2020–2027.
61 Esteve-Lanao, J., et al., *Impact of training intensity distribution on performance in endurance athletes.* The Journal of Strength & Conditioning Research, 2007. **21**(3): p. 943–949.
62 Lovell, R. and G. Abt, *Individualization of time–motion analysis: A case-cohort example.* International Journal of Sports Physiology and Performance, 2013. **8**(4): p. 456–458.
63 Rago, V., et al., *Application of individualized speed zones to quantify external training load in professional soccer.* Journal of Human Kinetics, 2020. **72**: p. 279–289.
64 Bangsbo, J., *The physiology of soccer--with special reference to intense intermittent exercise.* Acta Physiologica Scandinavica. Supplementum, 1994. **619**: p. 1–155.
65 Bangsbo, J., L. Nørregaard, and F. Thorsø, *Activity profile of competition soccer.* Canadian Journal of Sport Sciences = Journal canadien des sciences du sport, 1991. **16**(2): p. 110–116.
66 Dwyer, D.B. and T.J. Gabbett, *Global positioning system data analysis: Velocity ranges and a new definition of sprinting for field sport athletes.* Journal of Strength and Conditioning Research, 2012. **26**(3): p. 818–824.
67 Modric, T., et al., *Analysis of the association between running performance and game performance indicators in professional soccer players.* International Journal of Environmental Research and Public Health, 2019. **16**(20): p. 4032.
68 Anderson, L., et al., *Quantification of seasonal-long physical load in soccer players with different starting status from the English Premier League: Implications for maintaining squad physical fitness.* International Journal of Sports Physiology and Performance, 2016. **11**(8): p. 1038–1046.

69 Malone, S., et al., *Wellbeing perception and the impact on external training output among elite soccer players.* J Sci Med Sport, 2018. **21**(1): p. 29–34.
70 Rago, V., et al., *Methods to collect and interpret external training load using microtechnology incorporating GPS in professional football: A systematic review.* Research in Sports Medicine, 2020. **28**(3): p. 437–458.
71 Varley, M.C., et al., *Methodological considerations when quantifying high-intensity efforts in team sport using global positioning system technology.* International Journal of Sports Physiology and Performance, 2017. **12**(8): p. 1059–1068.
72 Delaney, J.A., et al., *Importance, reliability and usefulness of acceleration measures in team sports.* The Journal of Strength & Conditioning Research, 2017. **32**(12): p. 3485–3493.
73 Varley, M.C., I.H. Fairweather, and Aughey1, Robert J, *Validity and reliability of GPS for measuring instantaneous velocity during acceleration, deceleration, and constant motion.* Journal of Sports Sciences, 2012. **30**(2): p. 121–127.
74 Rago, V., et al., *Relationship between external load and perceptual responses to training in professional football: Effects of quantification method.* Sports, 2019. **7**(3): p. 68.
75 Oliva-Lozano, J.M., et al., *Acceleration and sprint profiles of professional male football players in relation to playing position.* Plos one, 2020. **15**(8): p. e0236959.
76 Varley, M.C. and R.J. Aughey, *Acceleration profiles in elite Australian soccer.* International Journal of Sports Medicine, 2013. **34**(01): p. 34–39.
77 Bradley, P.S., et al., *High-intensity activity profiles of elite soccer players at different performance levels.* The Journal of Strength & Conditioning Research, 2010. **24**(9): p. 2343–2351.
78 Thornton, H.R., et al., *Interunit Reliability and Effect of Data-Processing Methods of Global Positioning Systems.* International Journal of Sports Physiology and Performance, 2019. **14**(4): p. 432–438.
79 Johnston, R.D., A. Hewitt, and G. Duthie, *Validity of real-time ultra-wideband global navigation satellite system data generated by a wearable microtechnology unit.* The Journal of Strength & Conditioning Research, 2020. **34**(7): p. 2071–2075.
80 Barrett, S., A. Midgley, and R. Lovell, *PlayerLoad™: Reliability, convergent validity, and influence of unit position during treadmill running.* International Journal of Sports Physiology and Performance, 2014. **9**(6): p. 945–952.
81 Nicolella, D.P., et al., *Validity and reliability of an accelerometer-based player tracking device.* PloS one, 2018. **13**(2): p. e0191823.
82 Delaney, J.A., et al., *Acceleration-based running intensities of professional rugby league match play.* International Journal of Sports Physiology and Performance, 2016. **11**(6): p. 802–809.
83 Delaney, J.A., et al., *Modelling the decrement in running intensity within professional soccer players.* Science and Medicine in Football, 2017. **2**(2): p. 86–92.
84 Calder, A. and T. Gabbett, *Influence of tactical formation on average and peak demands of elite soccer match-play.* International Journal of Strength and Conditioning, 2022. **2**(1). p. 1–10.
85 Rampinini, E., et al., *Accuracy of GPS devices for measuring high-intensity running in field-based team sports.* International Journal of Sports Medicine, 2015. **36**(01): p. 49–53.
86 Osgnach, C., et al., *Energy cost and metabolic power in elite soccer: a new match analysis approach.* Medicine & Science in Sports & Exercise, 2010. **42**(1): p. 170–178.
87 Buchheit, M., et al., *Monitoring locomotor load in soccer: Is metabolic power, powerful?* International Journal of Sports Medicine, 2015. **36**(14): p. 1149–1155.
88 Brown, D.M., et al., *Metabolic power method: underestimation of energy expenditure in field-sport movements using a global positioning system tracking system.* International Journal of Sports Physiology and Performance, 2016. **11**(8): p. 1067–1073.
89 Akubat, I. and G. Abt, *Intermittent exercise alters the heart rate–blood lactate relationship used for calculating the training impulse (TRIMP) in team sport players.* Journal of Science and Medicine in Sport, 2011. **14**(3): p. 249–253.

90 Stagno, K.M., R. Thatcher, and K.A. van Someren, *A modified TRIMP to quantify the in-season training load of team sport players.* Journal of Sports Sciences, 2007. **25**(6): p. 629–634.
91 Torreño, N., et al., *Relationship between external and internal loads of professional soccer players during full matches in official games using global positioning systems and heart-rate technology.* International Journal of Sports Physiology & Performance, 2016. **11**(7): p. 940–946.
92 Arrones, L.S., et al., *Match-play activity profile in professional soccer players during official games and the relationship between external and internal load.* Journal of Sports Medicine and Physical Fitness, 2014. **55**: p. 1417–1422.
93 Coutts, A.J., et al., *Heart rate and blood lactate correlates of perceived exertion during small-sided soccer games.* Journal of Science and Medicine in Sport, 2009. **12**(1): p. 79–84.
94 Rampinini, E., et al., *Factors influencing physiological responses to small-sided soccer games.* Journal of Sports Sciences, 2007. **25**(6): p. 659–666.
95 Alexandre, D., et al., *Heart rate monitoring in soccer: interest and limits during competitive match play and training, practical application.* The Journal of Strength & Conditioning Research, 2012. **26**(10): p. 2890–2906.
96 van Ravenswaaij-Arts, C.M., et al., *Heart rate variability.* Annals of Internal Medicine, 1993. **118**(6): p. 436–447.
97 Michael, S., K.S. Graham, and G.M. Davis, *Cardiac autonomic responses during exercise and post-exercise recovery using heart rate variability and systolic time intervals—a review.* Frontiers in Physiology, 2017. **8**:301.
98 D'Agosto, T., et al., *Cardiac autonomic responses at onset of exercise: Effects of aerobic fitness.* International Journal of Sports Medicine, 2014. **35**(10): p. 879–885.
99 Stanley, J., J.M. Peake, and M. Buchheit, *Cardiac parasympathetic reactivation following exercise: Implications for training prescription.* Sports Medicine, 2013. **43**(12): p. 1259–1277.
100 Buchheit, M., *Monitoring training status with HR measures: Do all roads lead to Rome?* Frontiers in Physiology, 2014. **5**: p. 73.
101 Djaoui, L., et al., *Monitoring training load and fatigue in soccer players with physiological markers.* Physiology & Behavior, 2017. **181**: p. 86–94.
102 Perrotta, A.S., et al., *Validity of the elite HRV smartphone application for examining heart rate variability in a field-based setting.* The Journal of Strength & Conditioning Research, 2017. **31**(8): p. 2296–2302.
103 Halson, S.L., *Monitoring training load to understand fatigue in athletes.* Sports Medicine, 2014. **44**(2): p. 139–147.
104 Torres-Ronda, L., et al., *Tracking systems in team sports: A narrative review of applications of the data and sport specific analysis.* Sports Medicine-Open, 2022. **8**(1): p. 1–22.
105 Buchheit, M., *Want to see my report, coach.* Aspetar Sports Medicine Journal, 2017. **6**: p. 36–43.
106 Nosek, P., et al., *Feedback of GPS training data within professional English soccer: A comparison of decision making and perceptions between coaches, players and performance staff.* Science and Medicine in Football, 2021. **5**(1): p. 35–47.
107 Hopkins, W.G., *Measures of reliability in sports medicine and science.* Sports Medicine, 2000. **30**(1): p. 1–15.
108 Malone, J.J., et al., *Seasonal training load and wellness monitoring in a professional soccer goalkeeper.* International Journal of Sports Physiology and Performance, 2018. **13**(5): p. 672–675.
109 Sainz De Baranda, P., E. Ortega, and J.M. Palao, *Analysis of goalkeepers' defence in the World Cup in Korea and Japan in 2002.* European Journal of Sport Science, 2008. **8**(3): p. 127–134.

110 Chambers, R., et al., *The use of wearable microsensors to quantify sport-specific movements.* Sports Medicine, 2015. **45**(7): p. 1065–1081.

111 Ziv, G. and R. Lidor, *Physical characteristics, physiological attributes, and on-field performances of soccer goalkeepers.* International Journal of Sports Physiology and Performance, 2011. **6**(4): p. 509–524.

112 Moreno-Pérez, V., et al., *Activity monitoring in professional soccer goalkeepers during training and match play.* International Journal of Performance Analysis in Sport, 2020. **20**(1): p. 19–30.

113 Owen, A.L., et al., *A contemporary multi-modal mechanical approach to training monitoring in elite professional soccer.* Science and Medicine in Football, 2017. **1**(3): p. 216–221.

114 Gabbett, T.J., *The training-injury prevention paradox: Should athletes be training smarter and harder?* British Journal of Sports Medicine, 2016. **50**(5): p. 273–280.

115 Ehrmann, F.E., et al., *GPS and injury prevention in professional soccer.* The Journal of Strength & Conditioning Research, 2016. **30**(2): p. 360–367.

116 Cross, R., et al., *Scheduling of training and recovery during the in-season weekly micro-cycle: Insights from team sport practitioners.* European Journal of Sport Science, 2019. **19**(10): p. 1287–1296.

117 Hopkins, W., *How to interpret changes in athletic performance test in Sports Science* 2004. p. 1–7.

118 Martín-García, A., et al., *Quantification of a professional football team's external load using a microcycle structure.* The Journal of Strength & Conditioning Research, 2018. **32**(12): p. 3511–3518.

119 Oliva-Lozano, J.M., et al., *Effect of training day, match, and length of the microcycle on the worst-case scenarios in professional soccer players.* Research in Sports Medicine, 2021. **30**(4): p. 1–14.

120 Oliva-Lozano, J.M., et al., *Impact of contextual variables on the representative external load profile of Spanish professional soccer match-play: A full season study.* European Journal of Sport Science, 2021. **21**(4): p. 497–506.

121 Grünbichler, J., P. Federolf, and H. Gatterer, *Workload efficiency as a new tool to describe external and internal competitive match load of a professional soccer team: A descriptive study on the relationship between pre-game training loads and relative match load.* European Journal of Sport Science, 2020. **20**(8): p. 1034–1041.

122 Ellens, S., et al., *Interchangeability of player movement variables from different athlete tracking systems in professional soccer.* Science and Medicine in Football, 2021. **6**(1): p. 1–6.

8 Recovery and nutrition

Francisco Tavares, António Pedro Mendes, Francisco Pereira, Brett Singer, Michael Watts and Hannah Sheridan

Overview of nutrition and recovery

One of the main objectives of an elite soccer player is to create positive adaptations in order to give themselves a greater chance to enhance team success; through a carefully periodized training plan which creates an overload to develop athleticism, mindset, and/or technical ability. A well-considered training plan also factors in time to recover between sessions and training phases. Alongside a structured training plan, nutritional recommendations need align with the training phases to allow players to have energy for the demands, as well as recovery accordingly. The objective of most training phases is to create enough stress followed by a period of recovery to create a status known as 'super compensation' [1]. The training stimulus promotes a disturbance to homeostasis leading to a biological response and a temporary impairment to an athlete's performance, a phenomenon frequently described as *fatigue* [2]. The planned state of stress and the fatigue that follows may be referred to *functional overreaching* (FOR). Furthermore, it is possible that too much stress without recovery can lead to feelings of tiredness, fatigue, and a lack of motivation. Excess fatigue is often unplanned and can require an extended period off to help recover the athlete. This unwanted adaptation is known as *non-functional overreaching* (NFOR). Additionally, in some extreme cases, athletes are pushed so hard physically and/or mentally until they reach an unsought state known as *overtraining syndrome* (OTS). In exercise, recovery is often described as the period of time when the biological responses to re-establish homeostasis and performance occur [2].

Soccer, being an intermittent multiple-sprint sport characterized by repeated bouts of short duration high-intensity sprints in an endurance context, may result in players having significant depletion of muscle glycogen stores, muscle damage, dehydration, and central fatigue. Hence, a careful planning of nutritional strategies is crucial for elite soccer players. Nutritional prescriptions should be periodized alongside recovery modalities in an elite soccer environment. Players competing at the elite level should be applying all necessary, and valid, approaches to avoid unwanted training stimulus and promote readiness leading into games. For the purpose of this chapter, recovery will be defined as the time frame between the end of a training unit and the beginning of the next training unit.

DOI: 10.4324/9781003200420-8

The overtraining syndrome

Overtraining can be divided into three different categories: *overload*, *overreaching*, and *stages* [3]. Overload is referred to a planned systematic and progressive increase in training to improve performance. Whereas, overreaching has been categorized under two terms: FOR and NFOR [4]. These states are defined as either planned FOR or unplanned NFOR. Lastly, OTS refers to an untreated state of overreaching that causes long-term decreased performance and ability to train. Other descriptions or terms for these states may include burnout, staleness, under recovery, or chronic fatigue [5]. Research states that effective conditioning and positive adaptation requires a balance of training or stress (volume and intensity) mixed with dedicated phases of recovery [6, 7]. A situation resulting in too much load or stress and not enough recovery can lead to physiological and psychological symptoms which may indicate FOR, NFOR, or even OTS. Coaches and practitioners who don't plan or do not place an importance on recovery lead to limitations on performance, a suboptimal adaptation, and in extreme cases can result in missed training sessions or even competition [4].

An imbalance between training and recovery can be amplified or worsened due to poor nutrition, immune health, psychological stress, movement efficiency, and poor sleep [8, 9]. These factors all impact and may contribute to states of overreaching which not only lead to a reduction in performance or maladaptation but can lead to immune dysfunction, inflammation, neurological issues, and hormonal and metabolic dysfunction [10].

The nervous system and its role in recovery

The Sympathetic branch of the ANS is also referred to as the 'Fight of Flight Response' and is the body's natural stress response, linked to the release of hormones such as Cortisol and Norepinephrine [11]. The Parasympathetic branch or the 'Rest and Digest Response' is linked to a lowering in the heart rate, increase in salivary glands function and dilation of the arteries [12]. Both play an important role in the functioning of an individual or athlete. It was found that if an athlete experiences NFOR, a decline in HRV was found which correlated to poor performance in an event [13].

Parasympathetic alterations include fatigue, depression, bradycardia, and a loss of motivation. Whereas, sympathetic alterations include insomnia, irritability, agitation, tachycardia, hypertension, and restlessness [5]. Interestingly, Parasympathetic alterations were more common in aerobic sports, whereas sympathetic alterations were more common in anaerobic sports. Furthermore, it has been reported that over 125 signs and symptoms have been acknowledged in the literature which adds to the complexity of each condition [5].

Recovery in elite soccer

Success in recovery will be highly dependent on the key components of recovery (i.e. training load planning, rest, sleep, hydration, and nutrition). Sleep has been regarded as the single most effective recovery strategy for athletes [14]. Alongside sleep, nutritional habits are integral for athletes in the recovery process. Numerous nutritional factors directly affect the quality of sleep. Therefore, sleep and nutrition alterations go hand in hand as the best interventions to enhance recovery and athletic performance.

Additionally, recovery sessions are popular within soccer clubs and are sometimes done as a stand-alone session on a separate day or prescribed at the commencement of a field training session. Many different modalities are now available, such as compression, stretching, foam rolling, massage, cold water immersion (CMI), electrical muscle stimulation, and cryotherapy. However, it has been suggested that more research is needed to quantify the effectiveness of each modality [2].

Sleep

Sleep plays a critical role in the recovery of athletes, as it is linked to a number of processes that facilitate restoration and recovery of both the brain and the body [15]. A wide range of performance benefits have been associated with adequate sleep, including both physiological and psychological aspects [15, 16]. In essence, 'sleep provides a restorative function to the body to recover from prior wakefulness and fatigue by repairing processes and restoring energy' [15]. Specifically, deep sleep allow for recovery via hormone activity, restoring immune, and metabolic expenditure [14, 16].

On the contrary, sleep deprivation has been associated with many detrimental effects on the human body, specifically sport-specific and physical performance [17]. In relation to the physical demands required to compete in elite soccer, sleep deprivation has been linked with decreased time to exhaustion, decreased aerobic or anaerobic contribution, decreased fitness testing results, and decreases in mean and peak power [17]. Therefore, it is recommended that athletes require seven to nine hours of quality sleep per night in order to recover and yield the desired adaptations expected by the coaches and practitioners [18]. However, young players or players exposed to higher training loads, such as pre-season, are recommended to sleep for a minimum of eight to ten hours per night [16, 19]. Furthermore, if these prescriptions are not feasible due to non-modifiable aspects, such as travel, elite athletes have also seen benefits from napping during the day [20]. Although sleep seems like a rudimentary concept for discussion in elite soccer, practicing good sleep-hygiene can excel players' ability to perform and could be the small margin contributing to overall team success. Aside from sleep, athletes at the elite level may have the luxury of applying a variety of modalities that have been shown to encourage recovery.

Nutrition and recovery

The intense training and competition schedule inherent to elite football, combined with regular travel, can pose a considerable challenge to the recovery, performance, and immune function of players throughout a ten-month season [21, 22]. Players have limited recovery time in-between matches and disturbed sleeping patterns as a result of varying kick-off times and international travel [23]. Throughout the season, there is additional pressure for players to maintain an optimal body composition; this can be difficult to achieve consistently as players must prioritize fueling and recovery for match performance, often without the knowledge of the starting line-up or their potential contribution to the match ahead. In addition, sleep deprivation and fatigue can alter eating habits and appetite, creating further challenges for maintaining optimal body composition [24].

A tailored nutrition strategy can play a key role in recovery from training, preparation, and recovery from match play, optimization of immune function, body composition, sleep quality, and circadian adaptation when travelling across time-zones [23, 25, 26]. It is always advised that the foundations of a player's diet are based on a varied, whole-food intake in which they should achieve the majority of their macro- and micro-nutrient targets [27, 28]. However, the demands of elite sport can pose challenges to optimal eating behaviors during which supplementation may be advantageous to a player's recovery, performance, and/ or wellbeing [29].

Training load and recovery

In soccer, players frequently have multiple daily training sessions during consecutive days. The high density of training and competition load associated with

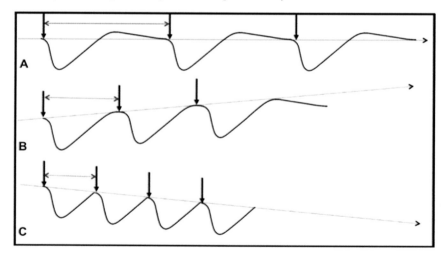

Figure 8.1 Schematic representation of hypothetical training capacity/preparedness to train (vertical axis), according to the three different intervals between training stimulus (blue arrow). (a) The interval is too long and no adaptation occurs (undertraining); (b) the interval is appropriate and desired adaptations will occur; and (c) the interval is too short and the training capacity decreases as the accumulated fatigue increases (overreaching) (Adapted from Bishop et al. [6]).

limited time to recovery may lead to a decrease in performance (i.e. fatigue) and an increased risk of injury [30]. Theoretically, one can draw three possible scenarios from *training load–recovery* relationship, where time to recovery is too long (Figure 8.1a), time to recovery is adequate (Figure 8.1b) or time to recovery is too short (Figure 8.1b) [6, 31, 32].

Although the scenario B (Figure 8.1b) is the one the performance staff is aiming for, a shifting from B to C is frequently observed, especially at the highest levels of practice. For this reason, coaches and practitioners need to be aligned and work together to maintain each player is balanced in the training load–recovery paradigm. Together with the planification of the training load, factors such as rest, sleep, nutrition, and hydration have been recognized as the key components to recovery from training [8, 9].

Nutritional intake and associated challenges

Despite the suggested benefits of certain nutritional strategies in soccer performance, evidence has been revealing some concerns regarding soccer players' food habits. While one might assume professional soccer players consistently follow evidence-based nutrition recommendations for training and recovery to support optimal performance, evidence suggests that might not always be the case. A study done with English Premier League players showed that in a congested fixture period, average carbohydrate intake at training and recovery days was 4.2 g·kg·day, which may well be short of recommendations for higher volume training and match days [33]. Food habits of soccer players can often be non-compatible with peak physical performance [34]. Fat intake appears to be too high when compared to evidence-based recommendations, as it is the most proportionally over-consumed macronutrient [35–37]. While protein intake generally meets the total daily recommendations, distribution and timing often falls sort of best practice [38]. When it comes to carbohydrates, a review indicated that senior soccer players had an intake of 4.3–5.0 g·kg of carbohydrate per day, which may be adequate in some cases, but not others, in comparison to the UEFA recommendations [39, 40]. Furthermore, research has revealed that increasing deficits of just 10% in glycogen replenishment can elicit decrements in performance over a period of time [39, 41]. Another common, undesirable practice among players is the tendency to have infrequent meals that may lead to muscle catabolism and reductions in muscle mass [35, 42]. As players get older, the tendency to skip meals, especially breakfast and snacks, also increases [35, 37]. Thus, the above-mentioned factors combined present a worrisome scenario when recovery time between matches is limited in elite soccer environments.

It is difficult to understand why carbohydrate is systematically below recommendations in an array of studies. It might be related to weight-related concerns, individual tolerance, or warnings about carbohydrate overuse in the general population [35]. Long-term carbohydrate restriction regimens can be harmful for player's performance, as they might impair cognitive performance, perceptions of fatigue, and/or increased susceptibility to skeletal muscle damage while training or competing [43–45]. Players should be taught that performance improvements occur as a result of long-term changes to diet and training and not through instant solutions as nutritional product manufacturers might suggest [46]. Besides the deficits in nutritional intake, deficits in nutritional knowledge by staff and players shouldn't be overlooked, as they represent a barrier to change. Combatting nutrition misinformation, shared by coaches and players, based on their past experiences, can be particularly challenging for practitioners [47]. Cultural issues can also be a hurdle for changing behaviors, with implications for a culturally diverse team [48]. Although a delicate situation to navigate, practitioners should be open to learning from players about their previous experiences, while also seeking out opportunities to teach and incorporate more evidence-based nutrition behavioral changes.

General macronutrient requirements

While some athletes may seek out ergogenic aids as their first opportunity for performance improvement, meeting overall dietary needs through food should be prioritized first [39]. Macronutrients (carbohydrates, protein, and fat) serve as the primary energy sources, thus placing a large emphasis on the requirements for elite soccer players.

Carbohydrates

Although several recommendations have been made, current reviews indicate that macronutrient intake in soccer is not consistently adequate to fulfil players' needs [39]. Additionally, the lack of evidence regarding muscle glycogen utilization during field-based soccer training sessions make it difficult to outline carbohydrate recommendations for training, other than to suggest that they might differ from match play [49]. Based on an investigation with English Premier League players, during a seven-day microcycle – with two matches and five training sessions – the mean daily carbohydrate intake was 6.4 and 4.2 g·kg on match and training days, respectively [33]. Given that muscle glycogen stores are a determining factor for preparation and recovery from match play, it is advised to increase carbohydrate intake to 6–8 g·kg·bodyweight (BW) on MD-1, MD, and MD+1 [50]. In turn, during periods of lower daily loads (one match per week), considering that players do not perform any additional training outside the club, a daily intake of 3–6 g·kg may be sufficient to promote fueling and to optimize recovery [40].

Recent evidence has provided new insights into the enhancement of adaptive responses to training and recovery in environments with low carbohydrate availability, which may increase mitochondrial biogenesis and oxidative metabolism [51, 52]. Thus, glycogen can be considered not only an energetic substrate but also a regulator of signaling responses, which has led to a growing interest on a 'periodized' approach [51]. Periodizing the consumption of carbohydrates can be done by soccer players, alongside the season calendar, coaches' training models, athletes body composition, and performance goals [53]. Although there is evidence showing that soccer players might naturally practice some type of nutrition periodisation plan, they are usually not qualified to self-develop an adequate strategy in this sense, hence the importance of being closely monitored by a nutritionist [53].

Protein

Besides depleting glycogen stores, frequent training and matches can induce stress on tendinous and musculoskeletal tissues, so repairing and remodelling these structures to improve and maintain their integrity is necessary for optimized recovery and adaptations, hence the importance of protein [54]. According to the recommended dietary allowance, the general protein requirement for a sedentary person is 0.8 g·kg·BW/day [55, 56]. However, there is a good rationale to recommend higher protein intakes to athletes in the range of 1.6–2.2 g·kg/day [40]. In this sense, soccer players may require protein for more than just alleviation of the risk for deficiency, but also to aid in an elevated level of functioning and possibly adaptation to the exercise stimulus [57].

Although distribution and timing of protein intake often falls sort of best practice, recent dietary surveys suggest that most professional players meet the overall daily recommended protein intake [38, 54]. Nevertheless, they usually exhibit a skewed pattern of protein intake – similar to the general population – with the highest intakes observed at dinner and sub-optimal intakes at breakfast and snacks, which may not optimally stimulate muscle protein synthesis on each meal occasion [38, 58]. The suggested 'ideal' recommendation is four-to-five protein containing meals, with at least 0.4 g·kg/meal. With the intake of four meals, this recommendation would result in roughly 1.6 g·kg of protein consumed per day (Figure 8.2) [40, 59].

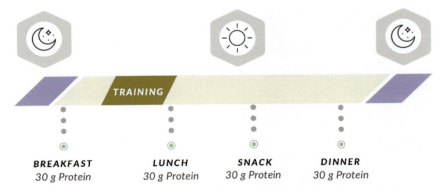

Figure 8.2 Representation of a possible protein distribution throughout the day for a 75 kg player.

Fat

Fat is the most concentrated source of energy in human nutrition, as well as a vehicle for the intake and absorption of fat-soluble vitamins. Although considered the most proportionally over-consumed macronutrient, athletes are often misinformed on the importance of fat intake and, in some cases, limited the amount of fat in their nutritional habits. There is current debate on the intake of fat in the athletic population; however, the expert group recommendation suggests that fat intake, for soccer players, should account for 20%–35% of total dietary energy [40, 60, 61]. Over-restricting fat intake to less than 20% may result in missing out on a range of food with valuable nutrient profiles [62]. Furthermore, a high-fat, low-carbohydrate diet has been shown to impair performance in elite endurance athletes [60, 63]. In summary, there are varied noted outcomes with altered fat-carbohydrate ratios. It is strongly recommended that practitioners remain with evidence-based suggestions in relation to fat intake, without compromising other macronutrients.

Match nutrition: from preparation to recovery

Pre-match day/MD -1

The primary focus on pre-match day is to ensure that muscle and liver glycogen stores are at their maximum, since it's known that athletes who begin a game with low muscle glycogen stores are more likely to cover less distance and at slower speeds, particularly in the second half [64, 65].

Typically, MD-1 training session consist of brief tactical work and short high intensity exercises. Nutritionally, evidence emphasizes the need to load with 6–8 g·kg·BW of carbohydrate starting 24 h before the match [33]. For a 75 kg player, this would be equivalent to 450–600 g of carbohydrates (Figure 8.3).

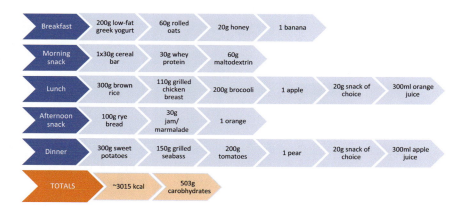

Figure 8.3 Example of a carbohydrate loading day for a 75 kg player.

In practical terms, it is quite possible to distribute this amount by four to five meals. For example, at lunch and at dinner, it is not unreasonable to suggest 2 g·kg, plus 1 g·kg at breakfast and the remaining carbohydrates may be distributed at the afternoon snack and supper, through easily digestible snacks and drinks. Notwithstanding, achieving an intake of 6 g·kg can be challenging, and the reality is that players' daily intake may be closer to about 4 g·kg [39]. In this regard, a conscious intake of carbohydrate-rich foods is needed, by increasing carbohydrate intake at the cost of fat intake to ensure glycogen restoration [40]. If the match schedule consists of congested fixtures, carbohydrate intake should be maintained within the recommendations (6–8 g·kg) for the 48–72 h between games [40].

The day before the match also represents an opportunity to access and optimize player's hydration for the following day. Urinary indices of hydration such as daily body mass measurements, urine-specific gravity and osmolality, urine color, or degree of thirst may be useful indicators to measure hydration status [66]. Besides every methods limitations, urine specific gravity, osmolality, and urine color are the most effective methods in determining and monitoring hydration status. Therefore, values for specific gravity and osmolality of <1.020 and <700 mOsmol·kg, respectively, should be assured as they indicate euhydration. Urine color should appear light yellow on MD-1 [67]. Body weight measurements taken on MD-1 should be kept within 1% of typical daily body weight, as a starting weight outside of this range is associated with dehydration. Similarly, player's fluid consumption should be monitored before and after training. This way, the amount of fluid lost during training can be determined [67].

Nutritionists, coaches, and other specialized team members educate players on hydration needs, and encourage them to meet their daily requirements [39]. Monitoring training loads and players' dietary intake may be helpful to determine individual nutritional needs and establish tailored interventions [68].

Game/match day (MD)

On match day, carbohydrate intake continues to be one of the most determinant factors to improve performance. Glycogen stores can drop drastically during a match, with almost half of the muscle fibers being empty or almost empty once it finishes [69]. Therefore, athletes should adopt nutritional strategies to maximize pre-game muscle glycogen levels through the manipulation of carbohydrate intake, during and after match play. Within an overall intake guideline of 6–8 g·kg·BW·day, players should be encouraged to consume a carbohydrate-rich meal (1–3 g·kg·BW) three to four hours before kick-off, to ensure that glycogen stores are sufficient to endure match demands (Figure 8.4).

Besides the carbohydrate intake guidelines, gastrointestinal comfort is also an aspect to consider in the meals that precede the match. In this sense, it is advised that players ingest easy digestible foods. These foods should be aligned with players' preferences and rituals, so carbohydrate intake guidelines don't override their intrinsic taste for certain foods. Unfamiliar foods can lead to

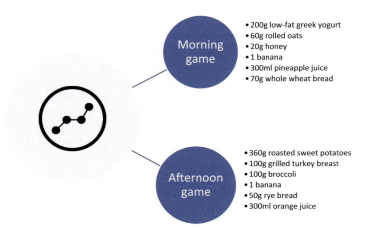

Figure 8.4 Two examples of meeting MD nutrition requirements (three hours before kick-off) for a 75 kg player.

nausea, stomach cramps, and diarrhea, so keeping meals choices simple is essential for a successful pre-event fueling [70]. Within 60 minutes before the match until warm-up, light snacks high in carbohydrates may further increase its availability, thus sparing liver glycogen during activity [70]. To this respect, the quantity and timing of feeding within 1 h before the game should be up to the players' preference.

As the beginning of the match gets closer, caffeine intake arises as an additional nutritional strategy to be considered. Specifically, ingesting 3–6 mg·kg of caffeine 20–60 minutes prior to the match can improve performance [71]. Depending on the caffeine source, individual response can vary. Some players might prefer to ingest caffeine in a gel form and others as a pill. Therefore, personalized strategies should take place beforehand in order to test individual responses. When it comes to hydration, the main goal is to begin the game in a euhydrated state and with normal plasma electrolyte levels. Hydration recommendations consist of ingesting 5–7 ml·kg·BW of fluid in the two to three hours before the match, which gives time for excess fluid to be voided prior to exercise [72, 73]. During this period, monitoring hydration status presents as a difficult task. Given the difficulty and impracticality of monitoring hydration status on game day, players should be educated and reminded of the importance of adequate fluid intake.

Before kick-off and during warm-up, it is advised to drink small amounts of fluids, as fluid ingestion is the only way to replace sweat losses and thereby reduce the risk of dehydration [74, 75]. The mechanism by which sweating-induced hypohydration may impair soccer performance includes impaired cognitive and thermoregulatory function, increased perception of effort, increased cardiovascular strain, and reduced technical skills [76]. The magnitude of these effects has been shown to be correlated to the degree of dehydration [77]. Although some individuals may be more or less sensitive to hypohydration during exercise, the level needed to induce a decrease in performance is around > 2% decrease in body mass [78]. Therefore, players should aim to drink enough fluids to prevent a deficit of 2%–3% of pre-exercise body weight during the match, while avoiding signs of hyperhydration (e.g. increased body weight) and ensuring their needs are met.

During match-play

Nutritional strategies during match-play usually include the 30 minutes preceding kick-off plus the 90-min match [74]. Here, the main goals are to ensure sufficient carbohydrate and fluid intake. Research shows performance benefits in protocols that simulate soccer matches when consuming 30–60 grams of carbohydrate per hour [79]. In some cases, it might not be easy to achieve these recommendations despite the advantages in doing so, such as improving the ability to perform high intensity intermittent actions [80, 81]. Potential rationale to scenarios of under-fueling during match play are limited feeding opportunities and/or the fear of gastrointestinal distress. Thus, unveiling the importance of sports foods as carbohydrate drinks or gels, that can provide a preferred delivery option and help to reach match-play recommendations. Stoppages during match play present an opportunity for players to replenish some of the fluids lost and to consume some carbohydrates. Carbohydrate mouth-rinsing during breaks of match play has also shown to be able to enhance performance in situations where carbohydrate ingestion is limited due to gastrointestinal concerns [82]. Carbohydrate mouth rinses can be utilized by swilling a carbohydrate solution in the mouth periodically for 5–10 seconds [83]. This is related to receptors in the oral cavity that may exert central effects when carbohydrate is consumed during exercise, thereby reducing the perception of effort [84].

Another practice that has been considered novel in professional soccer is the use of pickle juice in relation to players that report muscle cramps. The mechanism of action is still not well understood, but studies suggest that its ingestion triggers a reflex in the oropharyngeal region, which reduces the activity of the alpha neuron pool [85]. Regardless the lack of related studies, pickle juice can be used for the potential acute relief of exercise-associated muscle cramps [85]. All off the mentioned nutrition strategies mentioned above should be implemented in training, in order for the players to become accustomed to potential adverse effects, with minimal impact on match performance.

Post-match recovery

The consumption of carbohydrates immediately after a game is important for optimum glycogen resynthesis, given that glycogen synthesizing enzymes are most active during this period [86]. Delaying carbohydrate feeding 2 h after exercise can, in fact, result in lower muscle glycogen concentration by 45% compared to immediate carbohydrate ingestion [87]. During the 4 h post exercise, the consumption of 1–1.2 g·kg·h carbohydrate has shown to induce maximal glycogen resynthesis [87]. This can be considered a significantly large amount of food for most players. Also, their appetite can be suppressed following the match, so liquid protein, and carbohydrate supplements, as an alternative to solid foods, can be useful for enhancing recovery mainly during periods with a high number of fixtures. In the following 24 h after a game, carbohydrate intake of 6–8 g·kg·BW should be maintained up to 48–72 h during congested fixture schedules [74].

Rehydration is an important part of the post-exercise recovery process, and it can be seen as one of the first to be put in practice. Inadequate rehydration may have negative effects on glycogen restoration and protein synthesis rates, so post-exercise is a period where rehydration strategies should be implemented in order to aid these mechanisms and to replace the volume of the fluids lost [88]. Ideally, players should replace 150% of what have they lost. That means that for every kg of weight lost during exercise, 1.5 L of ingested fluid is required [89]. Beverages containing sodium (with a content greater than 600 mg/L) induce lower urine production and helps stimulating thirst and retaining the ingested fluids, thus re-establishing water balance [75]. On the contrary, rehydrating with just water might take three times longer to restore plasma volume [90]. The addition of carbohydrate, sodium, and protein, such as milk or carbohydrate-protein recovery beverages, can also enhance rehydration in comparison to plain water or even sports drinks alone [91]. When consumed with food, water can be an effective rehydration beverage as the addition of macronutrients and sodium from food should slow the absorption and improve retention of fluid [92].

The optimal sodium level during rehydration can be as high as 50–80 mmol/L, which exceeds the amounts found in a typical sports drink. Therefore, drinks with a high electrolyte content (40–50 mmol/L of sodium chloride) and with a high carbohydrate content to help with glycogen restoration can be more suitable for rehydration purposes [90]. The consumption of carbohydrates immediately after a game is important for optimum glycogen resynthesis, given that glycogen synthesizing enzymes are most active during this period [86]. Delaying carbohydrate feeding 2 h after exercise can, in fact, result in lower muscle glycogen concentration by 45% compared to immediate carbohydrate ingestion [87].

Optimizing muscle protein synthesis rates is also crucial, and meals should reach 0.4 g·kg·meal of high-quality protein, scheduled every three to four hours, to maximally repair tissues [93–95]. Nutrition strategies towards the end of the day are often overlooked by athletes. This time of the day, however, represents an additional feeding opportunity for overnight recovery. For instance, a 40 g dose of casein, 30 minutes prior to sleep, accelerates functional recovery and, therefore, provides means of attenuating performance deficits in the following days after a match [96, 97]. This is due to its slow-release properties over a prolonged sleeping period [98]. Professional players typically report an intake of 0.1 g·kg·BW of protein at this time, highlighting an opportunity to improve nutritional choices [33, 58]. As it would be expected, the absence of this pre-sleep feed will not improve overnight protein balance and will possibly compromise muscle protein synthesis rates over the 24h period [98].

Supplements

Despite the heterogeneous definition of the term supplement, it is indisputable that the prevalence of supplement use is far greater in athletes than in the general population [99]. Supplements are the largest group of products marketed to athletes. However, only a few have good evidence of benefits, namely creatine, caffeine, specific buffering agents (beta-alanine and bicarbonate) and nitrates, which may be included in a supplementation protocol (especially when food intake or food choice is restricted) [100]. It is not unusual for dietary supplements to be used without a full understanding of its potential benefits and risks by athletes. In addition, given the potential costs of its use and doping concerns, a complete nutritional assessment should be considered before decisions regarding supplement use are made.

Creatine

Creatine is produced from the amino acids glycine, methionine and arginine by the liver. It can also be obtained from exogenous sources, predominantly from meat and fish, with a typical diet supplying around 1–2 grams of creatine per day [101]. Around 95% of all creatine in the body is stored in the skeletal muscle and 60% of it is in the phosphorylated form (phosphocreatine) [102]. In a rapid one-step process, phosphocreatine donates a phosphate to ADP resulting in ATP synthesis. This energy system is relied on heavily for high intensity exercise such as sprinting, jumping, or resistance training. Supplementation with creatine increases muscle creatine, allowing the athlete to depend on this rapid energy system for a few seconds longer [103]. In more general terms, the athlete can sustain high-intensity outputs longer, while recovering quicker between bursts of activity. This would be especially beneficial for soccer, as high-intensity running, repeated sprinting, jump ability, and other intermittent efforts are crucial elements of performance [104]. Creatine supplementation may also lead to chronic adaptations which include lean mass gains and improvements in muscular and strength power [100]. On the other hand, aerobic-oriented activities do not appear to benefit from creatine supplementation [105].

Regarding the traditional supplementation protocols, most studies have employed a 'loading phase' that consists of taking 5 g of creatine, four times daily for 5–7 days [106]. A more recent approach suggests a lower dose of 3 g per day which has shown to increase muscle total creatine to the same values. However, it takes longer (about 30 days) [107]. In both strategies, a maintenance phase of 3–5 g·day or 0.03 g·kg·day should be followed for the rest of the supplementation period [108]. To maximize its storage in the muscle, it is recommended that creatine is consumed with a carbohydrate or protein source, given the role of insulin in increasing muscle creatine uptake [108]. The only expected side effect with creatine supplementation is weight gain (1–1.5kg), which is more evident in men compared to women, and is likely due to intracellular water accumulation [104].

Beta-alanine

Beta-alanine is an amino acid produced in the liver and it can be obtained through the consumption of foods such as poultry and meat. Although it doesn't have direct ergogenic properties, it acts as a substrate for the synthesis of carnosine, which is an intracellular dipeptide found in high concentrations in the skeletal muscle. It exerts its function by sequestering hydrogen ions (H^+) that result from the conversion of lactic acid to lactate and are responsible for acidifying muscles during exercise [109]. Since muscle acidosis contributes to the onset of fatigue, a higher concentration of carnosine increases this ability to sequester hydrogen ions, delaying the onset of fatigue [109]. Nevertheless, supplementation of carnosine is inefficient in augmenting its levels, as it is metabolized before reaching skeletal muscle. Therefore, the most effective way to increase endogenous synthesis of carnosine is through the intervene of beta-alanine intramuscular availability [110].

Improvement in performance from beta-alanine supplementation depends on the level of acidosis that the exercise itself generates [111]. When an exercise protocol elicits high-acidosis, improvement in performance is more likely to take place. Beta-alanine has been linked to improved performance in high-intensity exercise activity lasting between 30 seconds to 10 minutes in duration or where there may be repeated bouts of high intensity exercise, such as soccer drills and match-play [100]. Time until maximal muscle carnosine levels are reached from chronic beta-alanine supplementation appears to be variable between individuals [112, 113]. Despite a multitude of studies, there is still no exact recommendation regarding dosing or exact duration, though recommendations are currently for somewhere between 3.2 and 6.4 g per day over the course of 4–24 weeks. This total amount should further be split into smaller doses between 0.8 and1.6 per dose every 3–4 h which should alleviate the potential side effect linked to beta-alanine, paresthesia, which is a harmless short term tingling sensation in the hands and face briefly following supplementation [113]. Additionally, doses should be combined with meals which may further enhance muscle carnosine levels [114].

Caffeine

Caffeine is the world's most consumed psychoactive substance, and it occurs naturally in several plant species, including coffee, tea, and cocoa [115]. Its study has been a longstanding topic of interest, as it continues to be a compound of concern, not only in the public health field but also in the sports context. It is believed that caffeine acts on the central nervous system via the antagonism of adenosine receptors [116]. By suppressing these receptors, its intake leads to an increased neurotransmitter release and motor unit firing rates [117]. Caffeine use is correlated with increased performance in endurance activities as well as in intermittent and strength activities [118]. Considering soccer, there is robust evidence that caffeine intake leads to improved performance through the enhancement of different parameters such as: repeated sprint performance, increased countermovement jump and jumping ability, increased number of sprints and total distance covered at high intensity, improvement of reactive agility, and reduced decline in the ability to perform mental tasks towards the end of the game [119, 120].

Based on existing research, most studies use the administration of dosages around 6 mg·kg·BW [121, 122]. However, ergogenic effects of caffeine can occur with a variety of caffeine doses and timings as it is the case of the evidence demonstrating the beneficial effects of the ingestion of lower amounts of caffeine on performance [123]. Several studies suggest that there is no dose-response between caffeine intake and increased performance during endurance exercise. According to the latest position stand from the international society of sports nutrition, caffeine is ergogenic when consumed in doses of 3–6 mg·kg·BW [118]. In healthy adult populations, moderate daily caffeine intakes of up to 400 mg·day or 6 mg·kg are not associated with adverse effects. On the contrary, higher doses (>6–9 mg·kg) may be associated with side effects such as jitters, increased heart rate and performance impairment [115]. Regarding the timing of ingestion, caffeine is rapidly absorbed peaking after about 60 minutes in blood plasma. Given that is slowly catabolized, concentration in circulation is maintained near the maximum in 3–4 h following administration, so its intake 1 h before the game enables an ergogenic effect during the entire game [117, 124]. Some of the alternative sources of caffeine such as caffeinated chewing gums or gels may promote a faster absorption than caffeine-containing capsules. Therefore, timing of ingestion should be considered by individuals who are interested in supplementing with caffeine [115, 125].

Nitrates

Nitrates have become increasingly popular for their potential role as an ergogenic aid [126]. Nitric oxide (NO) is a signaling molecule produced through endogenous and exogenous pathways by dietary nitrate ingestion [126]. Increased nitric oxide availability can affect numerous vascular and cellular functions, namely in increasing efficiency of mitochondrial respiration and muscle blood flow by promoting vasodilatation during physical activity, which consequently reduces ATP consumption during muscle contraction [127, 128]. Leafy green and root vegetables like rocket, celery, beetroot, and spinach are the primary source of dietary nitrate, although beetroot juice is the most used supplemental nitrate source in exerciseinterventions [127, 129]. As nitrate needs are likely to be met by ingesting around 250–500 g of these vegetables per day, dietary supplements represent a more convenient way of covering the athlete's needs [126]. In addition, the content of nitrate rich vegetables varies greatly, and depends on many factors such as the origin of the vegetable, quality, and pH of the soil, type, and frequency of nitrogen fertilizers.

Performance benefits can manifest acutely, following a bolus of 310–560 mg, taken 2–3 h before exercise [100, 127]. Recent work also highlights a cumulative influence of repeated intake (more than three days) on performance [127, 130, 131]. However, chronic intake of more than three consecutive days before the event seems to reap greater benefits for well-trained athletes [126, 132]. The increase in plasma nitrite after a nitrate load is highly dependent on nitrate reduction in the oral cavity by commensal bacteria as the usage of antibacterial mouthwash to remove these bacteria will impair this recycling process. As such, this may be an important implication for athletes, who should refrain from mouthwash usage [126]. Supplementation effects are less pronounced in athletes with a higher VO_{2MAX} [126, 133]. Nevertheless, the effect of nitrates shouldn't be neglected as it is regarded by the International Olympic Committee as one of a handful dietary supplements with a direct positive effect on performance [100, 126]. As differences between competitors are marginal, it may be desirable to use nitrates in a supplementation protocol that might include other supplements as well.

The injured athlete

There is irrefutable evidence that regular physical activity is effective in the prevention of several chronic diseases and, by consequence, is associated with a longer health span [134]. However, despite its health benefits, the demand and competitiveness generated around professional soccer and other sports have made the risk of developing sports injuries very high [135]. To counter this trend, the knowledge about the factors that are at the genesis of sports injuries, the commitment to the rehabilitation plan as well as the communication between the multidisciplinary team and the athletes is essential. It is common for injured athletes to resort to different methods that allow them to recover faster, namely electrical stimulation, ice, heat, and acupuncture, among others. However, an often-overlooked aspect of recovery is nutrition. An adequate and planned nutritional approach should also be seen as a recovery strategy during all stages of the injury [136].

At this time, studies in this field are scarce, with most recommendations based on studies utilizing subjects on bed rest or with limb immobilization rather than an injury per se. Despite this, recommendations can be drawn based on this evidence to devise nutritional interventions that may be appropriate for the injured player. In this section, we will consider the exercise-induced injuries that are more severe, which can be categorized by two main stages, both influenced by nutrition [136]. The first is called the 'immobilization' or 'atrophy stage'. Depending on the type and severity of the injury, the length of time for immobilization will vary, from a few days to several months. During this stage, if there is a partial or full immobilization of the injured limb, the progressive loss of skeletal muscle is the main effect caused by muscle disuse (see *Chapter 9*). Besides the loss of muscle, other tissues, such as tendons, may also be impacted. The second stage — rehabilitation phase — follows the return to mobility. In this phase, the primary nutritional goal is to support muscle growth and strength-induced return to activity. Generally, nutritional recommendations aimed at rehabilitation are, in a way, like non-injured athletes who aim to increase muscle mass [137]. Thus, the main nutritional focus should be on energy and protein intake recommendations.

Energy

Energy intake must be considered when carrying out a food plan aimed to recover from an injury. Recommendations in these cases are sometimes counterintuitive. Given the decrease in activity and, in turn, the energy expenditure, reducing energy intake seems to be the most obvious recommendation [136]. Nevertheless, during prolonged periods of reduced activity, as is the case with sports injuries, energy expenditure might not be as low as expected. In fact, a case study done with players from the Premier League showed that the mean daily energy intake and energy expenditure was 2,765 ± 474 and 3,178 kcal·day, respectively [33]. Depending on the severity of the injury, this can be explained by a 15–50% increase in basal metabolic rate during recovery, which is related to its impact on muscle protein synthesis [136]. Athletes and practitioners should strive to maintain energy balance, as an excessive caloric surplus or deficit have both been associated with accelerated muscle atrophy [138, 139].

Protein

The most frequently associated macronutrient to the recovery from an injury is protein, which can be explained for its role in muscle, tendon, and other soft tissues' function and structure. During immobilization, muscle protein synthesis is suppressed, causing a decreased response to protein and an increase in muscle atrophy. This suppression of muscle protein synthesis has also been noted during age-related sarcopenia, and muscle loss during times of significant weight loss. Higher protein intakes have been linked to higher protein synthesis within older populations where anabolic resistance is expected, thus it is thought higher protein intakes may also have a sparing effect within injured athletes as well [140]. A protein intake upwards of 2.0–2.5 g·kg per day has been recommended to preserve muscle mass during immobilization [136]. Regarding the amount of protein, in an active muscle, a dose of 0.25–0.40 g·kg is sufficient to maximize a resting and/or exercised muscle protein synthesis [141, 142]. However, given the anabolic resistance that occurs with immobilization and/or reduced activity, it is expected that the amount needed to optimize muscle protein synthesis in an immobilized muscle would be higher. Injured athletes may then need to consume as much as 0.4–0.55 g kg protein each meal to achieve the higher total protein intake while maximizing muscle protein synthesis as best as possible [143].

As aforementioned, protein should be distributed into four to five feedings across the day if feasible. Bearing this in mind, it makes sense to recommend injured athletes to plan their meals in a way that stimulates muscle protein synthesis and, and the same time, mitigates muscle mass loss. Reaching this quantity of protein through food alone may prove to be challenging for some athletes.

Particularly early on after an injury, when appetite may be suppressed, the use of whey protein may assist the athlete in achieving their total protein needs in a high quality and low volume source of protein.

Creatine, omega-3, and collagen

As aforementioned, one of the main reasons why creatine is used in an array of sports is related to its effect on enhancing muscular hypertrophy which is amplified by resistance exercise [102]. In the scope of sports injuries, the use of creatine in muscle mass loss mitigation has been investigated. During immobilization, creatine within skeletal muscle decreases significantly [144]. It has also shown to have a positive effect on the increase of the expression of 'glucose transporters type 4' (GLUT4) located in the skeletal muscle which is related to increased insulin sensitivity [145]. Results are mixed regarding whether creatine supplementation can reduce muscle atrophy during times of immobilization. More studies are needed to determine its impact on muscle mass loss in different muscle groups before definitive recommendations can be made so that an adequate dosage is established. Despite this, it may be advisable to supplement with creatine since it is affordable, may help preserve muscle in some cases, and is likely to be beneficial once the athlete initiates the resistance training portion of their rehabilitation.

Omega-3 fatty acids are often related with treatment of sports injuries for its anti-inflammatory and immunomodulatory properties. Its supplementation seems to be particularly important in cases where inflammation is excessive and prolonged [137]. Recently, omega-3 has gained interest related to its potential for sparing muscle mass during times of increased atrophy risk. As aforementioned, during immobilization, muscle protein synthesis appears to be suppressed. Omega-3 is believed to potentially enhance muscle protein synthesis at times when it would usually be suppressed, such as injury or age-related sarcopenia [140]. Research indicated that those who supplemented 5 g of omega-3 daily for four weeks (prior to two weeks of leg immobilization), resulted in muscle protein synthesis and partially protected quadriceps volume compared to the placebo trial [146]. Omega-3 may require as many as four weeks in order to increase omega-3 composition within skeletal muscle [146]. Recognizing that muscle atrophy can occur within days after an injury, and that the full benefits of omega-3 may take several weeks to occur, it may be advisable for athletes to take omega-3 persistently throughout the season in preparation just an in case an injury were to occur [140].

Collagen is the most abundant protein in the human body, being responsible for the elasticity and firmness of tendons, ligaments, connective tissues, and it represents the most predominant compounds in the extracellular matrix of skeletal muscle. Collagen seems to be highly sensitive to mechanical load resulting from the practice of sports that involve frequent accelerations and decelerations or that are characterized by constant moments of impact, which, in turn, can translate into structural damage to muscle fibers and the surrounding extracellular matrix. In this sense, a study demonstrated that the ingestion of

10 g of collagen resulted in increased collagen synthesis in the knee's cartilage of athletes with a history of pain and discomfort due to mechanical stress, injury, or in the postoperative period [147]. It has been noted that amino acids, in conjunction within collagen, peak approximately one hour after consumption [148]. By exercising during this window, it is suggested that these amino acids can be directed toward the area of need while at their peak. The underlying mechanism is not fully understood, but it is speculated that it is related to increased collagen synthesis in the connective tissues around the muscle and the modulation of the inflammatory response to exercise, which appears to result in the early remodelling of the injured structure [149]. Although studies on nutritional interventions aimed at sports injuries recovery are scarce, some advances in the understanding of the mechanism of collagen action are being published. In addition, there is adequate evidence from other non-athlete populations that can be applied to athletes, as is the case of the literature associated with wound healing models, trauma, surgery, and sarcopenia. Currently, collagen recommendations are for 15–20 g of either gelatin, hydrolysed collagen or collagen peptides approximately one hour prior to activity. Vitamin C is required for the cross-linking of collagen, so players should either incorporate approximately 50 mg of Vitamin C with the collagen supplement if fasted, or should consume Vitamin C through food sources sometime prior to supplementation. More work in the area of collagen needs to be performed, and we still lack data comparing collagen to other forms of protein, such as whey, in relation to tendon, ligament, and bone health.

Recovery modalities

As aforementioned, the importance of sleep and nutrition have been heavily prioritized for enhancing performance and recovery in elite soccer. Given the high density of training sessions and fixtures, in addition to adequate nutrition and sleep strategies, coaches and practitioners often implement recovery modalities to enhance recovery [9]. Cold modalities such as contrast therapy (CWT) and cold-water immersion (CWI) are the most common recovery strategies implemented in most team sports [150, 151], including soccer [7]. Additionally, massage therapy is often implemented in elite soccer environments. Massage methods have now been presented in multiple variations in elite soccer. Alongside passive modalities for enhancing recovery, active recovery sessions are often implemented and programmed in elite soccer settings.

Cold water and physiology

Physiological responses to cold therapies are well described in the literature [151–153]. The exposure to cold decreases skin, core, and muscle temperatures, leading to vasoconstriction and decreasing swelling and acute inflammation from muscle damage [154]. A reduction in tissue temperature is also associated with a decreased nerve conduction properties and muscle spasm and pain [155]. In addition, cold modalities involving immersion in water lead to hydrostatic pressure-induced changes in blood flow, with some research studies suggesting a beneficial effect by promoting metabolic waste removal [156, 157]. When athletes alternate between cold and hot water immersion (contrast water therapy; CWT), the hot water increases vasodilation, leading to an increase in blood flow and facilitation of oxygen and antibody supply, metabolite clearance, and a reduction in muscle spasm and pain [9, 156, 158]. Although the scientific literature suggests a beneficial effect of CWI and CWT improving recovery, some authors observed that chronically exposing subjects to may blunt anabolic responses from training, which, in turn, affects muscle size adaptations [159]. Nevertheless, several limitations have been raised regarding previous research investigating the chronic effects of cold modalities and their practical application to athletes. For example, the training frequency (two to three training sessions per week) used in these studies potentially allow for full recovery between sessions, limiting the rationale for the inclusion of cold modalities [160].

When designing and implementing cold water immersion protocols, the paradox between the implementation of cold modalities to acutely (i.e. 24–48 h post-exercise) enhance recovery and readiness to train, and the potential harmful effects on the long-term adaptations to training (i.e. decreases in muscle size) need to be contemplated.

Factors affecting cold water immersion methodology

The factors contributing to water-immersion recovery protocols designing have been reviewed elsewhere [158]. These factors can be divided in protocol characteristics, individual and external factors (Table 8.1).

Protocol characteristics

The intensity of a protocol can be determined by the effect that protocol has reducing core and muscle temperature (Table 8.1). The body area in contact with water, the water temperature, and duration of immersion can be manipulated in order to increase or decrease the protocol intensity [158]. Recent literature suggests the water temperature to range between 10°C and 15°C to promote a decrease in core and deep muscle temperature, with lower temperatures

Table 8.1 Protocol characteristics and individual and external factors to be considered when designing a water immersion recovery protocol

Protocol characteristics	Individual factors	External factors
Duration of exposure to cold Immersion depth Temperature used	Physique traits Sex	Phase of the season Density of the weekly schedule Goals of the athlete (long-term and short-term)

Source: Adapted from Tavares et al. [158].

representing an increase in the protocol intensity [151, 153, 161]. In terms of duration, a total time of 5–15 minutes is normally used with longer immersion times being associated with a greater decrease in body temperature. Given that body temperature occurs in a gradual manner, as opposed to instantaneously, and superficial tissue temperatures reduce and rewarm significantly quicker than deeper tissues, dividing the total time (i.e. 12 min) in two to three sets may be more tolerable while having similar effects on deep tissue temperature. The immersion depth is another variable that can be manipulated. The area of the body that is submersed affects the intensity as a larger surface area in contact with the cold represents more heat transfer from the body to the water and vice-versa, resulting on a greater thermal stress. Furthermore, the deeper the immersion, the greater the impact of hydrostatic pressure on the body.

Internal characteristics

When compared to muscle and skin, fat provides a greater thermal transfer insulation. For this reason, differences in body composition (i.e. muscle mass and body fat) seem to justify individual responses to cold modalities [162]. The ratio between body surface area and body mass (BSA:BM) also affects thermal responses as a larger BM increases heat production and retention, and a larger BSA increases evaporation, convection, and conduction of heat. Therefore, athletes with high fat mass and/or lower BSA:BM require more severe cold protocols to reduce muscle and core temperature to a same extend than athletes with a greater BSA:BM. Although these characteristics are of upmost importance in sports such as American Football or Rugby, this individualization can also be important when considering athletes from different positions in soccer. Furthermore, given the association between sex and body fat or BSA:BM (i.e., females > males), different responses to water immersion recovery protocols can be expected.

External characteristics

When considering the implementation of CWI/CWT, there are a few questions about the training content and weekly density that should be addressed in order to help practitioners deciding *how* and *when* to implement cold modalities:

- How physically demanding was the training sessions – Was the player exposed to a training session that is likely to lead to significant levels of delayed onset muscle soreness?
- When will the next training session occur – Will the next training session occur within 36h?
- What are the goals of the next training session – In the subsequent training sessions players will be required to produce high mechanical outputs?

If the answer to all these three questions is *yes*, there is potentially a rational to include cold modalities protocols during the training week. For example, there is a clear distinction between the density of the training week of professional

Table 8.2 Example of a cold recovery scheme for elite and amateur team-sport athletes during an in-season week

		Match day	Off	Day 1	Day 2	Day 3	Day 4	Day 5	Match Day
Elite	Training load	Very high	Day off	Low to moderate	High	Low	Moderate to high	Low	Very high
	Intensity of cold modalities	Recovery from damage		Recover to adapt			Recover to perform		
		+++			+		++	+++	
	Example	CWI: 2 × 5 min (8–10°C); full body			CWT: 3× (1 min cold:2 min hot); lower body		CWT: 3× (2 min cold:1 min hot); full body	CWI: 2 × 5 min (11–15°C); lower body	
Amateur	Training load	Very high	Day off	Low	Moderate to high	Day off	Moderate to low	Low or day off	Very high
	Intensity of cold modalities	Recovery from damage		Recover to adapt				Recover to perform	
		+++					+	++	
	Example	CWI: 2 × 5 min (11–15°C); full body					CWT: 3× (1 min cold:2 min hot); lower body	CWT: 3× (2 min cold:1 min hot); lower body	

Source: Adapted from Tavares et al. [158].

adult soccer players and young amateur soccer players, with the last being likely to have lower physical demands during training and competition with longer periods to recovery from load due to a lower number of training sessions. For this reason, it seems reasonable to appropriate alter cold modality prescriptions to each scenario. An example of the intensities that can be used in the amateur and elite scenarios can be seen in Table 8.2.

As aforementioned, exposing athletes to cold modalities may interfere with muscle mass adaptations. Thus, during non-competition periods that involve training designed for increases in muscle mass, it seems counterproductive to reduce the inflammatory response from exercise by exposing athletes to CWI or CWT. It is important to mention that even during periods without competition, the type of training is adjusted according to individual needs. For example, some athletes can be aiming to increase peak power output, therefore, requiring for athletes to perform in a non-fatigued state. Given this, during non-competition training phases, such as pre-season, CWI or CWT can aid in training quality, resulting in an increased potential for training adaptations. For the aforementioned reason, it is important to understand that the advice to completely avoid cold modalities within preseason or another preparatory period is not conclusive.

Similarly, during the in-season period, the inclusion and manipulation of cold modalities protocols need to be adjusted according to the individual training goals, including potential selection to play on game day, training age, and competitive goals. For example, it is common to observe age-group athletes training within elite senior squads. Normally, these athletes have lower training ages and therefore have lower body weight and muscle mass in comparison with senior players. Therefore, it might be reasonable to pursue further gains in muscle mass even during competitive periods, resulting in the need to limit cold exposure in less experienced athletes. Furthermore, if an athlete is less likely to be selected for some weeks, and increases in muscle mass are desirable, practitioners may want to limit the use of cold modalities. On the contrary, more experienced and older athletes, that are regularly exposed to greater training loads and match time, may benefit from an increase in the intensity of the cold protocols.

Massage therapy

While the application of massage therapy has been around for decades, there has been a lack of comparable methods in research, resulting in mostly anecdotal accounts [163]. Massage therapy can often be applied via manual (or manipulative) therapy, or percussion massager [164].

Manual massage

Manual massage therapy refers to a variety of techniques that a licensed massage therapist (LMT) applies in order to help reduce the severity of fatigue. Although an LMT has the ability to vary techniques and approaches, research suggests that Effleurage and Petrissage are the most effective in terms of reducing exercise-induced fatigue for athletes after training sessions and/or sport [165]. The most common durations for manual massage application in sport are 10–30 minutes [166]. However, some evidence suggests that shorter durations (5–12 minutes) have shown superior outcomes in performance markers compared to those exposed to longer massage therapy sessions (>13 minutes) [167]. With little consensus on the methods, and durations, for manual massage application in sport, the largest analysis of sports massage (to date) concluded that there is no evidence that sports massage improves performance directly [168]. Due to the popularization of massage in elite soccer, it is suggested that massage therapy should not be avoided, presuming practitioners abide by the notion to 'do no harm' [169].

Percussion massager

A novel application to massage therapy has been the use of a percussion massage, or massage gun. Due to the novel innovation of these apparatuses, the validity of results remains unclear. However, similar to manual massage therapy, massage guns have shown to increase range of motion (ROM) and potentially reduce the perception of muscle soreness [170]. Therefore, with no added negative repercussions associated with the use of massage guns, it is advised that practitioners can recommend the use of percussion massage prior to warm-ups [171].

Active recovery

While often viewed as tradition in elite soccer, active recovery sessions have been prescribed for decades. Despite the lack of evidence surrounding the efficiency of active recovery sessions in the athlete population, it seems as though the majority of professional soccer teams are allocating training days around active recovery [7, 172]. Although no significant evidence (to date) has been noted between the effectiveness of active vs passive recovery sessions in soccer, it has still been advised that practitioners place high importance on recovery [173]. In elite soccer, regeneration (regen) sessions are often implemented within 24 h post-game (Match-day plus one; MD+1). From a practical perspective, planning for players to attend the training facility on MD+1 allows the coaching staff to conduct video sessions to reflect on team and individual performance. Therefore, practitioners have the ability to utilize a variety of resources to enhance recovery within that time-period. If active recovery sessions are not favoured by the practitioner, the MD+1 recovery can be catered towards additional modalities, such as CWI, CWT, and/or massage. Preference of recovery prescription is often individual; therefore, given the mixed evidence on active recovery procedures, practitioners should cater recovery modalities individually [173].

Compression

Compression garments are readily available to players for a variety of body areas. Many of the compression garment manufacturers offer different types of garments, catering for activity type. Specifically, some common types of compression garments are labelled 'running', 'recovery', and even 'flight'. With more wearable compression gear available to players, begs the question to their effectiveness and practicality. While the idea of compression garments for lower extremities is to increase femoral blood flow, the use of compression for mid-activity or post-activity, for recovery still remains questioned [174]. For use in the recovery process, compression garments have not shown to benefit repeat-sprint performance, peak power outputs, isokinetic strength, sprint, agility, or countermovement jump performance [7]. Additionally, compression garments have not shown any additional recovery benefits, compared to other modalities [7]. However, some research in elite soccer has shown that players who wear compression garments in games could potentially reduce perceived muscle soreness and increase physical outputs [175]. Due to having no associated negative outcomes, it is suggested that lower limb compression garments are made available to players to wear during games, dependent on their comfort level. There have been several proposed benefits associated with wearing compression garments, such as thermal effects, venous return, and decrease of muscle oscillation [176]. Therefore, it is suggested that practitioners investigate the use of compression garments for their players when exposed to long flights.

Conclusion

With the high physical demands of elite soccer, it is integral that practitioners understand how positive and negative responses occur from training stimulus. More importantly, understanding how to enhance positive adaptations from training is vital. Sleep and nutrition have been identified as the best recovery strategies for elite soccer players. However, practitioners also have the ability to prescribe additional modalities to aid the recovery process. Overall, it is suggested that practitioners have knowledge of the training load and how to periodize recovery strategies to better prepare soccer players to withstand training and matches.

References

1 Bompa, T.O. and C. Buzzichelli, *Periodization-: Theory and methodology of training*. 6 ed. 2019, Champaign: Human Kinetics. 381.
2 Barnett, A., *Using recovery modalities between training sessions in elite athletes*. Sports Medicine, 2006. **36**(9): p. 781–796.
3 McArdle, W.D., *Sports and exercise nutrition*. 2018: Lippincott Williams & Wilkins.

4 Roy, B.A., *Overreaching/overtraining: More is not always better.* ACSM's Health & Fitness Journal, 2015. **19**(2): p. 4–5.
5 Kreher, J.B. and J.B. Schwartz, *Overtraining syndrome: A practical guide.* Sports Health, 2012. **4**(2): p. 128–138.
6 Bishop, P.A., E. Jones, and A.K. Woods, *Recovery from training: A brief review: Brief review.* The Journal of Strength & Conditioning Research, 2008. **22**(3): p. 1015–1024.
7 Nédélec, M., et al., *Recovery in soccer.* Sports Medicine, 2013. **43**(1): p. 9–22.
8 Kenttä, G. and P. Hassmén, *Overtraining and recovery.* Sports Medicine, 1998. **26**(1): p. 1–16.
9 Tavares, F., T.B. Smith, and M. Driller, *Fatigue and recovery in rugby: A review.* Sports Medicine, 2017. **47**(8): p. 1515–1530.
10 Cadegiani, F.A. and C.E. Kater, *Hormonal aspects of overtraining syndrome: A systematic review.* BMC Sports Science, Medicine and Rehabilitation, 2017. **9**(1): p. 1–15.
11 Lee, Y.-H., B.N.R. Park, and S.H. Kim, *The effects of heat and massage application on autonomic nervous system.* Yonsei Medical Journal, 2011. **52**(6): p. 982–989.
12 Shaffer, F. and J.P. Ginsberg, *An overview of heart rate variability metrics and norms.* Frontiers in Public Health, 2017: **5**: p. 258.
13 Plews, D.J., et al., *Heart rate variability in elite triathletes, is variation in variability the key to effective training? A case comparison.* European Journal of Applied Physiology, 2012. **112**(11): p. 3729–3741.
14 Halson, S.L., *Nutrition, sleep and recovery.* European Journal of Sport Science, 2008. **8**(2): p. 119–126.
15 Halson, S.L. and L.E. Juliff, *Sleep, sport, and the brain.* Progress in Brain Research, 2017. **234**: p. 13–31.
16 Marshall, G.J. and A.N. Turner, *The importance of sleep for athletic performance.* Strength & Conditioning Journal, 2016. **38**(1): p. 61–67.
17 Fullagar, H.H., et al., *Sleep and athletic performance: The effects of sleep loss on exercise performance, and physiological and cognitive responses to exercise.* Sports Medicine, 2015. **45**(2): p. 161–186.
18 Vitale, K.C., et al., *Sleep hygiene for optimizing recovery in athletes: Review and recommendations.* International Journal of Sports Medicine, 2019. **40**(08): p. 535–543.
19 Walsh, N.P., et al., *Sleep and the athlete: Narrative review and 2021 expert consensus recommendations.* British Journal of Sports Medicine, 2021. **55**(7): p. 356–368.
20 Halson, S.L., *Sleep and the elite athlete.* Sports Science, 2013. **26**(113): p. 1–4.
21 Lastella, M., G.D. Roach, and C. Sargent, *Travel fatigue and sleep/wake behaviors of professional soccer players during international competition.* Sleep Health, 2019. **5**(2): p. 141–147.
22 Nédélec, M., et al., *Stress, sleep and recovery in elite soccer: A critical review of the literature.* Sports Medicine, 2015. **45**(10): p. 1387–1400.
23 Fullagar, H.H., et al., *Sleep, travel, and recovery responses of national footballers during and after long-haul international air travel.* International Journal of Sports Physiology and Performance, 2016. **11**(1): p. 86–95.
24 Zimberg, I.Z., et al., *Short sleep duration and obesity: Mechanisms and future perspectives.* Cell Biochemistry and Function, 2012. **30**(6): p. 524–529.
25 Dickstein, J.B. and H. Moldofsky, *Sleep, cytokines and immune function.* Sleep Medicine Reviews, 1999. **3**(3): p. 219–228.
26 Weingarten, J.A. and N.A. Collop, *Air travel: Effects of sleep deprivation and jet lag.* Chest, 2013. **144**(4): p. 1394–1401.
27 Casazza, G.A., et al., *Energy availability, macronutrient intake, and nutritional supplementation for improving exercise performance in endurance athletes.* Current Sports Medicine Reports, 2018. **17**(6): p. 215–223.
28 Maurer, J., *Nutrition for the Athlete*, in R. Donatelli (Eds.) Sports-Specific Rehabilitation. 2007, Churchill Livingstone. p. 279–292.

29 Beck, K.L., et al., *Role of nutrition in performance enhancement and postexercise recovery.* Open Access Journal of Sports Medicine, 2015. **6**: p. 259.
30 Julian, R., R.M. Page, and L.D. Harper, *The effect of fixture congestion on performance during professional male soccer match-play: A systematic critical review with meta-analysis.* Sports Medicine, 2021. **51**(2): p. 255–273.
31 Padua, D.A. and J.A. Oñate, *Training load, recovery, and injury: A simple or complex relationship?* Journal of Athletic Training, 2020. **55**(9): p. 873–873.
32 Polman, R. and K. Houlahan, *A cumulative stress and training continuum model: A multidisciplinary approach to unexplained underperformance syndrome.* Research in Sports Medicine, 2004. **12**(4): p. 301–316.
33 Anderson, L., et al., *Energy intake and expenditure of professional soccer players of the English Premier League: Evidence of carbohydrate periodization.* International Journal of Sport Nutrition and Exercise Metabolism, 2017. **27**(3): p. 228–238.
34 Rico-Sanz, J., *Body composition and nutritional assessments in soccer.* International Journal of Sport Nutrition and Exercise Metabolism, 1998. **8**(2): p. 113–123.
35 Caruana Bonnici, D., et al., *Nutrition in soccer: A brief review of the issues and solutions.* Journal of Science in Sport and Exercise, 2019. **1**(1): p. 3–12.
36 García-Rovés, P.M., et al., *Nutrient intake and food habits of soccer players: Analyzing the correlates of eating practice.* Nutrients, 2014. **6**(7): p. 2697–2717.
37 Ruiz, F., et al., *Nutritional intake in soccer players of different ages.* Journal of Sports Sciences, 2005. **23**(3): p. 235–242.
38 Brinkmans, N.Y., et al., *Energy expenditure and dietary intake in professional football players in the Dutch Premier League: Implications for nutritional counselling.* Journal of Sports Sciences, 2019. **37**(24): p. 2759–2767.
39 Steffl, M., et al., *Macronutrient intake in soccer players—A meta-analysis.* Nutrients, 2019. **11**(6): p. 1305.
40 Collins, J., et al., *UEFA expert group statement on nutrition in elite football. Current evidence to inform practical recommendations and guide future research.* British Journal of Sports Medicine, 2021. **55**(8): p. 416–416.
41 Zehnder, M., et al., *Resynthesis of muscle glycogen after soccer specific performance examined by 13C-magnetic resonance spectroscopy in elite players.* European Journal of Applied Physiology, 2001. **84**(5): p. 443–447.
42 Jonnalagadda, S.S., C.A. Rosenbloom, and R. Skinner, *Dietary practices, attitudes, and physiological status of collegiate freshman football players.* Journal of Strength and Conditioning Research, 2001. **15**(4): p. 507–513.
43 Moore, D.R., et al., *Protein ingestion to stimulate myofibrillar protein synthesis requires greater relative protein intakes in healthy older versus younger men.* Journals of Gerontology Series A: Biomedical Sciences and Medical Sciences, 2015. **70**(1): p. 57–62.
44 Levenhagen, D.K., et al., *Postexercise nutrient intake timing in humans is critical to recovery of leg glucose and protein homeostasis.* American Journal of Physiology-Endocrinology and Metabolism, 2001. **280**(6): p. E982–E993.
45 Moore, D.R., et al., *Differential stimulation of myofibrillar and sarcoplasmic protein synthesis with protein ingestion at rest and after resistance exercise.* The Journal of Physiology, 2009. **587**(4): p. 897–904.
46 Williams, J.H., *The science behind soccer nutrition.* 2012: CreateSpace.
47 Ono, M., et al., *Nutrition and culture in professional football. A mixed method approach.* Appetite, 2012. **58**(1): p. 98–104.
48 Flatt, J., *Carbohydrate balance and food intake regulation.* The American Journal of Clinical Nutrition, 1995. **62**(1): p. 155–157.
49 Jeong, T.-S., et al., *Acute simulated soccer-specific training increases PGC-1α mRNA expression in human skeletal muscle.* Journal of Sports Sciences, 2015. **33**(14): p. 1493–1503.

50 Shirreffs, S.M., et al., *The sweating response of elite professional soccer players to training in the heat.* International Journal of Sports Medicine, 2005. **26**(02): p. 90–95.
51 Marquet, L.-A., et al., *Enhanced endurance performance by periodization of Cho intake: 'sleep low' strategy.* Medicine and Science in Sports and Exercise, 2016. **48**(4): p. 663–672.
52 Hawley, J.A., et al., *Maximizing cellular adaptation to endurance exercise in skeletal muscle.* Cell Metabolism, 2018. **27**(5): p. 962–976.
53 Fernandes, H.S., *Carbohydrate Consumption and periodization strategies applied to elite soccer players.* Current Nutrition Reports, 2020. **9**(4): p. 414–419.
54 Lemon, P.W., *Protein requirements of soccer.* Journal of Sports Science, 1994. **12**: p. S17–22.
55 Wolfe, R.R. and S.L. Miller, *The recommended dietary allowance of protein: A misunderstood concept.* Jama, 2008. **299**(24): p. 2891–2893.
56 EFSA Panel on Dietetic Products, N. and Allergies, *Scientific opinion on dietary reference values for protein.* EFSA Journal, 2012. **10**(2): p. 2557.
57 Phillips, S.M., *Dietary protein for athletes: From requirements to metabolic advantage.* Applied Physiology, Nutrition, and Metabolism, 2006. **31**(6): p. 647–654.
58 Anderson, L., et al., *Daily distribution of macronutrient intakes of professional soccer players from the English Premier League.* International Journal of Sport Nutrition and Exercise Metabolism, 2017. **27**(6): p. 491–498.
59 Morton, R.W., et al., *A systematic review, meta-analysis and meta-regression of the effect of protein supplementation on resistance training-induced gains in muscle mass and strength in healthy adults.* British Journal of Sports Medicine, 2018. **52**(6): p. 376–384.
60 Burke, L.M., et al., *Low carbohydrate, high fat diet impairs exercise economy and negates the performance benefit from intensified training in elite race walkers.* The Journal of Physiology, 2017. **595**(9): p. 2785–2807.
61 Rodriguez, N.R., N.M. DiMarco, and S. Langley, *Position of the American dietetic association, dietitians of Canada, and the American college of sports medicine: Nutrition and athletic performance.* Journal of the American Dietetic Association, 2009. **109**(3): p. 509–527.
62 Potgieter, S., *Sport nutrition: A review of the latest guidelines for exercise and sport nutrition from the American College of sport nutrition, the international Olympic committee and the international society for sports nutrition.* South African Journal of Clinical Nutrition, 2013. **26**(1): p. 6–16.
63 Burke, L., *Low carb high fat (LCHF) diets for athletes–Third time lucky?* Journal of Science and Medicine in Sport, 2017. **20**: p. S1.
64 Saltin, B., *Metabolic fundamentals in exercise.* Medicine and Science in Sports, 1973. **5**(3): p. 137–146.
65 Hulton, A.T., et al., *Energy requirements and nutritional strategies for male soccer players: A review and suggestions for practice.* Nutrients, 2022. **14**(3): p. 657.
66 Armstrong, L.E., et al., *Urinary indices during dehydration, exercise, and rehydration.* International Journal of Sport Nutrition and Exercise Metabolism, 1998. **8**(4): p. 345–355.
67 Ersoy, N., G. Ersoy, and M. Kutlu, *Assessment of hydration status of elite young male soccer players with different methods and new approach method of substitute urine strip.* Journal of the International Society of Sports Nutrition, 2016. **13**(1): p. 34.
68 Larson-Meyer, D.E., K. Woolf, and L. Burke, *Assessment of nutrient status in athletes and the need for supplementation.* International Journal of Sport Nutrition and Exercise Metabolism, 2018. **28**(2): p. 139–158.

69 Krustrup, P., et al., *Muscle and blood metabolites during a soccer game: Implications for sprint performance.* Medicine and Science in Sports and Exercise, 2006. **38**(6): p. 1165–1174.
70 Oliveira, C.C., et al., *Nutrition and supplementation in soccer.* Sports, 2017. **5**(2): p. 28.
71 Guest, N.S., et al., *International society of sports nutrition position stand: Caffeine and exercise performance.* Journal of the International Society of Sports Nutrition, 2021. **18**(1): p. 1.
72 Armstrong, L.E., et al., *Human hydration indices: Acute and longitudinal reference values.* International Journal of Sport Nutrition & Exercise Metabolism, 2010. **20**(2): p. 145–153.
73 Collins, J. and I. Rollo, *Practical considerations in elite football.* Sports Science Exchange, 2014. **27**(133): p. 1–7.
74 Abreu, R., et al., *Portuguese football federation consensus statement 2020: Nutrition and performance in football.* BMJ Open Sport & Exercise Medicine, 2021. **7**(3): p. e001082–e001082.
75 Adams, W.M. and D.J. Casa, *Hydration for football athletes.* Sports Science Exchange, 2015. **28**(141): p. 1–5.
76 Nuccio, R.P., et al., *Fluid balance in team sport athletes and the effect of hypohydration on cognitive, technical, and physical performance.* Sports Medicine, 2017. **47**(10): p. 1951–1982.
77 Kiitam, U., et al., *Pre-practice hydration status in soccer (Football) players in a cool environment.* Medicina, 2018. **54**(6): p. 102.
78 Sawka, M.N., et al., *American college of sports medicine position stand. Exercise and fluid replacement.* Medicine and Science in Sports and Exercise, 2007. **39**(2): p. 377–390.
79 Baker, L.B., et al., *Acute effects of carbohydrate supplementation on intermittent sports performance.* Nutrients, 2015. **7**(7): p. 5733–5763.
80 Nilsson, L.H., P. Fürst, and E. Hultman, *Carbohydrate metabolism of the liver in normal man under varying dietary conditions.* Scandinavian Journal of Clinical and Laboratory Investigation, 1973. **32**(4): p. 331–337.
81 Williams, C. and L. Serratosa, *Nutrition on match day.* Journal of Sports Science, 2006. **24**(7): p. 687–697.
82 Rollo, I., et al., *The influence of carbohydrate mouth rinse on self-selected intermittent running performance.* International Journal of Sport Nutrition and Exercise Metabolism, 2015. **25**(6): p. 550–558.
83 Jeukendrup, A.E., I. Rollo, and J.M. Carter, *Carbohydrate mouth rinse: Performance effects and mechanisms.* Sports Science Exchange, 2013. **26**(118): p. 1–8.
84 Carter, J.M., A.E. Jeukendrup, and D.A. Jones, *The effect of carbohydrate mouth rinse on 1-h cycle time trial performance.* Medicine and Science in Sports and Exercise, 2004. **36**(12): p. 2107–2111.
85 Miller, K.C., et al., *Reflex inhibition of electrically induced muscle cramps in hypohydrated humans.* Medicine and Science in Sports and Exercise, 2010. **42**(5): p. 953–961.
86 Ivy, J., et al., *Muscle glycogen synthesis after exercise: Effect of time of carbohydrate ingestion.* Journal of Applied Physiology, 1988. **64**(4): p. 1480–1485.
87 Burke, L., *Fueling strategies to optimize performance: Training high or training low?* Scandinavian Journal of Medicine & Science in Sports, 2010. **20**: p. 48–58.
88 J. Maughan, R. and S. Shirreffs, *Recovery from prolonged exercise: Restoration of water and electrolyte balance.* Journal of Sports Sciences, 1997. **15**(3): p. 297–303.
89 Shirreffs, S.M. and R.J. Maughan, *Volume repletion after exercise-induced volume depletion in humans: Replacement of water and sodium losses.* American Journal of Physiology-renal Physiology, 1998. **274**(5): p. F868–F875.
90 Shirreffs, S.M., *Restoration of fluid and electrolyte balance after exercise.* Canadian Journal of Applied Physiology, 2001. **26**(S1): p. S228–S235.

91 Desbrow, B., et al., *Comparing the rehydration potential of different milk-based drinks to a carbohydrate-electrolyte beverage.* Applied Physiology, Nutrition, and Metabolism, 2014. **39**(12): p. 1366–72.
92 Evans, G.H., et al., *Optimizing the restoration and maintenance of fluid balance after exercise-induced dehydration.* Journal of Applied Physiology (1985), 2017. **122**(4): p. 945–951.
93 Koopman, R., et al., *Nutritional interventions to promote post-exercise muscle protein synthesis.* Sports Medicine, 2007. **37**(10): p. 895–906.
94 Morton, R.W., C. McGlory, and S.M. Phillips, *Nutritional interventions to augment resistance training-induced skeletal muscle hypertrophy.* Frontiers in Physiology, 2015. **6**: p. 245.
95 van Loon, L.J., *Role of dietary protein in post-exercise muscle reconditioning,* in K,D, Tipton, & L.J, van Loon (Eds.), *Nutritional Coaching Strategy to Modulate Training Efficiency.* 2013, Karger Publishers. p. 73–83.
96 Beelen, M., et al., *Nutritional strategies to promote postexercise recovery.* International Journal of Sport Nutrition and Exercise Metabolism, 2010. **20**(6): p. 515–532.
97 Abbott, W., et al., *Presleep casein protein ingestion: Acceleration of functional recovery in professional soccer players.* International Journal of Sports Physiology and Performance, 2019. **14**(3): p. 385–391.
98 Ranchordas, M.K., J.T. Dawson, and M. Russell, *Practical nutritional recovery strategies for elite soccer players when limited time separates repeated matches.* Journal of the International Society of Sports Nutrition, 2017. **14**(1): p. 1–14.
99 Knapik, J.J., et al., *Prevalence of dietary supplement use by athletes: Systematic review and meta-analysis.* Sports Medicine, 2016. **46**(1): p. 103–123.
100 Maughan, R.J., et al., *IOC consensus statement: Dietary supplements and the high-performance athlete.* International Journal of Sport Nutrition and Exercise Metabolism, 2018. **28**(2): p. 104–125.
101 Poortmans, J.R., et al., *A-Z of nutritional supplements: Dietary supplements, sports nutrition foods and ergogenic aids for health and performance Part 11.* British Journal of Sports Medicine, 2010. **44**(10): p. 765–766.
102 Bemben, M.G. and H.S. Lamont, *Creatine supplementation and exercise performance.* Sports Medicine, 2005. **35**(2): p. 107–125.
103 Rawson, E.S. and P.M. Clarkson, *Scientifically debatable: Is creatine worth its weight.* Sports Science Exchange, 2003. **16**(4): p. 1–6.
104 Claudino, J.G., et al., *Creatine monohydrate supplementation on lower-limb muscle power in Brazilian elite soccer players.* Journal of the International Society of Sports Nutrition, 2014. **11**(1): p. 1–6.
105 Terjung, R.L., et al., *American college of sports medicine roundtable. The physiological and health effects of oral creatine supplementation.* Medicine and Science in Sports and Exercise, 2000. **32**(3): p. 706–717.
106 Kreider, R.B., et al., *International society of sports nutrition position stand: Safety and efficacy of creatine supplementation in exercise, sport, and medicine.* Journal of the International Society of Sports Nutrition, 2017. **14**(1): p. 18.
107 Robinson, T.M., et al., *Role of submaximal exercise in promoting creatine and glycogen accumulation in human skeletal muscle.* Journal of Applied Physiology, 1999. **87**(2): p. 598–604.
108 Cooper, R., et al., *Creatine supplementation with specific view to exercise/sports performance: An update.* Journal of the International Society of Sports Nutrition, 2012. **9**(1): p. 1–11.
109 Artioli, G.G., et al., *Role of beta-alanine supplementation on muscle carnosine and exercise performance.* Medicine and Science in Sports and Exercise, 2010. **42**(6): p. 1162–1173.
110 Perim, P., et al., *Can the skeletal muscle carnosine response to beta-alanine supplementation be optimized?* Frontiers in Nutrition, 2019. **6**: p. 135.

111 Hill, C., et al., *Influence of β-alanine supplementation on skeletal muscle carnosine concentrations and high intensity cycling capacity.* Amino Acids, 2007. **32**(2): p. 225–233.
112 Saunders, B., et al., *Twenty-four weeks of β-alanine supplementation on carnosine content, related genes, and exercise.* Medicine and Science in Sports and Exercise, 2017. **49**(5): p. 896–906.
113 Perim, P., et al., *Can the skeletal muscle carnosine response to beta-alanine supplementation be optimized?* Frontiers in Nutrition, 2019. **6**: p. 135.
114 Trexler, E.T., et al., *International society of sports nutrition position stand: Beta-Alanine.* Journal of the International Society of Sports Nutrition, 2015. **12**(1): p. 1–14.
115 Burke, L.M., *Caffeine and sports performance.* Applied Physiology, Nutrition, and Metabolism, 2008. **33**(6): p. 1319–1334.
116 Goldstein, E.R., et al., *International society of sports nutrition position stand: Caffeine and performance.* Journal of the International Society of Sports Nutrition, 2010. **7**(1): p. 1–15.
117 Graham, T.E., *Caffeine and exercise.* Sports Medicine, 2001. **31**(11): p. 785–807.
118 Guest, N.S., et al., *International society of sports nutrition position stand: Caffeine and exercise performance.* Journal of the International Society of Sports Nutrition, 2021. **18**(1): p. 1–37.
119 Duvnjak-Zaknich, D.M., et al., *Effect of caffeine on reactive agility time when fresh and fatigued.* Medicine and Science in Sports and Exercise, 2011. **43**(8): p. 1523–1530.
120 Russell, M. and M. Kingsley, *The efficacy of acute nutritional interventions on soccer skill performance.* Sports Medicine, 2014. **44**(7): p. 957–970.
121 Pickering, C. and J. Grgic, *Caffeine and exercise: What next?* Sports Medicine, 2019. **49**(7): p. 1007–1030.
122 Grgic, J., *Effects of caffeine on resistance exercise: A review of recent research.* Sports Medicine, 2021. **51**(11): p. 2281–2298.
123 Pickering, C. and J. Kiely, *Are the current guidelines on caffeine use in sport optimal for everyone? Inter-individual variation in caffeine ergogenicity, and a move towards personalised sports nutrition.* Sports Medicine, 2018. **48**(1): p. 7–16.
124 Hespel, P., R. Maughan, and P. Greenhaff, *Dietary supplements for football.* Journal of Sports Sciences, 2006. **24**(07): p. 749–761.
125 Ryan, E.J., et al., *Caffeine gum and cycling performance: A timing study.* The Journal of Strength & Conditioning Research, 2013. **27**(1): p. 259–264.
126 Macuh, M. and B. Knap, *Effects of nitrate supplementation on exercise performance in humans: A narrative review.* Nutrients, 2021. **13**(9): p. 3183.
127 Peeling, P., et al., *Evidence-based supplements for the enhancement of athletic performance.* International Journal of Sport Nutrition and Exercise Metabolism, 2018. **28**(2): p. 178–187.
128 Van De Walle, G.P. and M.D. Vukovich, *The effect of nitrate supplementation on exercise tolerance and performance: A systematic review and meta-analysis.* Journal of Strength and Conditioning Research, 2018. **32**(6): p. 1796–1808.
129 McMahon, N.F., M.D. Leveritt, and T.G. Pavey, *The effect of dietary nitrate supplementation on endurance exercise performance in healthy adults: A systematic review and meta-analysis.* Sports Medicine, 2017. **47**(4): p. 735–756.
130 Thompson, C., et al., *Dietary nitrate supplementation improves sprint and high-intensity intermittent running performance.* Nitric Oxide, 2016. **61**: p. 55–61.
131 Thompson, C., et al., *Dietary nitrate improves sprint performance and cognitive function during prolonged intermittent exercise.* European Journal of Applied Physiology, 2015. **115**(9): p. 1825–1834.
132 Senefeld, J.W., et al., *Ergogenic effect of nitrate supplementation: A systematic review and meta-analysis.* Medicine and Science in Sports and Exercise, 2020. **52**(10): p. 2250.
133 Salehzadeh, H., et al., *The nitrate content of fresh and cooked vegetables and their health-related risks.* PLoS One, 2020. **15**(1): p. e0227551.

134 Ruegsegger, G.N. and F.W. Booth, *Health benefits of exercise.* Cold Spring Harbor Perspectives in Medicine, 2018. **8**(7). p. a029694.
135 Lee, Y.-S., et al., *Sports injury type and psychological factors affect treatment period and willingness-to-pay: Cross-sectional study.* Medicine, 2020. **99**(50). p. e23647.
136 Tipton, K.D., *Nutritional support for exercise-induced injuries.* Sports Medicine, 2015. **45**(1): p. 93–104.
137 Tipton, K.D., *Nutrition for acute exercise-induced injuries.* Annals of Nutrition and Metabolism, 2010. **57**(Suppl 2): p. 43–53.
138 Biolo, G., et al., *Positive energy balance is associated with accelerated muscle atrophy and increased erythrocyte glutathione turnover during 5 wk of bed rest.* The American Journal of Clinical Nutrition, 2008. **88**(4): p. 950–958.
139 Wolfe, R.R., *The underappreciated role of muscle in health and disease.* The American Journal of Clinical Nutrition, 2006. **84**(3): p. 475–482.
140 Wall, B.T., J.P. Morton, and L.J. Van Loon, *Strategies to maintain skeletal muscle mass in the injured athlete: Nutritional considerations and exercise mimetics.* European Journal of Sport Science, 2015. **15**(1): p. 53–62.
141 Witard, O.C., et al., *Myofibrillar muscle protein synthesis rates subsequent to a meal in response to increasing doses of whey protein at rest and after resistance exercise.* The American Journal of Clinical Nutrition, 2014. **99**(1): p. 86–95.
142 Moore, D.R., et al., *Ingested protein dose response of muscle and albumin protein synthesis after resistance exercise in young men.* The American Journal of Clinical Nutrition, 2009. **89**(1): p. 161–168.
143 Schoenfeld, B.J. and A.A. Aragon, *How much protein can the body use in a single meal for muscle-building? Implications for daily protein distribution.* Journal of the International Society of Sports Nutrition, 2018. **15**(1): p. 1–6.
144 Rawson, E.S., M.P. Miles, and D.E. Larson-Meyer, *Dietary supplements for health, adaptation, and recovery in athletes.* International Journal of Sport Nutrition and Exercise Metabolism, 2018. **28**(2): p. 188–199.
145 Eijnde, B.O.t., et al., *Effect of oral creatine supplementation on human muscle GLUT4 protein content after immobilization.* Diabetes, 2001. **50**(1): p. 18–23.
146 McGlory, C., et al., *Fish oil supplementation suppresses resistance exercise and feeding-induced increases in anabolic signaling without affecting myofibrillar protein synthesis in young men.* Physiological Reports, 2016. **4**(6): p. e12715.
147 Clark, K.L., et al., *24-Week study on the use of collagen hydrolysate as a dietary supplement in athletes with activity-related joint pain.* Current Medical Research and Opinion, 2008. **24**(5): p. 1485–1496.
148 Shaw, G., et al., *Vitamin C-enriched gelatin supplementation before intermittent activity augments collagen synthesis.* The American Journal of Clinical Nutrition, 2017. **105**(1): p. 136–143.
149 Clifford, T., et al., *The effects of collagen peptides on muscle damage, inflammation and bone turnover following exercise: A randomized, controlled trial.* Amino Acids, 2019. **51**(4): p. 691–704.
150 Crowther, F., et al., *Team sport athletes' perceptions and use of recovery strategies: A mixed-methods survey study.* BMC Sports Science, Medicine and Rehabilitation, 2017. **9**(1): p. 1–10.
151 Higgins, T.R., D.A. Greene, and M.K. Baker, *Effects of cold water immersion and contrast water therapy for recovery from team sport: A systematic review and meta-analysis.* The Journal of Strength & Conditioning Research, 2017. **31**(5): p. 1443–1460.
152 Broatch, J.R., A. Petersen, and D.J. Bishop, *The influence of post-exercise cold-water immersion on adaptive responses to exercise: A review of the literature.* Sports Medicine, 2018. **48**(6): p. 1369–1387.

153 Machado, A.F., et al., *Can water temperature and immersion time influence the effect of cold water immersion on muscle soreness? A systematic review and meta-analysis.* Sports Medicine, 2016. **46**(4): p. 503–514.
154 White, G.E. and G.D. Wells, *Cold-water immersion and other forms of cryotherapy: Physiological changes potentially affecting recovery from high-intensity exercise.* Extreme Physiology & Medicine, 2013. **2**(1): p. 1–11.
155 Algafly, A.A. and K.P. George, *The effect of cryotherapy on nerve conduction velocity, pain threshold and pain tolerance.* British Journal of Sports Medicine, 2007. **41**(6): p. 365–369.
156 Cochrane, D.J., *Alternating hot and cold water immersion for athlete recovery: A review.* Physical Therapy in Sport, 2004. **5**(1): p. 26–32.
157 Halson, S.L., et al., *Physiological responses to cold water immersion following cycling in the heat.* International Journal of Sports Physiology and Performance, 2008. **3**(3): p. 331–346.
158 Tavares, F., et al., *Practical applications of water immersion recovery modalities for team sports.* Strength & Conditioning Journal, 2018. **40**(4): p. 48–60.
159 Roberts, L.A., et al., *Post-exercise cold water immersion attenuates acute anabolic signalling and long-term adaptations in muscle to strength training.* The Journal of Physiology, 2015. **593**(18): p. 4285–4301.
160 Tavares, F., et al., *Effects of chronic cold-water immersion in elite rugby players.* International Journal of Sports Physiology and Performance, 2019. **14**(2): p. 156–162.
161 Vieira, A., et al., *The effect of water temperature during cold-water immersion on recovery from exercise-induced muscle damage.* International Journal of Sports Medicine, 2016. **37**(12): p. 937–943.
162 Stephens, J.M., et al., *Cold-water immersion for athletic recovery: One size does not fit all.* International Journal of Sports Physiology and Performance, 2017. **12**(1): p. 2–9.
163 Hemmings, B.J., *Physiological, psychological and performance effects of massage therapy in sport: A review of the literature.* Physical Therapy in Sport, 2001. **2**(4): p. 165–170.
164 Best, T.M., et al., *Effectiveness of sports massage for recovery of skeletal muscle from strenuous exercise.* Clinical Journal of Sport Medicine, 2008. **18**(5): p. 446–460.
165 Zhong, H., et al., *The techniques of manual massage and its application on exercise-induced fatigue: A literature review.* Frontiers in Sport Research, 2019. **1**(1): p. 43–50.
166 Moraska, A., *Sports massage. A comprehensive review.* Journal of Sports Medicine and Physical Fitness, 2005. **45**(3): p. 370–380.
167 Poppendieck, W., et al., *Massage and performance recovery: A meta-analytical review.* Sports Medicine, 2016. **46**(2): p. 183–204.
168 Davis, H.L., S. Alabed, and T.J.A. Chico, *Effect of sports massage on performance and recovery: A systematic review and meta-analysis.* BMJ Open Sport & Exercise Medicine, 2020. **6**(1): p. e000614.
169 Sriwongtong, M., et al., *Does massage help athletes after exercise?* The Ochsner Journal, 2020. **20**(2): p. 121–122.
170 Konrad, A., et al., *The acute effects of a percussive massage treatment with a hypervolt device on plantar flexor muscles' range of motion and performance.* Journal of Sports Science & Medicine, 2020. **19**(4): p. 690–694.
171 Martin, J., *A critical evaluation of percussion massage gun devices as a rehabilitation tool focusing on lower limb mobility: A literature review.* 2021.
172 Field, A., et al., *The use of recovery strategies in professional soccer: A worldwide survey.* International Journal of Sports Physiology and Performance, 2021. **16**(12): p. 1804–1815.
173 Rey, E., et al., *Practical active and passive recovery strategies for soccer players.* Strength & Conditioning Journal, 2018. **40**(3): p. 45–57.

174 Sigel, B., et al., *Type of compression for reducing venous stasis. A study of lower extremities during inactive recumbency.* Archives of Surgery, 1975. **110**(2): p. 171–175.
175 Gimenes, S.V., et al., *Compression stockings used during two soccer matches improve perceived muscle soreness and high-intensity performance.* The Journal of Strength & Conditioning Research, 2021. **35**(7): p. 2010–2017.
176 Valle, X., et al., *Compression garments to prevent delayed onset muscle soreness in soccer players.* Muscles, Ligaments and Tendons Journal, 2014. **3**(4): p. 295–302.

9 Return to play

Ryan Timmins, John Hartley, Risto-Matti Toivonen, Alexander Mouhcine and Alex Calder

Overview of common injuries

Winning matches and trophies in soccer is the ultimate goal and marker of success. However, injuries can wreak havoc on title winning chances by the limited number of players available for training and matches. Injuries negatively impact performance, with evidence showing teams with lower injury rates have more success than those with higher incidences [1–3]. Therefore, understanding the burden of injuries in soccer can assist in limiting the incidence of injury and potentially support success.

Over the past 18 years in elite soccer, there has been a reduction in injury incidence of 3% per season [4]. Most of this change is associated with a decrease in ligament injuries (approximately 4% per season) with no change in the rate of muscle injuries over the past 18 years. The incidence of re-injury has also progressively improved, with ligament-based recurrences decreasing by 6% per season, whilst muscle re-injuries are declining by 4% per season. Whilst the incidence has reduced, the severity of injuries has risen. Overall injury severity has increased 1% per season, with ligament injuries being approximately 4% more severe each season [4]. This highlights the significant improvements in injury prevention and rehabilitation over almost two decades of elite soccer.

Whilst the incidence of injury (how many injuries per a specific time e.g. 1,000 hours) is a key variable to monitor, the severity (number of days lost) of these injuries is sometimes overlooked. The product of incidence and severity is defined as 'injury burden' [5, 6]. Figure 9.1 highlights the intricate nature of the 14 most reported injuries in elite soccer [5]. When interpreting Figure 9.1, it is noted that hamstring muscle injuries have the highest incidence (alongside lower leg contusions), whilst anterior cruciate ligament (ACL) tears don't occur as often but have a higher severity. As such, practitioners undertaking risk assessments should consider the total burden of injury and not just how often it occurs (Figures 9.2 and 9.3).

Common muscle injuries

Muscle-based injuries are the most common injury to result in time lost in elite soccer. For every 1,000 hours of soccer, there are approximately five muscle injures. Whilst muscle injuries occur often in elite soccer, the average amount

DOI: 10.4324/9781003200420-9

224 Ryan Timmins et al.

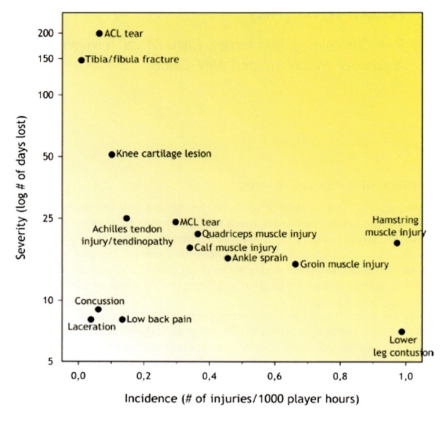

Figure 9.1 Matrix indicating the relationship between incidence and severity when determining injury burden (Extracted from Bahr [5]).

of days absent from training is moderate, with approximately 18 days missed on average [4]. Of these muscle injuries, the most frequently occurring are hamstring strains, followed by groin muscle concerns and then by quadriceps and calf muscle group injuries.

Hamstring injuries

Of all muscle-based injuries, hamstring strain injuries (HSIs) have been the greatest burden to elite soccer clubs for over 30 years [7]. Their high prevalence in both training and matches has led to an extensive field of research being developed to attempt to reduce the high incidence of injury. Despite this concerted research effort, hamstring injuries have increased by 4% annually since 2001 in elite soccer. In more recent times, greater clarity has been developed around the diagnosis and management of different types of hamstring injuries, specifically those which involve the intramuscular tendon [8]. This section will

Return to play 225

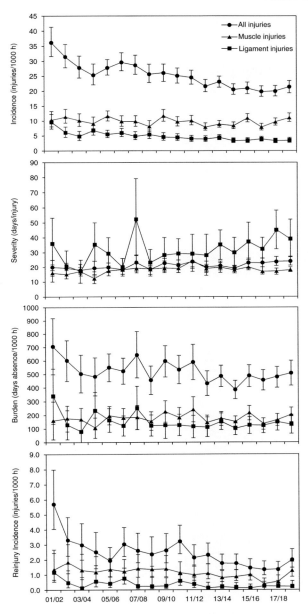

Figure 9.2 Match injuries. Development of injury incidence, injury severity, injury burden and re-injury rate for all injuries, muscle injuries and ligament injuries in matches over the study period. Injury incidence is defined as the number of injuries per 1,000 hours of match exposure with 95% CI. Injury severity is defined as the average number of absence days following match injuries with 95% CI. Injury burden is defined as the number of absence days caused per 1,000 hours of match exposure with 95% CI. Re-injury rate is defined as the number of re-injuries per 1,000 hours of training exposure with 95% CI (Extracted from Ekstrand et al. [4]).

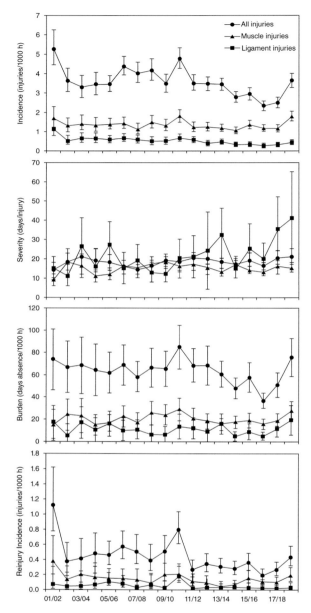

Figure 9.3 Training injuries. Time course of injury incidence, injury severity, injury burden and re-injury rate for all injuries, muscle injuries and ligament injuries over the study period. Injury incidence is defined as the number of injuries per 1,000 hours of training exposure with 95% CI. Injury severity is defined as the average number of absence days following training injuries with 95% CI. Injury burden is defined as the number of absence days caused per 1,000 hours of training exposure with 95% CI. Re-injury rate is defined as the number of re-injuries per 1,000 hours of training exposure with 95% CI (Extracted from Ekstrand et al. [4]).

highlight the incidence and recurrence of these injuries, providing information around which of the hamstring muscles are most commonly injured, along with more information of the differing types of hamstring injuries, specifically those involving the intramuscular tendon.

Incidence of injury

Hamstring injuries are the most common injury in elite soccer, representing ~12% of all injuries [9]. In a squad of approximately 25 players, typically there will be five to six hamstring injuries each season. Of these injuries, a first time incident will take around 18 days on average to return to play (RTP), with re-injuries typically taking a little longer at 22 days [10]. As a result, upwards of 100 days can be missed per club, per season due to HSIs, potentially costing organizations more than 2 million USD($) per season [11].

The most commonly involved muscle is the biceps femoris long head (BFLH), with up to 84% of all first-time injuries being reported in this muscle [12]. Across the other hamstring muscles, the semimembranosus (SM) and semitendinosus (ST) make up for approximately 12% and 4%, respectively [12]. Whilst the BFLH is injured the most, there are no large differences in the number of days taken to RTP, with BFLH injuries averaging 20 days, SM 18 days and ST 23 days. Finally, injuries involving the BFLH have a higher rate of recurrence (18%), compared to incidents involving the medial hamstrings (SM/ST) (2%).

The intramuscular tendon — what does the evidence say

Injuries involving the intramuscular tendon of the hamstrings have recently become a controversial topic within sports medicine [8, 13, 14]. Recent evidence has shown that injuries involving the intramuscular tendon of the hamstrings can take almost 50 days longer to recover than those which are considered 'normal' injuries [15, 16]. Once returned to play, those with a history of a prior intramuscular tendon injury have a greater rate of re-injury, with approximately 60% of these going on to reoccur, compared to 18% in 'normal' hamstring injuries. Considering these statistics and the significant time lost as a result, researchers and practitioners have begun paying more attention to the magnetic resonance imaging (MRI) results once an injury occurs.

Whilst these findings are worrying statistics, they should be considered alongside alternative reports. In the studies mentioned above, the researchers and clinicians involved in the decision for RTP were not blinded to the MRI findings. Therefore, the modification of the time taken to rehabilitate and a potential RTP timeframe could have been artificially inflated due to a precautionary approach being taken as a result of the MRI findings showing intramuscular tendon involvement. This phenomenon is sometimes referred to as a 'self-fulfilling prophecy', where it is hypothesized that an injury will take longer to heal and as such the practitioners decision to clear them to RTP is based on this, prolonging the time undertaking rehabilitation as a result [17]. An alternative approach recently suggested performing rehabilitation independent of the MRI findings, as such removing the capacity for this potential bias to lengthen the time taken to RTP, with clearance given based on clinical markers of recovery [14]. To put evidence to this theory, researchers undertook rehabilitation whilst blinded to the MRI findings. After all participants completed their rehabilitation, all MRI findings were reviewed and those which involved the intramuscular tendon were compared to those which did not. Overall, the average RTP time was approximately one week longer in injuries that involved the intramuscular tendon compared to those which did not. Interestingly, this additional week was only evident when the MRI identified 100% of the intramuscular tendon cross-sectional area being damaged. Otherwise, it was only two to three days longer to complete rehabilitation in injuries that included <100% of the intramuscular tendon involved when compared to injuries where it wasn't (Figure 9.4). In addition to this, utilizing a similar blinded approach, researchers compared the rate of re-injury within 12 months of returning to play for those which had intramuscular tendon involvement to those which didn't [13]. There was no difference in the re-injury rates between the two groups, with approximately 20% of athletes in each group suffering a recurrent incident.

Considering the findings presented above, practitioners should consider the environment they are in, the athlete involved, the manager, and all the subsequent pressures that come with these decisions, when choosing to accept or ignore the MRI findings during rehabilitation. These contrasting findings may provide comfort to some practitioners that rehabilitation can progress using normal approaches when these intramuscular injuries occur, without the need to have athletes out for months on end. However, it does take a brave person

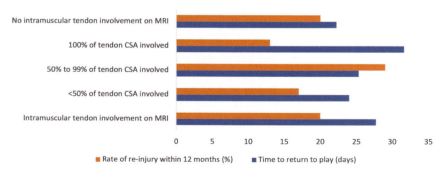

Figure 9.4 Time to return to play and rate of re-injury for injuries without intramuscular tendon involvement and injuries with varying degrees of intramuscular tendon involvement (Adapted from Van der Made et al. [13, 14]).

to ignore the MRI findings in favour of all the clinical and performance data and should be considered as part of a more holistic approach to rehabilitation.

Hip and groin injuries

Hip and groin injuries are second to HSI as the most frequently occurring muscle injuries in elite soccer [5]. Between 2001 and 2016, hip and groin injuries contributed 14% of all injuries. This equated to around one injury per 1,000 hours, with more injuries occurring during match play (3.1/1,000hrs) than training (0.6/1,000hrs) [18]. Whilst over this period there was a reduction in the number of hip and groin injuries, the average severity (time lost per injury) increased, resulting in no change of the overall burden of these injuries. The most common of all hip and groin injuries are adductor-related injuries, which occur twice as frequently as all other hip and groin concerns such as iliopsoas-related, pubic-related, and inguinal-related injuries. As time progressed over the years, the incidence of femoroacetabular impingement (FAI) increased, potentially owing to the greater evidence guiding its effective diagnosis [19]. Of all hip and groin injuries, 11% go on to suffer a subsequent re-injury in the same season. On an individual level, this calculates to approximately 24% of all athletes who suffer an adductor-related injury will go on to have another incident in that same season, which is comparable to the 20% of iliopsoas-related injuries which will reoccur at some point throughout the season.

This evidence is derived from the diagnosed hip and groin injuries reported in elite soccer players. There is a range of unrecorded hip and groin complaints which are managed individually with each athlete. This is mainly due to the pain associated with these concerns being insidious and the soccer player playing through a certain level of discomfort. This is different say to an HSI, where continuing to play could hinder progression due to the associated decline in function. Whereas with hip and groin injuries, whilst being reported at a lower rate compared to hamstrings, soccer players can push through these periods of discomfort and have their load subsequently managed, resulting in avoiding time lost from training and matches. This phenomenon should be considered when comparing these injuries to others in the lower limb which may have a more acute onset (e.g. hamstrings and quadriceps), with more functional decrements, leading to a greater inability to 'push' through compared to hip and groin complaints.

Other muscle injuries

QUADRICEP INJURIES

Quadricep injuries account for approximately 4.6% of all muscle injuries in elite soccer [10]. Whilst not occurring frequently, they do have a moderate level of severity, with the average injury requiring approximately 19 days before being cleared to RTP. This is comparable to HSI which result in a similar time out per injury, yet occur at a much higher rate, leading to a more significant burden than quadriceps injuries. This is a similar relationship when considering the rate of recurrence, with 4% of athletes who suffer a quadriceps injury going on to have another incident in that same season. Subsequent incidents tend to be more severe, resulting in almost an additional week out of action than the initial injury.

CALF INJURIES

Calf complex injuries are the next most common injury in elite soccer, accounting for approximately 4% of all muscle injuries. The average time until being cleared to RTP is 17 days, which is comparable to the time lost on average due to hamstring or quadricep injuries. This is a similar story to quadricep strains, where the injury tends to be as severe as the hamstring injuries (days lost), but due to the low rate of injury, the burden placed on organizations is not as high.

COMMON LIGAMENT INJURIES

Whilst not as common as muscle-based injuries, ligament injuries have a far greater severity, leading to a greater number of days lost on average per injury. A ligament injury will result in, on average 27 days unavailable, compared to 18 days for muscle injuries. Whilst the severity is much greater than muscle injuries, the incidence of ligament injuries is approximately half that of muscle injuries, with approximately 2.5 ligament injuries occurring for every 1,000 hours of soccer. Of these ligament injuries, the most frequently occurring are lateral ankle ligament injuries, followed by medial collateral ligament (MCL) injuries. Whilst not a frequently occurring injury, ACL injuries are the most severe.

Knee injuries

ACL injuries

Whilst missing from the 30 most commonly occurring injuries in elite soccer [10], ACL injuries are by far the most severe. Contributing less than 1% of all injuries, they make up for their lack of frequency with their significant severity, with an average ACL injury resulting in 210 days (approximately 7.5 months) unavailable. Of all first time ACL injuries, around 6% to 7% go on to re-injure upon returning to play.

MCL injuries

Injuries involving with the MCL contribute approximately 3.5% of all injuries in elite soccer, making it the most common of the knee ligaments injured. Whilst a more frequently occurring injury, their severity on average is around one tenth that of ACL injures, with the average MCL injury resulting in 24 days unavailable.

Of all MCL injuries, around 10% will go on to re-injure their MCL in the same season. Despite having an incidence rate almost double that of ACL injuries, MCL injuries don't provide anywhere near the same burden due to the significantly lower time unavailable [10].

Lateral ankle ligament injuries

Of all ligament injuries in elite soccer, the most frequent to occur are those in the lateral ankle compartment. Injuries to this region of the body account for approximately 6% of all injuries in elite soccer. Whilst the most frequent, their moderate severity of 14 days unavailable results in them not having such a burden compared to other ligament injuries such as the MCL and ACL injuries in the knee joint. Of all lateral ankle ligament injuries, around 15% go on to re-injure at some point in the same season [10].

Head injuries

In recent years, there has been an increased focus on head injuries and sport-related concussion (SRC) across soccer and all sports from the medical profession and wider scientific community [20]. The most recent consensus statement for concussion in sport reflects current knowledge and acts as a guide to managing head injuries, but practitioners should always consider the individual and specific circumstances of the incident [21]. The consensus statement highlights the key sections of the '11 R's'; recognize, remove, re-evaluate, rest, rehabilitation, refer, recover, return to sport, reconsider, residual effects and sequelae, and risk reduction [21, 22] (Table 9.1).

Specific injury mechanisms

As the functional demands of muscles and ligaments across the lower limb vary during soccer, so do the potential mechanisms which may lead to injury.

Hamstrings

In general, hamstring injuries can be divided into *sprinting* and *stretching* type injuries (Table 9.2 and Figure 9.5) [23, 24].

When devising effective RTP protocols, it's imperative to consider that sprinting type injuries show significantly shorter RTP times compared with stretching type injuries [23, 24]. It is possible, this is due to the significant structural damage caused by some of these stretching type injuries, which sometimes require surgical interventions to correct.

The late swing phase of sprinting is considered to be the critical moment in the gait cycle where the hamstrings produce significant biomechanical and neuromuscular processes to slow down the forward-swinging shank [25]. Comparing kinematics and electromyographic (EMG) activities during different

Table 9.1 Stages of a head injury in elite soccer

	Enhanced care setting pathway		Standard return to play pathway	
	Adult	Under 19	Adult	Under 19
STAGE 1 – Initial Rest Period	**24 hours** minimum rest period after which the player must be symptom free before progressing	**7 days** minimum initial rest period after which the player must be symptom free before progressing	**14 days** beginning at midnight on the day of injury. The player must be symptom free at the end of this period before progressing	**14 days** beginning at midnight on the day of injury. The player must be symptom free at the end of this period before progressing
		Return to academic studies or work		
	Clearance by Doctor Recommended			
STAGE 2 – Light Exercise	Minimum duration **24 hours**	Minimum duration **24 hours**	Minimum duration **24 hours**	Minimum duration **48 hours**
STAGE 3 – Football-Specific Exercise	Minimum duration **24 hours**	Minimum duration **24 hours**	Minimum duration **24 hours**	Minimum duration **48 hours**
STAGE 4 – Non-contact Training	Minimum duration **24 hours**	Minimum duration **24 hours**	Minimum duration **24 hours**	Minimum duration **48 hours**
	Clearance by Doctor Recommended	Clearance by Doctor Recommended	Clearance by Doctor Recommended	Clearance by Doctor Recommended
STAGE 5 – Full-contact Practice	Minimum duration **24 hours**	Minimum duration **24 hours**	Minimum duration **24 hours**	Minimum duration **48 hours**
STAGE 6 – Return to Play (Minimum Return to Play Time, Dependent on individualized recovery programme)	**Day 6** – **Earliest** Return to Play	**Day 12** – **Earliest** Return to Play	**Day 19** – **Earliest** Return to Play	**Day 23** – **Earliest** Return to Play

(Minimum 4 days if symptom free between stages for Enhanced care Adult, Enhanced care Under 19, Standard Adult; Minimum 8 days if symptom free for Standard Under 19)

Note: The colors represent the stage of rehab: red = initial stage and green = RTP.

parts of the sprint (acceleration vs maximum velocity), research has shown that the functional demands of the medial and lateral hamstrings muscles differ between these portions [26]. The ST typically produces higher activation patterns during mid to late swing phase when undertaking acceleration, whereas the lateral hamstrings greatest activation tends to occur during the terminal swing phase at maximum speed [27]. During maximum sprinting efforts, the

Table 9.2 Mechanisms of hamstring injury strains in elite soccer

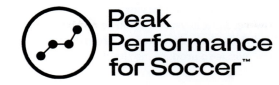

Stretching	Sprinting

• Reaching
• Kicking
• Decelerating
• Re-stabilizing
	• Accelerating
	    ◦ Rolling Start
	    ◦ Deadstop
	• Max Sprint (and sub-max)

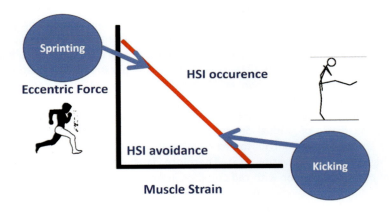

Figure 9.5 An illustration of the relationship between muscle strain and eccentric force in HSI occurrences. The red line represents the theoretical maximum capacity of the muscle. If we have an eccentric force that exceeds this (e.g. sprinting) then we have injury. If we have strain that exceeds this (e.g. kicking, stretching), an injury often occurs.

biceps femoris undergoes the greatest amount of length change, with it elongating to 10% its length in neutral stance. Comparably, semitendinosus (~8%) and the semimembranosus (~7.5%) show lesser changes in length during maximum sprinting [27]. This difference in length change during maximum sprinting could potentially account for some of the variance in the number of injuries experienced in the biceps femoris when compared to the medial hamstrings. Understanding these intricate relationships while considering the principles of synergism is key to a differentiated approach and adequate exercise selection during the RTP process [28].

Rectus femoris

Regarding injuries to the rectus femoris, three specific mechanisms have been highlighted: acceleration, deceleration, and kicking [29]. Acceleration and kicking actions require excessive eccentric activation combined with high angular velocities at the hip and knee [30, 31]. Similarly, decelerations are characterized by high braking forces and require the muscle to produce high levels of eccentric force [32].

Calf

Research of RTP strategies for the calf complex is limited. Regarding specific therapeutic regimes and interventions, it's essential to consider the epidemiology of the triceps surae complex, which is formed by the gastrocnemius and the soleus muscle. Both muscles show differences concerning injury mechanisms, RTP-times and re-injury rates [33]. Almost half of the calf injuries don't have a specific identifiable incident, with multiple being induced by a gradual onset of muscle tension [34]. Of those non-insidious injuries, the common mechanisms described are acceleration or steady state running. When comparing the two muscles of the triceps surae, the soleus is more at risk of injury during steady state running, whereas the gastrocnemius is more susceptible to injury during high-intensity efforts [33]. Therefore, it is imperative that practitioners acknowledge these risks when programming conditioning interventions (see *Chapter 5 for more detail*).

The biomechanical characteristics of the calf complex may partially explain the high incidence of gradual-onset induced calf injuries. The calf muscle complex is an important contributor to running at a range of steady state speeds with high levels of activation [35]. Therefore, fatigue tolerance could be one crucial point to consider with calf complex interventions.

Hip and groin

As was the case with the calf complex, evidence surrounding the mechanisms of injury across the hip and groin is limited. Some authors have highlighted that the kicking action was one potential injury mechanism [36]. It was stated that the structures of the hip and abdomen are stressed substantially during kicking and shooting, potentially increasing their risk of injury [37]. Consequently, kinematics and nervous system activation patterns while kicking could be altered after hip and groin related injuries, potentially increasing the risk of a future-injury [38].

Due to their function as stabilizers of the hip in different planes, it could be hypothesized that the muscles surrounding the groin complex play a highly important role in multidirectional actions (e.g. change of directions) [39]. Whilst it is suggested, it has not been explicitly studied and might be a key concept to consider regarding the specific injury mechanisms for the hip and groin complex in practice.

Rehabilitation process

Designing a framework

Taking the healing process into account, one can determine four phases of rehabilitation in the management of sports soft tissue injuries: (1) acute inflammatory phase, (2) re-conditioning phase, (3) controlled sport-specific phase, and (4) return to play phase [40]. Regardless of the type or region of injury, the basic phases of rehabilitation should always be considered in the process. Decisions and progressions made during any phase of the RTP protocol should be driven by considerations to tissue type, pathological presentation, and required tissue adaptation, with specific criteria in each segment. The duration of these different phases will differ depending on the severity of the injury [41]. There is a lack of validated criteria and consensus regarding which clinical measurements are useful to predict the time to RTP. Although a combination of clinical findings initially following an injury and at the day 7 could provide some guidance in determining the duration of rehabilitation until RTP, this model is of linear nature and has limitations [42]. Therefore, it is suggested that practitioners conduct daily, ongoing examinations of subjective and objective measures, to truly understand the non-linear nature of progression [43]. Key variables to consider daily when projecting the time to RTP are change in strength from initial assessment, pain, palpation, flexibility (if applicable), delay in starting treatment, and other specific movement patterns (demanding the injured tissue) [43, 44]. The rehabilitation process of an injury should be initiated by the etiology, i.e., the cause of the injury. The rehabilitation should then follow a progressive criteria-based continuum where the athlete progresses through different stages until fit to RTP. The different stages of the process need to be structured and progressive to prepare the athlete and the injured tissue to withstand the physical and physiological demands at the highest level of the sport [45]. The rehabilitation progress should be performance-based instead of the traditional time-based criteria which may overlook individual variation. Performance-based process focuses on identifying and resolving neuromuscular and cognitive deficits of the injured athlete and should aim to return the athlete with greater capability than pre-injury [46]. In order for the practitioner to develop the specific performance-based programme, a careful needs analysis investigating the physiological and biomechanical requirements of the sport is required (see Chapter 3 for more detail). Most common periodisation models adapted to the rehabilitation process follow either linear or non-linear periodisation. Where linear models emphasize training adaptations on only one parameter (e.g. endurance, hypertrophy, strength) at a time, a non-linear approach incorporates the ability to train more than one of these parameters simultaneously [41]. In most settings, a non-linear model can be considered a more modern approach in developing a RTP framework, for the variable nature of super compensations of metabolic, neural, and motor functions of the athlete [43, 47].

Acute inflammatory phase

Once the mechanism of the injury has been discovered, the anatomy and the function of the injured structure should be considered next. Exercise selection and programming following an injury should be based on optimal loading concept to maximize the physiological adaptation of the involved structures [46]. Mechanical load to the tissues can be influenced by variety of different factors, such as magnitude, direction, intensity, frequency, and duration. Where tendons are known to response well to increased magnitude of load with slower frequency, increased bone density and alteration tissues active stiffness qualities are seen after rapid movements such as jumping and running [48]. The most common exercise frequencies presented in the literature (Table 9.3) vary between three and seven sessions per week per body part [49].

When it comes to choosing appropriate exercises for the rehabilitation process, practitioners need to consider contraction type with regard to the mechanism. In the acute phase, the rehabilitation programme should consider all exercise variables (i.e. Frequency, intensity, duration, and tempo) and progress appropriately as the healing process progresses [41]. Eccentric exercises should be incorporated immediately following the injury to prepare the body for the high eccentric demands of elite soccer [50, 51]. Studies have identified that programmes not utilizing eccentric exercises can lead to higher re-injury rates and lower return to the previous level of performance, compared to including eccentric-biased exercises [52]. Eccentric-biased or eccentric-only strength training programmes offer a clear protective effect against injuries when compliance is high, therefore should be incorporated into rehabilitation as soon as possible [53–55]. Where eccentric exercises are very useful for the high amounts of force that they generate, concentric exercises should be utilized to create force with much higher velocities [56]. Additionally, isometric contractions can be used to bridge the gap between concentric and eccentric exercises, by creating force through the system but requiring no length change in the muscle [57]. Moreover, isometric-biased exercises can be prescribed

Table 9.3 Optimal loading approach following a soft tissue injury

Mobility	Running mechanics	Isometrics	Plyometrics and power	Strength (neural)	Strength (intermuscular)
3–7 times a week	3–5 times a week	3–7 times a week	3–5 times a week	3–5 times a week	3–5 times a week
2–3 sets of 8–15 reps	2–3 sets of 3–4 reps 10–15meters per rep	2–4 sets of 3–6reps 3-5sec per rep	3–5 sets 3–5 reps of power-based exercises or 10–30 hops	3–5 sets Early rehab: 6–12 reps Mid > end rehab: 1–6 reps	3–5 sets Early rehab: 6–12 reps Mid > end rehab: 4–8 reps

Note: Variables listed here may differ based on epidemiology and different phases of RTP.
Source: Adapted from Glasgow et al. [46] and Taberner et al. [48]

to reduce pain and motor inhibition, and provide an important option to offer for athletes for painful tendons that are difficult to load for example in the presence of tendinopathy [58]. Effective rehabilitation programmes should incorporate all contraction modes (isometric, concentric, and eccentric), where appropriate. In conjunction with developing strength capacities via all contraction modes, practitioners should also incorporate a plyometric continuum early in the rehabilitation process. Plyometric training utilizes the stretch-shortening cycle (SSC) to develop power. The rapid deceleration to acceleration mechanism exhibits the production of maximum force in the shortest period of time [59, 60]. Maximum acceleration and sprinting are considered plyometric actions, therefore, the early onset of plyometric development in a rehabilitation setting will allow the athlete to safely transition to running-specific activities [61].

Re-conditioning phase

The main objective of the re-conditioning phase is to develop capacities of the tissue to tolerate the load of training. These capacities include muscular strength, conditioning, tendon compliance, joint stress tolerance, etc. Mechanical loading, from resistance exercises alone, does not address the motor component of the muscle-tendon complex. Plyometric exercises should be incorporated in the programme as soon as possible to introduce high neuromuscular load and a progression towards sport-specific movements. Plyometric exercises are most effective at producing force at very high speeds and altering the stiffness qualities of the muscle-tendon complex. As with resistance exercises, a proper progression of plyometric exercises minimizes the risk of re-injury and builds the capacity for the athlete to perform intense movements later in the process [60]. Plyometric exercises consisting of altered variables (intensity, volume, load) to elicit low impact, with high repetitions, should be initiated immediately after the acute stage, due to the low level of physical and neural demand [60]. Although intensity of plyometric exercises can be difficult to measure, a careful consideration should be placed on impact velocity, contact time and distribution of load on contact when planning the appropriate progression of plyometric exercises [62].

Metabolic conditioning should be programmed alongside the resistance exercises to keep the athlete maintaining and improving soccer-specific energy system capacity (see *Chapter 5 for more detail on conditioning prescriptions*). To make the transition from rehabilitation to RTP easier and more efficient, the metabolic conditioning workouts can be programmed using the same periodisation structure that the rest of the team is following. For example, on an intensive-biased conditioning day, the practitioner can prescribe a non-running conditioning session consisting of 4 × 4 min at high intensity intervals (>85% maxHR) with 2 min of rest to stimulate the same heart rate response as seen from small-sided games from rest of the team, with the same work:rest prescription.

Many variables (Figure 9.6) can be manipulated within the rehabilitation process. When designing the RTP protocol, practitioners need to use clinical reasoning with a combination of scientific and professional theories [47]. The exercise variables

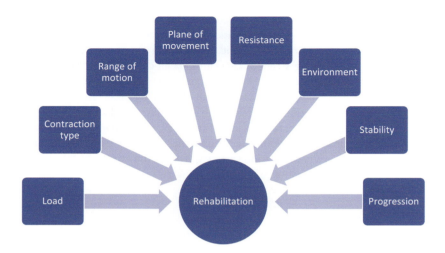

Figure 9.6 An example of manipulative variables of rehabilitation.

prescribed need to be diligently thought out, with a clear objective of desired adaptation. A thorough RTP protocol, involving multiple members of the performance staff, will ensure successful progression within your environment, regain confidence with the players, and avoid monotony (and other injury risks) throughout the process. The exercise prescription can be thought more as an art form, than science [63]. The selection of the exercises should be guided by clear goals of restoring strength and power qualities across the force-velocity spectrum around the injured site.

Controlled sport-specific and return to play phase

The return to training, and subsequently RTP, phase must be planned and adapted accordingly with continuous estimation of the risks and benefits of reintegrating the athlete back to full team training. When designing the framework for this phase, quantification and monitoring the on-field training load through global positioning system (GPS) metrics is most effective. Ensuring the athlete successfully completes the set exit criteria is vital in this final stage of the rehabilitation (Figure 9.7). The on-field training load must be accumulated gradually while the athlete continues to re-develop strength and rate of force development. Studies have shown the likelihood of injuries to rise significantly when training load increases were greater than 15% per week [64]. Changes in training load, however, must be interpreted in relation to the athlete's chronic load. Therefore, dependent on how long the player has missed on-field sessions, the time taken to incrementally build training must be calculated. Appropriately accumulated high training loads, ultimately leading to high chronic load, will eventually result in greater physical output in performance and increased robustness and resilience against injuries, compared to those with lower chronic loads and/or accumulating too fast [65, 66].

Hamstring RTP Exercise Menu/Progressions

Player #1

Position:	Wing	MAS:	4.5 m·s⁻¹
Age:	32	V_{MAX}:	8.92 m·s⁻¹
Height:	6'0"	Broad Jump:	260 cm
Weight:	185	CMJ:	55 "

NORD (L/R):	510 / 515	DOI:	05-Sep
Acc_{MAX}:	4.74 m·s⁻²	NOTES:	• BFLH Grade 2
Dec_{MAX}:	6.68 m·s⁻²		• Occurred during sprint (65' of game)
Trait:			

Initial screen

Exercises	Sets/Reps	Pain tol
Pain at Palpation	-	
Contraction sequencing		
- Straight leg	2 x 3e	
- Bent knee	2 x 3e	
Isometric positions for pain		
- Supine 90/90	1 x 5sec	
- Bench bent knee bridge	1 x 4	
- Hinge/RDL pattern	1 x 6	
- Sling/TRX Long lever bridge	1 x 4	
Notes:		

Early Stage

Exercises	Sets/Reps	Pain tol
Mini-Band Glute Bridge		
- Pilates style	3 x 5	
Supine Lying Extender	3 x 12e	
Cook hip lift	3 x 6e	
Supine Bridge + walk out	3 x 5	
SL Hip Bridge	3 x 6e	
BB RDL		
- ECC only	3 x 4	
Notes:		

Stage 1

Exercises	Sets/Reps	Pain tol
Valslide Supine slide outs		
- ECC only (5sec)	3 x 4	
SL Long Lever hip bridge	3 x 6e	
SL Diver (controlled)	3 x 6e	
BB RDL		
- ECC+ISO (4-2)	3 x 4	
Slide Glider	3 x 6e	
- 41x	3 x 4e	
Notes:		

Appropriate Distance accumulation

Stage 2

Exercises	Sets/Reps	Pain tol
TRX Supine slide outs		
- ECC + ISO (4-2)	3 x 4	
Valslide Supine SL slide outs	3 x 4e	
SL Diver (REI)	3 x 6e	
Banded Nordics		
- ECC only	3 x 3	
2-DB SL RDL		
- 41x	3 x 6e	
Notes:		

>80% GL HSR in single session
>20 MAS runs at 15:15

Stage 3

Exercises	Sets/Reps	Pain tol
TRX SL Supine Slide outs		
- ECC + ISO (4-2)	3 x 4e	
Nordics	3 x 3	
	4 x 2	
BB RDL		
- REI	3 x 3	
Banded Tantrums	3 x 20 sec	
Broad Jump	3 x 4	
SL Hop to Land	3 x 3e	
Notes:		

Broad Jump within 5%
SL Triple Hop within 5%
Nordic Force (N) within 10%
Nordic asymmetry within 15%
>2 Band 8 exposures
>2 Stage 3 strength session
>2 Full team training sessions

Figure 9.7 An example of a hamstring RTP exercise progression. Exit-criteria for each stage is listed below the exercise menu.

Although it has been suggested that between-limb strength asymmetries can increase the likelihood of injury [67, 68], there has been suggestion that strength symmetry is often functional for performance and not always associated with injury [69, 70]. Furthermore, it was noted that there is lack of evidence supporting the notion that asymmetries are detrimental to athletic performance [71]. Additionally, it has been illustrated that asymmetries can be found in a wide array of sports and potentially an adaptive outcome, dependent on the time spent playing the sport. Therefore, in an RTP setting, it is suggested that the practitioner take note of asymmetries within the injured player, but prioritize exercise prescriptions accordingly, based on the sport and epidemiology.

Once the athlete has successfully returned to normal team training, a modified exercise programme can be applied for the individual to avoid any dysfunctional adaptations or compensations and to regain any possible remaining deficits in strength, mobility, or rate of force development [72].

The athlete's integration back into normal team training can be done as a stepwise progression, such as the following: (1) return to team warm-up, (2) return to reduced team training (no contact; neutral [injury dependent]), (3) return to team training as neutral [injury dependent] with contact allowed, and finally, (4) return to full team training (Table 9.4).

Depending on how many on-field training days the player has missed, a practitioner should assess basic movement patterns prior to integrating the player to the team warm-up. Generally, if the player has missed minimal days (for example, 1–3), the player may be able to get involved in the team warm-up on the first day of being on the field. However, it is integral that practitioners have evaluated players thoroughly prior to any team activity, in order to reduce the risk of re-injury and/or avoid having to withdraw the player during the activity. It should also be noted that any advancement to team-related activities should involve all stakeholders of the process, i.e., practitioners, coaches, and the athlete themselves. If the player has passed criteria for clearance to participate in

Table 9.4 Progressions of integrating a player into team training during the return to play phase

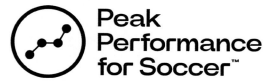

	Phase 1	Phase 2	Phase 3	Phase 4
Team warm-up	X	X	X	X
Non-contact ball drills (passing, rondos)		X	X	X
Team games as neutral			X	X
Full team training				X

X = ability to progress integration.

segments of training, yet still feels uncomfortable or not confident, practitioners must respect this notion and proceed once all stakeholders are synergetic.

Once the player has successfully progressed through the first two phases, the player can be incorporated into small-sided games as a neutral (3) for reduced cognitive and physical effort until returning to full team training (4). However, the need for a neutral (contact or no-contact) is strictly dependent on the mechanism. For example, a player returning from an HSI may not be exposed to any different physical demands on the posterior chain, when comparing neutral to playing in small-sided games. On the contrary, a player returning from an ankle injury may benefit from initial integration to small-sided games as a non-contact neutral, in order to adapt cognitively and physically before increasing the likelihood of direct contact and greater demands to the injured site (i.e. tackling and perturbation).

Key Performance Indicators

The main objective when constructing the RTP framework is to return the athlete to sport as quickly and safely as possible. Concurrently, the focus is to minimize the risk of future-injury whilst maximizing the robustness of the player [73].

In professional soccer, it is important to apply a structured, player-centred, criterion-based rehabilitation framework (Figure 9.8). This helps to manage the

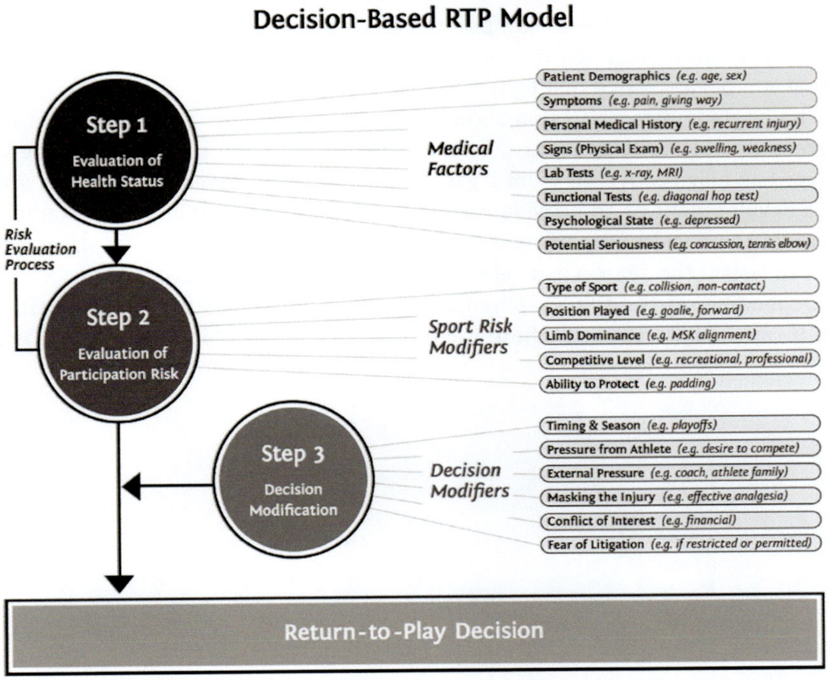

Figure 9.8 A decision-based RTP model (Extracted from Creighton et al. [74]).

external pressures placed upon staff and players to return as quickly as possible and to add control to the decision modifiers [74].

Consequently, a 'standardized approach' may not be adequate in the elite sporting environment and may need to be bespoke to both the player and their injury [74].

Testing in the RTP setting

Baseline measurements and ongoing objective data allow the performance and medical teams to have a point of reference when structuring the rehabilitation programme. Objective markers are important to allow the practitioner to apply structure to their clinical practice, identify any existing problems, compare injured to uninjured limbs, and build normative data for various player groups.

Historically, data collection on players is usually done at the onset of preseason and includes screening and performance testing (see *Chapter 3*). Each club will generally have its own battery of tests based on a needs analysis, sharing similarities, based on common injuries within the sport [4, 9]. It is now more common for experienced practitioners to perform ongoing testing and monitoring in season, rather than relying on a single preseason data point. This helps to produce valuable and reliable data on a longitudinal scale throughout the season, as opposed to relying on a single data point from preseason as reference post injury. These ongoing data points then act as a basis of the RTP process. Commonly used tests are outlined below in relation to ROM, strength, functional and performance testing (Figure 9.9).

The ongoing data collection allows the medical team to constantly monitor players throughout the season. This can be useful when assessing whether a player has fully recovered from a game, to re-evaluate baselines to assess athletic development or to provide recent data around a new injury. For example, it would be considered inefficient to rely on outdated testing data if a player was injured late in the season and relied on preseason testing data.

Depending on the fixture schedule, various approaches to planning testing can be applied. A couple of these recommendations are Match Day +2 (MD+2)

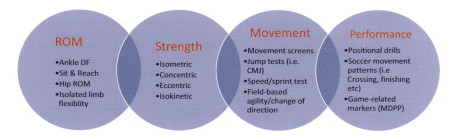

Figure 9.9 Commonly used performance tests throughout RTP procedures. CMJ = Countermovement jumps, MDPP = Most demanding passages of play.

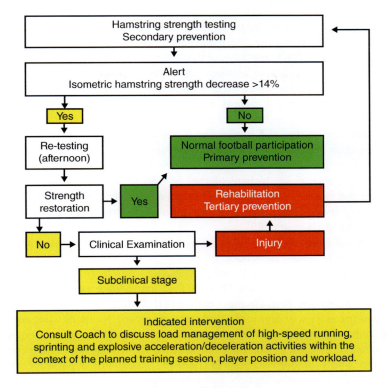

In-season secondary prevention and clinical process.

Figure 9.10 A decision-making tree examining progressions based on hamstring strength testing (Extracted from Wollin et al. [75]).

testing and Monthly monitoring. MD+2 testing looks at variability away from the baseline post game and return to those levels every week post game [75]. However, a congested schedule that requires shorter turnarounds (e.g. two to three days between games) may not fully benefit from the use of MD+2 testing protocols.

Figure 9.10 illustrates a holistic decision tree when examining a common HSI in elite soccer. This example is in relation to hamstring injury but can be applied to other monitoring tools.

Commonly used MD+2 tests include:

- ROM: knee to wall, sit & reach and hip range of motion
- Strength tests: Adductor/abductor squeeze & knee flexor isometric force outputs
- Force output tests: Counter movement jump (CMJ)

Application of testing in RTP

To increase specificity of key performance indicators (KPIs) for RTP post injury, it is vital to understand the injury mechanism and the specific demands for the injured structure. The knowledge of the kinematic and neuromuscular demands are crucial and can dictate appropriate areas of rehabilitation and KPIs. For example, regarding the relevance of high-speed running (HSR) concerning hamstring injuries (addressed earlier), exposing players to their maximum velocity prior to RTP should be one priority [76–78]. A prerequisite for exposure to HSR exposure is that the player has demonstrated the appropriate mobility and strength. Furthermore, once the player has the ability to develop HSR volume, practitioners must monitor and periodize appropriately [76]. The importance of maintaining higher volumes of HSR proceeding a hamstring injury, reduces the risk of re-injury [79]. Therefore, it is suggested that practitioners thoroughly investigate previous injury (etiology) when progressing with load management post injury [80].

Additional pain-tolerance KPIs can be monitored (where appropriate) to ensure that underlying restrictions of motion post injury have been monitored during rehabilitation and objectively measured using tests, such as ankle knee to wall, sit and reach, modified Thomas Test, active knee extension test, Jurdan Test, and Askling H Test, amongst others [81] (Figure 9.9).

Isometric tests are commonly used to assess strength initially using equipment such as hand-held dynamometers, the ForceFrame or Kangatech equipment, which are often used as objective markers for hamstring, hip flexion adductor/abductor and shoulder rotations in sport [82]. Isokinetic dynamometry is also regularly used in rehabilitation and testing to measure both concentric and eccentric strength. This allows objective data to be produced throughout the rehabilitation process to monitor a players' return to full strength and benchmark against normative data available for soccer. The NordBord is another valuable tool for this which is more conducive to field testing in the sporting environment [83].

Training and match data as KPIs

When practitioners are prescribing training loads in the RTP setting, it is integral that data from match-play is incorporated. It should be a main objective for practitioners to maximize fitness and locomotive capacities whilst the athlete is limited in training sessions. A RTP progression template should be established in order to proceed effectively and safely. For example, practitioners could categorize multiple stages with desired percentage ranges of match-play workloads (Figure 9.11). Although it may not be feasible for a practitioner to expose players to 100% of total game-load distance in a training (or rehabilitation) session, the intensity markers, such as high-speed running, sprint distance, and acceleration/deceleration can be carefully prescribed throughout. For example, a player returning from a hamstring injury can incrementally be exposed to reach

RTP Field Progressions

Intensive

Stage 1

Day	KPI	Date	Pain tol /10
Intro Acc/Dec	Acc/Dec (1m·s⁻²) exposure Acc/Dec (2m·s⁻²) exposure <=Acc/Dec (3m·s⁻²) exposure Multidirectional intro (COD)		
Intro +	15-25 Acc/Dec (3m·s⁻²) exposure Crossover progressions. Dense activity =>4m·s⁻²		
Totals	~15 Acc/Dec intro Density intro COD intro		

Stage 2

Day	KPI	Date	Pain tol /10
Mod Acc/Dec	60-70% GL Acc/Dec (3m·s⁻²) exposure Dense activity =>6m·s⁻² >Acc/Dec 4m·s⁻² exposure		
Mod +	70-80% GL Acc/Dec (3m·s⁻²) exposure MD movement =>7m·s⁻² >Dec 6m·s⁻² exposure		
Totals	60-80% GL Acc/Dec (3m·s⁻²) exposure >Dec 6m·s⁻² exposure Dead stop exposure		

Stage 3

Day	KPI	Date	Pain tol /10
High Acc/Dec	80-100% GL Acc/Dec (3m·s⁻²) exposure Dense activity =>8m·s⁻² >90% acc exposure		
High +	100% GL Acc/Dec (3m·s⁻²) exposure Shuttles =>1m·s⁻² >1min MDPP exposure		
Totals	>80% GL Acc/Dec (3m·s⁻²) Dense activity =>8m·s⁻² Shuttles		

Extensive

Stage 1

Day	KPI	Date	Pain tol /10
Intro Extensive	Continuous running >3mins Pace at 3.5-4m·s⁻¹		
Intro +	Continuous running >5mins Pace at 4-4.5m·s⁻¹ MAS Runs 2x8 @100%		
Totals	Continuous running block MAS 90-100 >3km total		

Stage 2

Day	KPI	Date	Pain tol /10
Mod Extensive	Interval running =>1:2 MAS Runs 2x10 @110%. 60-70% HSR GL		
Mod +	Interval running =>1:1. MAS Runs =>3sets @110%.+ 70-80% HSR GL Sprint intro ~100m		
Totals	HSR accumulation Interval conditioning Sprint intro		

Stage 3

Day	KPI	Date	Pain tol /10
High Extensive	80-100% HSR GL 60-80% Sprint GL Volume >5km		
High +	100% + HSR GL 80-100% Sprint GL >1min MDPP exposure		
Totals	HSR tolerance Sprint tolerance 45 min volume exposure		

Figure 9.11 An example of field-based progressions using GPS-related metrics from match-play. GL = Game Load, MDPP = Most demanding passage of play, extracted from match-play.

their 100% of total game-load high-speed running distances in a safe manner. Specifically, using Figure 9.7, a practitioner can plan an 'Extensive Stage 2' day where the optimal high-speed running exposure is 60–80% of their match load. Once that session has taken place, the performance and medical departments can evaluate how the player, and injured site, has tolerated the modified training load. This evaluation is a vital element of the exit criteria for the specific stage the player's RTP process.

It is common to build up the training load gradually post injury, particularly with long term injuries to build up the chronic workload for the player and reduce the risk of a spike in workload and potential subsequent injury [84]. This also allows the tissue to develop a tolerance to load as it continues to heal and remodel. When programming field-based progressions (Figure 9.11), sessions should also progress from a somewhat controlled to a more chaotic environment that mimics the game more closely and exposure to these elements should be gradual and progressive [84].

Considering all aspects mentioned, every RTP continuum should be bespoke and characterized by specific and individual KPI's instead of 'one-size-fits-all' approach (Figure 9.12).

Staff integration/continuum

It is important to have an athlete-centred, collaborative, multidisciplinary approach to the rehabilitation process, particularly when working in elite soccer. In elite soccer, rehabilitation of the athlete involves a variety of professionals and individuals using their expertise to create a shared experience for the athlete to return as quickly and as safely as possible (Figure 9.13). This is not always an easy process, as often practitioners within the multidisciplinary team (MDT) will undoubtedly have a varied experience and apply a divergent approach to dealing with the same problem. This acts to highlight that there can be many ways to achieve a successful rehabilitation, and, as we gain experience as practitioners and leaders in our environments, emphasizes the need for a truly integrated approach.

The primary focus for the athlete's support team is the shared common goal of providing the best possible care for the player. It is important that the leaders be facilitative in their approach to encourage different contributions whilst guiding the direction of the rehabilitation when needed. It is important that a collaborative approach is shown in the planning of the rehabilitation process and for individuals to not necessarily be concerned about exactly who delivers the prescription. Furthermore, it is important for all practitioners involved to have specific roles outlined within the process by the leadership team to ensure a streamlined and efficient rehabilitation process (this may differ from injury to injury and be dependent on the individual athlete preferences).

Not all members of staff will be involved during each phase of the RTP process, but it is important to keep key stakeholders informed of progress throughout the process. Throughout the injury, it is important to keep senior staff such

Return to play 247

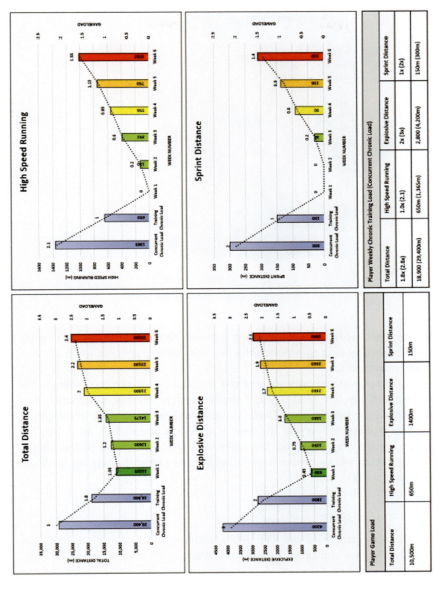

Figure 9.12 Example of weekly increments of volume and intensity markers in an RTP setting (Extracted from Taberner, Allen, and Cohen [84]).

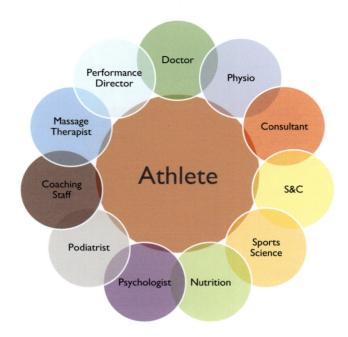

Figure 9.13 The various disciplines involved in an athlete-centred approach in elite soccer.

as the manager, sporting director, and performance director constantly up to date with developments to enhance the decision-making process when managing player movement.

It is also important to be aware of the social support systems, along with nutritional and psychological support the player has in place, particularly for those with a long-term injury. These systems will be continuous throughout the whole process to varying degrees at different stages but must not be forgotten for the player. During the acute and sub-acute phase of the injury, the rehabilitation will be predominantly led but the physiotherapy and medical team (Figure 9.14).

Acute inflammatory phase

During the acute stages of the RTP process, the main objective is to mitigate pain and swelling via modalities such as soft tissue mobilization, manual therapy, electrotherapy, and cryotherapy. A primary objective in the acute phase of the RTP process is to elicit optimal loading of tissue healing whilst increasing ROM. Depending on the needs analysis and epidemiology, strength prescriptions, BFR [85], and conditioning elements can still be targeted whilst acute management is taking place (Figure 9.15).

Return to play 249

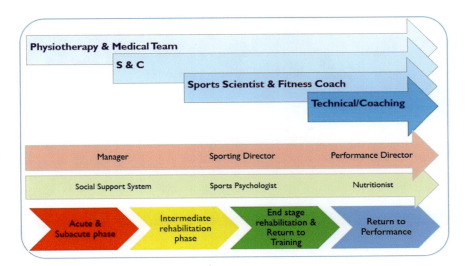

Figure 9.14 Return-to-play continuum outlining the overlap of involvement of practitioners throughout the process.

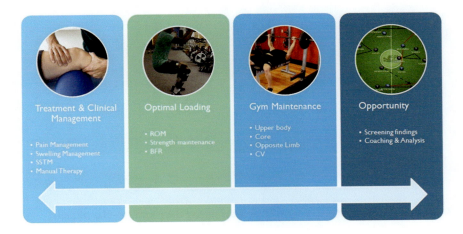

Figure 9.15 Elements of RTP process during the acute phase.

Re-conditioning

During the re-conditioning rehabilitation phase, the player will progress their loading and the strength & conditioning coaches will have more of an input to the RTP process, along with the collaboration of work with the sports scientists when the onset of on-field work commences (Figure 9.16).

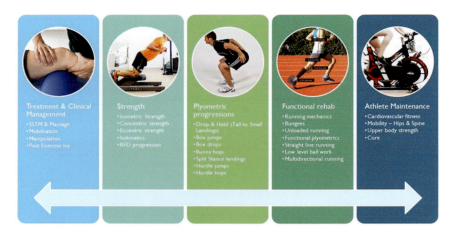

Figure 9.16 Elements of RTP process during the subacute phase.

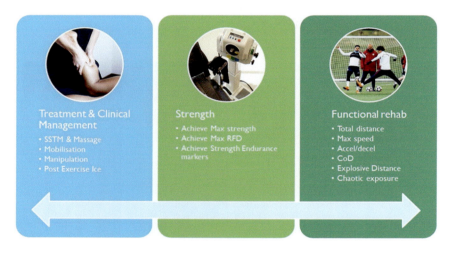

Figure 9.17 Elements of end-stage RTP process during the return-to-play phase.

Controlled sport-specific and return to play phases

During the end stage (RTP) rehabilitation phases, the input form the physiotherapy and medical department would reduce significantly to maintenance and on-going management of the player with an emphasis being placed on normalizing and maximizing strength work with the key focus being on achieving the on-field objective markers to RTP (Figure 9.17).

Novel approaches to assist in RTP

Pain free versus pain threshold rehabilitation

The majority of literature surrounding the criteria to progress through rehabilitation is largely based around the alleviation and avoidance of pain, with progression typically only allowed when pain-free on clinical assessments. As such, these clinical assessments prolong an athlete's progression through rehabilitation, despite not being related to the exercises being undertaken. The combination of both the avoidance of pain during rehabilitation and the need to be pain free to progress can lead to reduced loading of the injured muscle and may contribute to residual deficits that may elevate the risk of re-injury [50]. As such, alternative approaches should be considered to find this balance between returning an athlete to play as soon as possible, whilst ensuring the work undertaken during rehabilitation is sufficient to reduce the risk of re-injury.

Recent research within the HSI field has suggested the use of pain as a criterion to progress through rehabilitation and as something to avoid in these phases might actually be holding athletes back from making the most of their time on the road to RTP. In HSI rehabilitation, the use of eccentric loading and long-length exercises can reduce the risk of a future-injury and may also accelerate RTP time. However, introducing these beneficial exercises into a rehabilitation programme may be limited by the consistently implemented guideline to only perform and progress rehabilitation in the absence of pain. Recent muscle injury research [86] showed that delaying the start of exercise-based rehabilitation by nine days, compared to two days, prolonged the time taken to RTP. It is possible that delaying the exposure to eccentric and long-length exercises may limit the ability to achieve beneficial adaptations and also prolong time taken to obtain RTP clearance. Therefore, undertaking rehabilitation with the use of a pain threshold (4/10 or less), as well as using exercise tolerance to guide progress through rehabilitation, not clinical assessments, has been suggested as a contemporary approach to this conundrum.

When comparing this pain threshold approach to a group who undertook rehabilitation pain free, there was no accelerated time to RTP in the pain threshold group. Despite this, with the removal of pain as a criterion to progress through rehabilitation, individuals commenced eccentric training a week earlier on average. This means that using exercise tolerance and removing pain as a criterion during exercises and when assessed clinically can potentially allow practitioners to get an extra week of eccentric work into their injured athletes before returning to play at the same time they would have anyways. Whilst this novel approach to rehabilitation may not accelerate the time to RTP, it does have the capacity to improve outcomes for athletes following the successful completion of the rehabilitation and limiting their chance of re-injury risk.

BFR in RTP

The use of blood flow restriction (BFR) training has recently become a novel method to enhance the recovery process in various injures [87, 88]. BFR has shown to increase muscular strength, hypertrophy rates, rate of force development, and reduce the rate of atrophy in post-surgical patients [89]. Although the adaptations from BFR use have been compared to heavy resistance training [90], the prescription of BFR could potentially be used in conjunction with traditional resistance training to enhance the RTP process.

Depending on the etiology, players may achieve the desired physiological adaptations from BFR activities when resistance training is not feasible. Specifically, post-surgical players could utilize BFR in a passive manner to reduce atrophy [91]. Furthermore, if players illustrate minimal strength capacities, the use of BFR could potentially yield adaptations to shorten the re-strengthening phase [85, 89, 92].

The most researched protocol for BFR use is the '30-15-15-15' concept, where the individual completes 30 repetitions, followed by 3 sets of 15 repetitions, all with 30 seconds rest in-between [93]. This protocol can be applied to multi-joint and/or isolation movements, targeting a specific muscle group. Although the use of BFR can be advantageous in the RTP setting, certain injuries that benefit from avoiding concentric patterns (i.e. hamstring muscle group) may not benefit from BFR usage.

Platelet-Rich Plasma injections

The constant battle between reducing the risk of re-injury whilst accelerating an athlete's progress through rehabilitation has found new and novel ways to attempt to try and get players back as soon as possible whilst not getting injured again. One novel adjunct treatment to rehabilitation is platelet-rich plasma (PRP). These injections are autologous (taken from the person) platelets, growth factors, and alpha granules utilized with the desire to improve the healing process within injured muscle to accelerate RTP and reduce re-injury risk. As such, PRP injections have been a focus of recent research to try and push the boundaries of athlete injury recovery.

Numerous studies have reported the success of PRP injections to accelerate the time taken to RTP for various tendinopathies and muscle injuries [94–98]. The hamstring muscle group has been the focus of a range of controversies surrounding the use of PRP injections to aid in the rehabilitation process. Two of the most significant studies in this space found that PRP injections did not reduce the time taken to RTP anymore than placebo injections of isotonic saline [99] or an intensive rehabilitation protocol did [100]. Additionally, a recent systematic review stated that 'there is no evidence to suggest that PRP injections plus physical therapy reduced time to RTP or re-injury rates when compared to no treatment of physical therapy alone'. Whilst not entirely conclusive due to a range of quality and bias concerns, higher-quality studies in larger cohorts are needed to better support or disprove the use of PRP in accelerating the time to RTP.

Conclusion

A variety of injuries can occur in elite soccer, due to the uncontrolled chaotic nature of the sport. It is suggested that practitioners work cohesively amongst departments to develop a diligent, thorough RTP protocol. Many factors should be considered when designing a RTP framework, including etiology, exercise design/variables, cohort/environment, and training and match data. Key performance indicators should be identified throughout the RTP process to ensure that a safe and effective progression is being applied. Staff should divide tasks accordingly, whilst working cohesively to ensure best practice for RTP. Novel methods are encouraged but approached with guidelines and adjustments where necessary.

References

1. Arnason, A., et al., *Physical fitness, injuries, and team performance in soccer.* Medicine & Science in Sports & Exercise, 2004. **36**(2): p. 278–285.
2. Eirale, C., et al., *Low injury rate strongly correlates with team success in Qatari professional football.* British Journal of Sports Medicine, 2013. **47**(12): p. 807–808.
3. Hägglund, M., et al., *Injuries affect team performance negatively in professional football: An 11-year follow-up of the UEFA Champions League injury study.* British Journal of Sports Medicine, 2013. **47**(12): p. 738–742.
4. Ekstrand, J., et al., *Injury rates decreased in men's professional football: An 18-year prospective cohort study of almost 12,000 injuries sustained during 1.8 million hours of play.* British Journal of Sports Medicine, 2021. **55**(19): p. 1084–1091.
5. Bahr, R., B. Clarsen, and J. Ekstrand, *Why we should focus on the burden of injuries and illnesses, not just their incidence.* 2018, BMJ Publishing Group Ltd and British Association of Sport and Exercise Medicine.
6. Tabben, M., et al., *Injury and illness epidemiology in professional Asian football: Lower general incidence and burden but higher ACL and hamstring injury burden compared with Europe.* British Journal of Sports Medicine, 2021. **56**(1): p. 18–23.
7. Ekstrand, J., M. Waldén, and M. Hägglund, *Hamstring injuries have increased by 4% annually in men's professional football, since 2001: A 13-year longitudinal analysis of the UEFA Elite Club injury study.* British Journal of Sports Medicine, 2016. **50**(12): p. 731–737.
8. Brukner, P. and D. Connell, *'Serious thigh muscle strains': Beware the intramuscular tendon which plays an important role in difficult hamstring and quadriceps muscle strains.* British Journal of Sports Medicine, 2016. **50**(4): p. 205–208.
9. Ekstrand, J., M. Hägglund, and M. Waldén, *Epidemiology of muscle injuries in professional football (soccer).* The American Journal of Sports Medicine, 2011. **39**(6): p. 1226–1232.
10. Ekstrand, J., et al., *Time before return to play for the most common injuries in professional football: A 16-year follow-up of the UEFA elite Club injury study.* British Journal of Sports Medicine, 2020. **54**(7): p. 421–426.
11. Ekstrand, J., *Keeping your top players on the pitch: The key to football medicine at a professional level.* 2013, BMJ Publishing Group Ltd and British Association of Sport and Exercise Medicine.
12. Ekstrand, J., J.C. Lee, and J.C. Healy, *MRI findings and return to play in football: A prospective analysis of 255 hamstring injuries in the UEFA Elite Club Injury Study.* British Journal of Sports Medicine, 2016. **50**(12): p. 738–743.
13. Van Der Made, A.D., et al., *Intramuscular tendon injury is not associated with an increased hamstring reinjury rate within 12 months after return to play.* British Journal of Sports Medicine, 2018. **52**(19): p. 1261–1266.

14 van der Made, A.D., et al., *Intramuscular tendon involvement on MRI has limited value for predicting time to return to play following acute hamstring injury.* British Journal of Sports Medicine, 2018. **52**(2): p. 83–88.
15 Comin, J., et al., *Return to competitive play after hamstring injuries involving disruption of the central tendon.* The American Journal of Sports Medicine, 2013. **41**(1): p. 111–115.
16 Pollock, N., et al., *Time to return to full training is delayed and recurrence rate is higher in intratendinous ('c') acute hamstring injury in elite track and field athletes: Clinical application of the British athletics muscle injury classification.* British Journal of Sports Medicine, 2016. **50**(5): p. 305–310.
17 Reurink, G., R. Whiteley, and J. Tol, *Hamstring injuries and predicting return to play:'Bye-Bye MRI?'.* 2015, BMJ Publishing Group Ltd and British Association of Sport and Exercise Medicine.
18 Werner, J., et al., *Hip and groin time-loss injuries decreased slightly but injury burden remained constant in men's professional football: The 15-year prospective UEFA Elite Club Injury Study.* British Journal of Sports Medicine, 2019. **53**(9): p. 539–546.
19 Weir, A., et al., *Doha agreement meeting on terminology and definitions in groin pain in athletes.* British Journal of Sports Medicine, 2015. **49**(12): p. 768–774.
20 Putukian, M., et al., *Head injury in soccer: From science to the field; summary of the head injury summit held in April 2017 in New York City, New York.* British Journal of Sports Medicine, 2019. **53**(21): p. 1332–1332.
21 McCrory, P., et al., *Consensus statement on concussion in sport—the 5th international conference on concussion in sport held in Berlin, October 2016.* British Journal of Sports Medicine, 2017. **51**(11): p. 838–847.
22 Pusateri, M.E., B.J. Hockenberry, and C.A. McGrew, *Zurich to Berlin—'where' are we now with the concussion in sport group?* Current Sports Medicine Reports, 2018. **17**(1): p. 26–30.
23 Askling, C.M., N. Malliaropoulos, and J. Karlsson, *High-speed running type or stretching-type of hamstring injuries makes a difference to treatment and prognosis.* 2012, BMJ Publishing Group Ltd and British Association of Sport and Exercise Medicine.
24 Ekstrand, J., et al., *Hamstring muscle injuries in professional football: The correlation of MRI findings with return to play.* British Journal of Sports Medicine, 2012. **46**(2): p. 112–117.
25 Prince, C., et al., *Sprint specificity of isolated hamstring-strengthening exercises in terms of muscle activity and force production.* Frontiers in Sports and Active Living, 2021. **2**(211). p. 609–636.
26 Higashihara, A., et al., *Differences in hamstring activation characteristics between the acceleration and maximum-speed phases of sprinting.* Journal of Sports Sciences, 2018. **36**(12): p. 1313–1318.
27 Thelen, D.G., et al., *Hamstring muscle kinematics during treadmill sprinting.* Medicine & Science in Sports & Exercise, 2005. **37**(1): p. 108–114.
28 Giakoumis, M., *To Nordic or not to Nordic? A different perspective with reason to appreciate semitendinosus more than ever.* Sport Performance & Science Reports, 2020. **90**(1): p. 1–5.
29 Mendiguchia, J., et al., *Rectus femoris muscle injuries in football: A clinically relevant review of mechanisms of injury, risk factors and preventive strategies.* British Journal of Sports Medicine, 2013. **47**(6): p. 359–366.
30 Mendiguchia, J., et al., *Effects of hamstring-emphasized neuromuscular training on strength and sprinting mechanics in football players.* Scandinavian Journal of Medicine & Science in Sports, 2015. **25**(6): p. e621–e629.
31 Morin, J.-B., et al., *Sprint acceleration mechanics: The major role of hamstrings in horizontal force production.* Frontiers in Physiology, 2015. **6**: p. 404.
32 Chaabene, H., et al., *Change of direction speed: Toward a strength training approach with accentuated eccentric muscle actions.* Sports Medicine, 2018. **48**(8): p. 1773–1779.

33 Green, B., et al., *Calf muscle strain injuries in elite Australian football players: A descriptive epidemiological evaluation.* Scandinavian Journal of Medicine & Science in Sports, 2020. **30**(1): p. 174–184.
34 Green, B. and T. Pizzari, *Calf muscle strain injuries in sport: A systematic review of risk factors for injury.* British Journal of Sports Medicine, 2017. **51**(16): p. 1189–1194.
35 Dorn, T.W., A.G. Schache, and M.G. Pandy, *Muscular strategy shift in human running: Dependence of running speed on hip and ankle muscle performance.* Journal of Experimental Biology, 2012. **215**(11): p. 1944–1956.
36 Serner, A., et al., *Diagnosis of acute groin injuries: A prospective study of 110 athletes.* The American Journal of Sports Medicine, 2015. **43**(8): p. 1857–1864.
37 Charnock, B.L., et al., *Adductor longus mechanics during the maximal effort soccer kick.* Sports Biomechanics, 2009. **8**(3): p. 223–234.
38 Severin, A.C., D.B. Mellifont, and M.G. Sayers, *Influence of previous groin pain on hip and pelvic instep kick kinematics.* Science and Medicine in Football, 2017. **1**(1): p. 80–85.
39 Fox, A.S., *Change-of-direction biomechanics: Is what's best for anterior cruciate ligament injury prevention also best for performance?* Sports Medicine, 2018. **48**(8): p. 1799–1807.
40 Hunter, G., *Specific soft tissue mobilisation in the treatment of soft tissue lesions.* Physiotherapy, 1994. **80**(1): p. 15–21.
41 Reiman, M.P. and D.S. Lorenz, *Integration of strength and conditioning principles into a rehabilitation program.* International Journal of Sports Physical Therapy, 2011. **6**(3): p. 241.
42 Jacobsen, P., et al., *A combination of initial and follow-up physiotherapist examination predicts physician-determined time to return to play after hamstring injury, with no added value of MRI.* British Journal of Sports Medicine, 2016. **50**(7): p. 431–439.
43 Whiteley, R., et al., *Clinical implications from daily physiotherapy examination of 131 acute hamstring injuries and their association with running speed and rehabilitation progression.* British Journal of Sports Medicine, 2018. **52**(5): p. 303–310.
44 Wangensteen, A., et al., *Similar isokinetic strength preinjury and at return to sport after hamstring injury.* Medicine and Science in Sports and Exercise, 2019. **51**(6): p. 1091–1098.
45 Dhillon, H., S. Dhilllon, and M.S. Dhillon, *Current concepts in sports injury rehabilitation.* Indian Journal of Orthopaedics, 2017. **51**(5): p. 529–536.
46 Taberner, M., et al., *Physical preparation and return to performance of an elite female football player following ACL reconstruction: A journey to the FIFA Women's World Cup.* BMJ Open Sport & Exercise Medicine, 2020. **6**(1): p. e000843.
47 Blanchard, S. and P. Glasgow, *A theoretical model to describe progressions and regressions for exercise rehabilitation.* Physical Therapy in Sport, 2014. **15**(3): p. 131–135.
48 Glasgow, P., N. Phillips, and C. Bleakley, *Optimal loading: Key variables and mechanisms.* 2015, BMJ Publishing Group Ltd and British Association of Sport and Exercise Medicine. p. 278–279.
49 Wernbom, M., J. Augustsson, and R. Thomeé, *The influence of frequency, intensity, volume and mode of strength training on whole muscle cross-sectional area in humans.* Sports Medicine, 2007. **37**(3): p. 225–264.
50 Hickey, J., et al., *Pain-free vs pain-threshold rehabilitation for acute hamstring strain injury: A randomised controlled trial.* Journal of Science and Medicine in Sport, 2017. **20**: p. 11.
51 Timmins, R.G., et al., *Short biceps femoris fascicles and eccentric knee flexor weakness increase the risk of hamstring injury in elite football (soccer): A prospective cohort study.* British Journal of Sports Medicine, 2015. **50**(24): p. 1524–1535.
52 van Dyk, N., F.P. Behan, and R. Whiteley, *Including the Nordic hamstring exercise in injury prevention programmes halves the rate of hamstring injuries: A systematic review*

and meta-analysis of 8459 athletes. British Journal of Sports Medicine, 2019. **53**(21): p. 1362–1370.
53. Bourne, M.N., et al., *Impact of the Nordic hamstring and hip extension exercises on hamstring architecture and morphology: Implications for injury prevention.* British Journal of Sports Medicine, 2016. **51**(5): p. 469–477.
54. Bourne, M.N., et al., *An evidence-based framework for strengthening exercises to prevent hamstring injury.* Sports Medicine, 2018. **48**(2): p. 251–267.
55. Presland, J.D., et al., *The effect of Nordic hamstring exercise training volume on biceps femoris long head architectural adaptation.* Scandinavian Journal of Medicine & Science in Sports, 2018. **28**(7): p. 1775–1783.
56. Douglas, J., et al., *Chronic adaptations to eccentric training: A systematic review.* Sports Medicine, 2017. **47**(5): p. 917–941.
57. Hossain, M.Z., M. Pluta, and W. Grill. *In-vivo muscle length-force-joint angle relationship for quasi-static muscle action of the biceps muscle*, in *Health monitoring of structural and biological systems 2013.* 2013. International Society for Optics and Photonics.
58. Rio, E., et al., *Isometric exercise induces analgesia and reduces inhibition in patellar tendinopathy.* British Journal of Sports Medicine, 2015. **49**(19): p. 1277–1283.
59. Wathen, D., *Explosive/plyometric exercises.* Training, 1993. **25**(2): p. 122.
60. Davies, G., B.L. Riemann, and R. Manske, *Current concepts of plyometric exercise.* International Journal of Sports Physical Therapy, 2015. **10**(6): p. 760.
61. Chmielewski, T.L., et al., *Plyometric exercise in the rehabilitation of athletes: Physiological responses and clinical application.* Journal of Orthopaedic & Sports Physical Therapy, 2006. **36**(5): p. 308–319.
62. Ebben, W.P., et al., *Kinetic quantification of plyometric exercise intensity.* The Journal of Strength & Conditioning Research, 2011. **25**(12): p. 3288–3298.
63. Moore, G.E., *The role of exercise prescription in chronic disease.* British Journal of Sports Medicine, 2004. **38**(1): p. 6–7.
64. Gabbett, T.J., *The training-injury prevention paradox: Should athletes be training smarter and harder?* British Journal of Sports Medicine, 2016. **50**(5): p. 273–280.
65. Drew, M.K., J. Cook, and C.F. Finch, *Sports-related workload and injury risk: Simply knowing the risks will not prevent injuries: Narrative review.* British Journal of Sports Medicine, 2016. **50**(21): p. 1306–1308.
66. Windt, J. and T.J. Gabbett, *The workload—injury aetiology model.* 2016, BMJ Publishing Group Ltd and British Association of Sport and Exercise Medicine.
67. Fousekis, K., et al., *Intrinsic risk factors of non-contact quadriceps and hamstring strains in soccer: A prospective study of 100 professional players.* British Journal of Sports Medicine, 2011. **45**(9): p. 709–714.
68. Bourne, M.N., et al., *Eccentric knee flexor strength and risk of hamstring injuries in rugby union: A prospective study.* The American Journal of Sports Medicine, 2015. **43**(11): p. 2663–2670.
69. Afonso, J., et al., *Injury prevention: From symmetry to asymmetry, to critical thresholds,* in *Asymmetry as a Foundational and Functional Requirement in Human Movement.* 2020, Springer. p. 27–31.
70. Ueberschär, O., et al., *Measuring biomechanical loads and asymmetries in junior elite long-distance runners through triaxial inertial sensors.* Sports Orthopaedics and Traumatology, 2019. **35**(3): p. 296–308.
71. Maloney, S.J., *The relationship between asymmetry and athletic performance: A critical review.* The Journal of Strength & Conditioning Research, 2019. **33**(9): p. 2579–2593.
72. Dionyssiotis, Y., et al., *Physical rehabilitation of muscles, tendons and ligaments.* MOJ Orthopedics & Rheumatology, 2016. **6**(2): p. 2–6.
73. Hickey, J.T., et al., *Hamstring strain injury rehabilitation.* Journal of Athletic Training, 2022. **57**(2): p. 125–135.

74 Creighton, D.W., et al., *Return-to-play in sport: A decision-based model.* Clinical Journal of Sport Medicine, 2010. **20**(5): p. 379–385.
75 Wollin, M., et al., *A novel hamstring strain injury prevention system: Post-match strength testing for secondary prevention in football.* 2020, BMJ Publishing Group Ltd and British Association of Sport and Exercise Medicine. p. 498–499.
76 Duhig, S., et al., *Effect of high-speed running on hamstring strain injury risk.* British Journal of Sports Medicine, 2016. **50**(24): p. 1536–1540.
77 Ingebrigtsen, J., et al., *Acceleration and sprint profiles of a professional elite football team in match play.* European Journal of Sport Science, 2015. **15**(2): p. 101–110.
78 Edouard, P., et al., *Sprinting: A potential vaccine for hamstring injury.* Sport Performance & Science Reports, 2019. **1**: p. 1–2.
79 Stares, J., et al., *How much is enough in rehabilitation? High running workloads following lower limb muscle injury delay return to play but protect against subsequent injury.* Journal of Science and Medicine in Sport, 2018. **21**(10): p. 1019–1024.
80 Gabbett, T.J., *The training-performance puzzle: How can the past inform future training directions?* Journal of Athletic Training, 2020. **55**(9): p. 874–884.
81 Gabbe, B.J., et al., *Risk factors for hamstring injuries in community level Australian football.* British Journal of Sports Medicine, 2005. **39**(2): p. 106–110.
82 O'Brien, M., et al., *A novel device to assess hip strength: Concurrent validity and normative values in male athletes.* Physical Therapy in Sport, 2019. **35**: p. 63–68.
83 Croisier, J.-L., et al., *Strength imbalances and prevention of hamstring injury in professional soccer players: A prospective study.* The American Journal of Sports Medicine, 2008. **36**(8): p. 1469–1475.
84 Taberner, M., T. Allen, and D.D. Cohen, *Progressing rehabilitation after injury: Consider the 'control-chaos continuum'.* 2019, BMJ Publishing Group Ltd and British Association of Sport and Exercise Medicine. p. 1132–1136.
85 Patterson, S.D., et al., *Blood flow restriction training: A novel approach to augment clinical rehabilitation: How to do it.* 2017, BMJ Publishing Group Ltd and British Association of Sport and Exercise Medicine. p. 1648–1649.
86 Bayer, M.L., et al., *Role of tissue perfusion, muscle strength recovery, and pain in rehabilitation after acute muscle strain injury: A randomized controlled trial comparing early and delayed rehabilitation.* Scandinavian Journal of Medicine & Science in Sports, 2018. **28**(12): p. 2579–2591.
87 Lambert, B.S., et al., *Blood flow restriction therapy for stimulating skeletal muscle growth: Practical considerations for maximizing recovery in clinical rehabilitation settings.* Techniques in Orthopaedics, 2018. **33**(2): p. 89–97.
88 Husmann, F., et al., *Impact of blood flow restriction exercise on muscle fatigue development and recovery.* Medicine & Science in Sports & Exercise, 2018. **50**(3): p. 436–446.
89 Patterson, S.D., et al., *Blood flow restriction exercise: Considerations of methodology, application, and safety.* Frontiers in Physiology, 2019. **10**: p. 533.
90 Mouser, J.G., et al., *High-pressure blood flow restriction with very low load resistance training results in peripheral vascular adaptations similar to heavy resistance training.* Physiological Measurement, 2019. **40**(3): p. 035003.
91 Lorenz, D.S., et al., *Blood flow restriction training.* Journal of Athletic Training, 2021. **56**(9): p. 937–944.
92 Centner, C., et al., *Effects of blood flow restriction training on muscular strength and hypertrophy in older individuals: A systematic review and meta-analysis.* Sports Medicine, 2019. **49**(1): p. 95–108.
93 Loenneke, J., R.S. Thiebaud, and T. Abe, *Does blood flow restriction result in skeletal muscle damage? A critical review of available evidence.* Scandinavian Journal of Medicine & Science in Sports, 2014. **24**(6): p. e415–422.
94 Dallaudière, B., et al., *Intratendinous injection of platelet-rich plasma under US guidance to treat tendinopathy: A long-term pilot study.* Journal of Vascular and Interventional Radiology, 2014. **25**(5): p. 717–723.

95 Filardo, G., et al., *Use of platelet-rich plasma for the treatment of refractory jumper's knee.* International Orthopaedics, 2010. **34**(6): p. 909–915.
96 Kon, E., et al., *Platelet-rich plasma (PRP) to treat sports injuries: Evidence to support its use.* Knee Surgery, Sports Traumatology, Arthroscopy, 2011. **19**(4): p. 516–527.
97 Mautner, K., et al., *Outcomes after ultrasound-guided platelet-rich plasma injections for chronic tendinopathy: A multicenter, retrospective review.* PM&R, 2013. **5**(3): p. 169–175.
98 Sheth, U., et al., *Does platelet-rich plasma lead to earlier return to sport when compared with conservative treatment in acute muscle injuries? A systematic review and meta-analysis.* Arthroscopy: The Journal of Arthroscopic & Related Surgery, 2018. **34**(1): p. 281–288. e1.
99 Reurink, G., et al., *Platelet-rich plasma injections in acute muscle injury.* The New England Journal of Medicine, 2014. **370**(26): p. 2546–2547.
100 Hamilton, B., et al., *Platelet-rich plasma does not enhance return to play in hamstring injuries: A randomised controlled trial.* British Journal of Sports Medicine, 2015. **49**(14): p. 943–950.

10 Periodisation

Mark Read, Rick Rietveld, Danny Deigan, Matt Birnie, Lorcan Mason and Adam Centofanti

Periodisation overview

Periodisation within a soccer framework is the strategic planning of training to enhance performance for each competitive match across the season. Understanding of all the key variables from a physical, tactical, technical, and psychological standpoint is essential to ensure appropriate planning throughout the days, weeks, and months that make up a competitive season. Numerous structured and fluid definitions exist for the term periodisation throughout athletic performance literature [1]. In essence, periodisation can be defined as a flexible framework for progressively planning short-term and long-term training variables and performance goals to achieve positive adaptations in response to periods of progressive overload, supplemented by periods of rest and recovery with the goal of ultimately improving performance [2–5]. Matveyev and Zdornyj were two of the pioneers of the theory of periodisation and offered a time-bound structure in which training planning should be sequenced from general to specific preparation [6–8]. This time-bound structure consists of three layers (Figure 10.1); the macro-layer: (one season long) which is the overall long-term plan for achieving the desired performance goal. This macro-layer consists of multiple meso-layers (one phase of the season) which aim to progressively lead to adaptations to achieve the desired long-term performance goal. Finally, these meso-layers consist of smaller micro-layers (one week of the phase) which are progressively sequenced to achieve session to session adaptations to achieve the long-term performance goals of each meso-layer [2, 7].

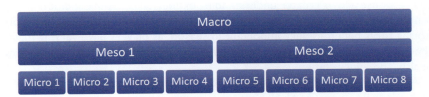

Figure 10.1 Visual representation of the structure of periodisation (Derived from Matveyev and Zdornyj [7]).

DOI: 10.4324/9781003200420-10

As a result of the complexity of planning in team sports such as soccer, it is imperative to minimize the catabolic responses [9, 10] and incidence of injury [11] during the season to facilitate peak performance through extended periods of unpredictable match-play demands and fixture schedules.

Assessing the variables

There are many ways to periodise physical performance and conditioning in elite soccer, with the main aim being to always achieve a positive training and performance effect, through manipulating the balance of training load and recovery. This is by planning and monitoring player response to the training programme to achieve an enhanced physical outcome, which will benefit holistic soccer performance across all the physical, technical, tactical, and mental elements of the game. The focus will change throughout microcycles (weekly), mesocycles (typically 3–6 weeks), and macrocycles (seasons). The season period (time of year), team and individual performances, and performance goals will guide targeted outcomes.

There is much greater control of periodisation through a pre-season period, as there are several other influences out of the practitioner's control during season. These influences include home and away matches, multiple competitions, training venues, travel schedules, possible altitude, environmental factors, international windows, and the greater possibility of injury that result from match play and competitive training situations. These factors also combined with the competing technical, tactical, and mental needs of training and the overall programme that are influenced by analysis and coach observation. The above-mentioned influences lend pre-season preparation to more traditional and planned models of periodisation which may include base, building, loading, and unloading microcycles. During season, training variables become more agile, however, in most cases, a weekly approach in soccer is to allow a two-day recovery focus following matches, two-day loading focus mid-week and two-day taper and preparation focus prior to the next match.

The overall planning and manipulation of training load can be achieved by monitoring several variables, such as the type of sessions, the number and frequency of each session type, and the volume and intensity of each session. The monitored training variables and responses can further be divided into external load and internal load (see Chapter 6). The combination and examination of dose and response allows greater understanding of individual player condition on the fitness-fatigue continuum. The individuality of player status, condition, and monitoring tools becomes very important in season, as players have varying match time and training participation that may be a result of team selection, tactics, health, and injury status.

A holistic view to planning and monitoring is needed to ensure that players have adequate exposure to all physical elements in preparation for match-play. This involves looking at the overall week, and periodically throughout the training week and in matches where elements may be overloaded.

- What are the training needs of the coach to instil his style of play?
- What are the game demands in the current competition?
- How many competitions may the players be involved in simultaneously?

Intensive and extensive

It is common to theme training sessions around the physical, technical, tactical, and mental elements of soccer. Themes may include an intensive (strength or resistance) session that incorporates smaller exercises and games, or an extensive (endurance) session that incorporates larger exercises and games. Utilizing monitoring tools such as global positioning system (GPS), heart rate, and RPE can assist in the fluid planning of training sessions, giving deeper insight to the training stimulus. The use of drill databases with good sample sizes of information from the relevant coach and players can assist in the planning and periodisation. Additionally, practitioners and coaches may analyse the objective/subjective markers from previous sessions and utilize drills from their database to elicit similar intensities in their ongoing planning and periodisation.

Periodizing resistance training

Power and strength training is also a key piece of the puzzle when periodising training load. Clubs traditionally schedule and perform separate weight training sessions following the field session, for various reasons (see *Chapter 4*). An alternative practice that is becoming more common is to utilize power and strength training in micro-doses, prior or following a pitch session to prime players for the physical demands and focus of these sessions. The monitoring and periodisation of power and strength training may be done around frequency, intensity, velocity-based targets, sets, reps, time under tension, or tonnage based on the aims of the programme. The focus of this work may mirror on-field adaptation aims to overload qualities and provide additional recovery on subsequent days or may be complementary to ensure all physical qualities are being addressed with exposure throughout the training cycle.

Periodising recovery/nutrition

An important part of the training programme is the periodisation of recovery. This includes the provision and advocation of nutrition and recovery interventions that accompany the planning and monitoring of the overall training programme (see *Chapter 8*). The most simple and beneficial components of recovery are sleep, nutrition, and the overall training programme itself. Recovery should be planned, monitored, and maintained to ensure optimal training objectives are met and physical performance maximised. There may be times during preseason or preparation phases, where strategies such as 'training low' to gain additional adaptations come the competitive season take place. In conjunction with training low, some recovery modalities are prescribed to potentially relieve muscle soreness and increase the likelihood of accelerated adaptations. However, certain recovery strategies may not be advised where players are expected to naturally adapt to the stimulus.

However, during season (or the competition phase), it is recommended to alter energy intake and use of recovery modalities in order to accelerate supercompensation [12, 13]. It is important that any nutritional modifications are monitored by a professional dietician with the understanding of individual player status. Additional recovery modalities that may be provided include contrast/cold water therapy, massage techniques, and compression garments. Recovery modalities should be implemented with consideration of all stressors players may experience. Some additional stressors that may trigger requirements for extra recovery strategies include considerations around family, contract, performance, travel, heat, and altitude. Variation in training type, intensity, and environment may also assist in enhancing the recovery process.

It is evident that periodisation in a soccer team setting needs to remain agile, with a focus on planning and monitoring team and individual player loads [1, 8, 14]. Whilst the concepts and theories of traditional periodisation are most definitely applicable to soccer, in particular preseason, there are several circumstances in season that these concepts cannot be applied. The nature of professional soccer means players are expected to physically peak weekly or even multiple times each week. However, careful consideration must be given to travel, potential altitude, and environmental conditions, which can influence the weekly periodisation. Increased attention to detail is integral to allow for appropriate planning and prescriptions.

Microcycles

The perfect training plan?

The design of a training structure is not only derived from the physical needs of a team, but rather is largely dependent on a wide array of factors which can be seen in the extensive table following. Ultimately there are multiple ways in which you can programme. However, it is evident that in order to construct the 'perfect' training plan, many key stakeholders are involved within the process, and an in-depth appreciation of all influences should be taken into account (Table 10.1).

Microcycle models

Training philosophies can be hugely varied in the modern game of soccer and the periodisation models to facilitate these philosophies can be differentiated from one another well, through the characteristics of how, what and when training is completed within the microcycles.

For some years now, many teams worldwide have been adopting a Tactical Periodisation approach, originating from Portugal [15]. This model can

Table 10.1 Planning considerations for developing a training structure

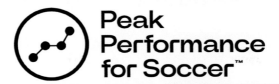

Physical performance	Technical/tactical	Social/ psychological	Environmental/ situational
Position in macrocycle	Coach philosophy	Long term	Competition level
Previous fixture	Coach experience	success of	Culture of club
Upcoming fixture	Tactical principles	team	Culture of country
Acute/chronic load of	Tactical	Short term	Religious beliefs
players	sub-principles	success of	Weather/climate
Position of strength/gym	Importance of	team	Pitch availability
work	next fixture	Team/staff	Staff availability
Position of conditioning	Standard of next	activities	Travel requirements
work	opposition	Health &	
Position of reserve/youth		wellbeing of	
games		team	
Starting vs non-starting		Family life	
players		Player/Individual	
Recovery philosophy		opinion	
Availability of players			

broadly be described as a method where the physical elements of soccer are being understood and adapted in parallel with the tactical dimensions. More specifically: it is thought that the Tactical Periodisation approach allows individuals to improve fitness levels at the same time as learning the 'game model'. It can be characterized as a model which has large fluctuating training loads and principles as a working week progresses. From a pure physical standpoint, this approach is 'daily undulating' whereby each day the body is being exposed to differing physical challenges and serves to mitigate the effect of repeated bouts of the same load. Ultimately, this type of periodisation is very inviting for a physical performance coach, as it presents a high quantity of 'acquisition days' as opposed to throwing the majority of training load on one single day.

In contrast, another periodisation method which can also be seen as a popular approach, especially within northern Europe, is the utilization of a 'High-Low' model. This methodology is essentially where a physical stimulus on any given training day is either 'bucketed' into a High Day, where players are exposed to larger quantities of training load, or a Low Day, which is essentially the opposite. The latter normally preceding and succeeding a 'High Day'. Including these two highlighted periodisation models, the below content addresses the positives and negatives of all the different approaches currently used within soccer.

Finally, it should be noted that the underlying theme with many successful training models is the ability to have variety in training load to:

a   work, when possible,
b   taper, when necessary, and
c   avoid monotony.

These should be seen to be a fundamentally essential concept in successful soccer training microcycles [16].

A 'prelude'

Given the development of professional soccer and the adoption of sport science over the past ten years, we can assume that many clubs now implement a similar approach in the two days succeeding a match day regardless of the club/coach philosophy. We can quite comfortably label these as 'recovery days'; however, the structure of the days is up for debate.

Active/passive recovery – (match day +1 or +2)

This day can be best described as a restoration day, whereby a variety of modalities can be implemented to speed up the recovery window and ensure that the players are in the process of reverting to their pre-competition 'homeostatic' state. In many situations, this will take place at the club. As aforementioned, this day could also take place on the second day after a game, but the principles will often remain the same. Situation- and environment-depending strategies can be inside or outside, with dedicated time focusing on; manual therapies, water immersion (hot/cold), and compression modalities, amongst many others (see Chapter 8) [13]. Overall, content of this training day is light from both physical and mental states.

'Switch off' – (match day +2 or +1)

Commonly a day off and a day away from the club. Essentially, this is not only an important physical restoration day but also a social/psychological restoration day.

'The lead-in'

A protocol of recovery, as stated above, will sequentially be followed by a new training phase leading into the next fixture. However, unlike the rather standardized recovery regimes used within the professional setting, the training models implemented in the next four to five days can differ greatly from club to club and country to country. Many clubs and teams will encounter situations with multiple games per week; however, the following 'lead-in' methods are only applicable to single-game weeks.

The 5-day

A 5-day 'lead-in' to a game is perhaps the most demanding from a social and psychological perspective, given the need to repeatedly 'load' on five consecutive days, albeit the first day being a lighter recovery focused day. When contrasted to all the other microcycles in Table 10.2, the 5-day 'lead-in' is the only method which utilizes a complete rest on the immediate day after a game. Although this method could be suitable for the players who have performed 60 min or more, it could be viewed as an opportunity missed to expose those players out of the squad or with limited playing time (<45 minutes) to a suitable training stimulus. This may subsequently result in the need to prescribe additional stimulus at a later date. However, it is recommended to approach with caution, as this specific microcycle is already long in nature with a consecutive load spread over many days without a period of rest. Another option would be to prescribe running-only conditioning after the match itself, but this can be extremely complex, and the practitioner may be severely restricted in what and how they can prescribe at this given point of time (see *Chapter 5*). For example, high-speed running can quite easily be implemented post-game; however, the ability to expose players to appropriate quantities of external loading values, such as total distance and accelerations/decelerations, is a little more challenging.

The characteristic of consecutive days of training should also be viewed with caution when planning for the normal training week, as to not induce chronic fatigue and/or increased risk of injury. Notice should be paid to how, when, and what overloading elements are implemented both on-and-off the pitch, given that unlike other methods, limited time is given to recover from such stimuli. As a result, there is a critical need to have suitable variation in training load between each day. In contract to the potential difficulties and complexities of planning and managing, all players from a physical perspective on this microcycle method, the 5-day 'lead-in' gives great opportunities to work with players from a technical and tactical perspective. As a result, this approach could be very effective for an academy setting, where contact time and development is prioritized over peak performance.

The 4-day

Although demanding, a 4-day 'lead in' remains strongly used in the modern game around the world [17]. In general, this model will allow for two distinct 'recovery/off days' immediately after a game, before then transitioning into a training phase of four days towards the following fixture. This model has almost exclusively been used in parallel with Tactical Periodisation models over recent years, and effectively spreads training load across several days rather than a very high day being followed by a period of rest [15]. Subjectively, it could be considered that four consecutive days of load may be too large to enable an athlete to perform optimally on match day. However, the opportunity to spread training load across several days is an inviting one for many, and certainly deserves to

Table 10.2 Four separate microcycles to approach a match day

Peak Performance for Soccer™

Match day code	Activity	| Match day lead in microcycles			
		5-day	4-day	2-day	1-day
MD+2	Session type	Recovery plus/build up	OFF/recovery	Recovery plus/build up	Recovery plus/build up
	Movement prep	Regeneration prehab (stretching, mobility, isometrics/core)	Rest day	Regeneration prehab (stretching, mobility, isometrics/core)	Regeneration prehab (stretching, mobility, isometrics/core)
	Pitch focus	Build up		Build up	Build up
	Strength & conditioning – on field	Hurdle mobility, coordination + Movement quality		Hurdle mobility, coordination + Movement quality	Hurdle mobility, coordination + Movement quality
	Strength & conditioning - gym	Optional upper body gym + core or extended recovery (yoga)		Optional upper body gym + core or extended recovery (yoga)a	Optional upper body gym + core or extended recovery (yoga)

Periodisation

Match day code	Activity	Match day lead in microcycles			
		5-day	4-day	2-day	1-day
MD-4	Session type	Intensive	Intensive	Intensive/extensive	Intensive
	Movement prep	Small-area prehab (glute, quad, adductor, knee/ankle, plyometrics)	Small-area prehab (glute, quad, adductor, knee/ankle, plyometrics)	Mixed-area prehab (glute, quad, adductor, hamstring, plyometrics)	Small-area prehab (glute, quad, adductor, knee/ankle, plyometrics)
	Pitch focus	Intensive practices	Intensive practices	Intensive/extensive practices	Intensive practices
	Strength & conditioning – on field	Acceleration, deceleration, change of direction, ball protection	Acceleration, deceleration, change of direction, ball protection	Acceleration, deceleration, change of direction, high-speed running	Acceleration, deceleration, change of direction, ball protection
	Strength & conditioning - gym	Upper body or total body	Upper body or total body	Lower body or total body	Upper body or total body
MD-3	Session type	Extensive	Extensive	OFF/recovery	
	Movement prep	Large-area prehab (glute, hamstring, psoas, calf)	Large-area prehab (glute, hamstring, psoas, calf)	Rest day	Large-area prehab (glute, hamstring, psoas, calf)
	Pitch focus	Extensive practices	Extensive practices		Extensive practices
	Strength & conditioning – on field	High-speed running + Large area prep	High-speed running + Maximum velocity		High-speed running + Maximum velocity
	Strength & conditioning – gym	Lower body or total body	Lower body or total body		Lower body or total body

(Continued)

| Match day code | Activity | \multicolumn{5}{c|}{Match day lead in microcycles} |
| | | 5-day | 4-day | 2-day | 1-day |

Match day code	Activity	5-day	4-day	2-day	1-day
MD-2	Session type	Speed	Speed	Speed	OFF/recovery
	Movement prep	Mixed area prehab (glute, hamstring, psoas, calf, knee/ankle)	Mixed area prehab (glute, hamstring, psoas, calf, knee/ankle)	Mixed area prehab (glute, hamstring, psoas, calf, knee/ankle)	Rest day
	Pitch focus	Tactical – speed/quality of action	Tactical – speed/quality of action	Tactical – speed/quality of action	
	Strength & conditioning – on field	Hurdle mobility + maximum velocity	Hurdle mobility + coordination/Agility	Hurdle mobility + maximum velocity	
	Strength & conditioning – gym	Power gym + individual extras	Power gym + individual extras	Power gym + individual extras	
MD-1	Session type	Pre-match	Pre-match	Pre-match	Pre-match
	Movement prep	MD-1 Prehab (stretching, mobility, reactions, neural priming)	MD-1 Prehab (stretching, mobility, reactions, neural priming)	MD-1 Prehab (stretching, mobility, reactions, neural priming)	MD-1 Prehab (stretching, mobility, reactions, neural priming)
	Pitch focus	Pre-match + priming	Pre-match + priming	Pre-match + priming	Pre-match + priming
	Strength & conditioning – on field	Reaction games + acceleration	Reaction games + acceleration	Reaction games + acceleration	Reaction games + acceleration
	Strength & conditioning – gym	Individual preparation	Individual preparation	Individual preparation	Individual preparation

Periodisation

Match day code	Activity		Match day lead in microcycles			
		5-day	4-day	2-day	1-day	
Match day	Session type	**Match Day**	**Match Day**	**Match Day**	**Match Day**	
	Movement prep	Match day prep – individual & team	Match day prep – individual & team	Match day prep – individual & team	Match day prep – individual & team	
	Pitch focus	Match	Match	Match	Match	
	Strength & conditioning – on field	Top-up conditioning for subs	Top-up conditioning for subs	Top-up conditioning for subs	Top-up conditioning for subs	
	Strength & conditioning – gym	Selected matches – gym for non-playing group	Selected matches – gym for non-playing group	Selected matches – gym for non-playing group	Selected matches – gym for non-playing group	
MD+1	Session type	OFF/Recovery	Recovery	Recovery	Recovery	
	Movement prep	Rest day	Structured recovery modalities + training group	Structured recovery modalities + training group	Structured recovery modalities + training group	
	Pitch focus		Top-up conditioning < 45 minutes players	Top-up conditioning <45 minutes players	Top-up conditioning <45 minutes players	
	Strength & conditioning – on field					
	Strength & conditioning – gym		Total body gym + optional UB gym for starters	Total body gym + optional UB gym for starters	Total body gym + optional UB gym for starters	

UB = Upper Body

be considered. Each day can be broken down into differing physical and tactical qualities to not heavily overload any specific entity. As a result, this gives practitioners a high volume of contact time with players to develop physical qualities, in line with what is delivered from a technical and tactical perspective. At this point, it is pertinent to outline how and what physical qualities could successfully be implemented effectively into a four day build in.

MATCH DAY (-4) – TIGHT AREA SESSION

Due to the smaller areas normally programmed into the first training day, it can be a great day to work on strength-demanding soccer components such as ball protection/shielding, 1v1's + 2v2's and smaller sided games (4v4–7v7). In parallel with this, change of direction, deceleration, stretch-shortening cycle, and lower body strength qualities fit very well alongside this type of a session and should be prioritized on such a day.

MATCH DAY (-3) – LARGE AREA SESSION

The second day into the training cycle and the third day before a game is a day where areas of use can be expanded, and longer durations can be implemented. On this day, physical qualities such as high-speed running are more easily obtained due to the availability of greater working areas. From a soccer perspective, this day should be used to repeatedly perform actions and gather volume from larger sided games (8v8–11v11s).

MATCH DAY (-2) – MODERATE AREA SESSION WITH SPEED

With two sessions left, prior to the match, this day can be considered a final acquisition day whilst being part of the taper process. Resulting in a moderate area session, whereby a greater focus is placed on speed of actions, with lower volumes compared to the preceding training days. Typically, this day is a great day to work with transitional based exercises and attacking focused drills, where the speed and quality of each action is essential. Due to the 'quicker' demands of the session, the physical qualities which could be developed in parallel with the technical/tactical elements are as follows; acceleration, absolute/maximal speed in addition to more powerful 'speed/strength' qualities off the pitch.

MATCH DAY (-1) – REACTIVE/PREPARATION SESSION

As with every soccer periodisation model, the day before the game will serve as a type of taper (or deload) towards the performance on the match day. This day will normally be reserved for final tactical elements and details and can be a great opportunity to work on reactive and priming activities to stimulate the nervous system. Cognitively challenging games with plenty of rest are perfect for this type of day and will also aid to build cohesion between the squad if implemented correctly.

CONSIDERATIONS FOR THE 4-DAY 'LEAD-IN'

Overall, due to the length and consistent nature of this type of training week, practitioners need to be very wary of the need for variation between sessions and how best to differentiate them from one another. The variation can come through a multitude of ways as outlined above; however, three stand out principles which can easily be manipulated to bring about this variation are Pitch Size, Playing Numbers and Work to Rest Ratios. As with all the microcycle examples presented in this chapter, the '4 day lead-in' approach has several pros and cons. However, when considering all the multifaceted layers of a training week, this specific approach certainly has more positives than negatives. In particular, the training day after a match day is a great opportunity to work with the players who have inadequate match minutes and load, whilst simultaneously allowing the high loaded players (>60 match minutes) to work specifically with the club's recovery interventions/protocols (see Chapter 8). In addition, this method facilitates large periods of time for the technical and tactical staff to work on the specific principles for each week, compared to other approaches with a lower number of training days.

One method which anecdotally has been suggested to be practically effective with the larger training weeks is to micro-dose various physical qualities into the warm-up phase of each session. Figure 10.2 outlines how a breakdown of such physical qualities may look on each given day. The suggestion is not to perform maximal speed within the first 15 minutes (typically allocated warm-up time) of a training session, but the final 4–5 minutes of any warm-up could be used with maximal effect to develop our players athletically (see Chapter 5).

The 2-day

A 2-day 'build-in' effectively works on the premise of keeping players fresh towards the back end of the week and allows them to be off and away from the club's facilities on MD-3. This approach allows for the initial days after a game to be part of a recovery cycle before introducing an overload training session in the middle of the week. Effectively, the model is a 'High/Low' approach and gives the players plenty of time to recover and crucially adapt from any applied stimuli. The 2-day 'lead-in' is a method which is favourable with players themselves, as it allows for a complete rest day mid-way through the microcycle to spend time away from the training ground, and subsequently recover both

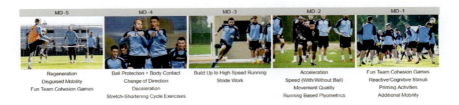

Figure 10.2 Utilizing the warm-up – the 4- and 5-day lead-in.

physically and mentally in preparation for the upcoming fixture. Nevertheless, practitioners should apply further precaution to the MD-2 session, where players are transitioning through a stage of recovery. This initial session back after an overload day must be prepared and planned carefully to not heighten any risk of injury. In particular, the MD-2 session on this microcycle approach would certainly be of a different nature to a MD-2 utilized in a four or five day lead-in method.

A further complexity of the 2-day build-in is the need to cram several physical qualities into the acquisition day (e.g. MD-4), which can cause some problems with the prescription of conditioning elements. For example, consideration around small- or large-sided games or exposure of change-of-direction of high-speed running qualities. Nevertheless, the ability to truly overload physical qualities on this 2-day 'lead-in' has many benefits, especially during season, when one high-loading training day within the week may be enough to elicit the maintenance of high levels of physical fitness, whilst also enhancing the likelihood of physical readiness towards the end of the week.

The 1-day

The final example of the four microcycles highlighted in Table 10.2 is based around a front-loaded week with a much-reduced load towards the end, due to a prescribed rest day on MD-2. From a comprehensive standpoint, the 1-day 'lead-in' has many positive attributes and is also well-balanced, compared to some of the other microcycles. From the beginning of the microcycle, the 1-day 'lead-in' has the option of an 'off-feet' recovery stimulus on the MD+1, or a conditioning opportunity for those requiring a physical stimulus. Therefore, this approach gives the possibility of two 'acquisition' days prior to a rest day, thus making the physical prescription of any on-field conditioning, or strength work, easier to navigate. Smaller area physical stimuli could be prescribed into the first acquisition day (MD-4), whilst bigger area and higher speed elements could fit suitably into the second day (MD-3). In parallel, due to the greater number of working days within this model, the warm-up 'micro dosing' process outlined in Figure 10.2 would also suit this approach. By having the second day before a game away from the training ground, there is a suggestion that all lower body strength and power work is potentially restricted to only MD-4 and MD-3, with MD+1/+2 being located within a recovery window and MD-1 being a preparation and taper session. However, most of the tactical work is also restricted to MD-1 or in the early phases of the week, which could present as an issue for technical staff (Table 10.3).

Multiple games per week

In many circumstances, teams across the world will face multiple games per week both domestically and internationally (Table 10.4). When reverting to the 'single game per week' model, it can be fair to assume that a squad is essentially

Table 10.3 Advantages and disadvantages to each match 'lead-in' approach

	5-day lead-in	4-day lead-in	2-day lead-in	1-day lead-in
Advantages	Allows more tactical preparation leading into a match	Provides a platform for full recovery before the start of a new training week	Provides opportunity for a true physical overload on MD-4	Accommodates for two distinct acquisition days + increased strength/power load due to rest day MD-2
	Allows psychological/physical switch off the day after a game	Allows more tactical preparation leading into a match	Ability to load from a strength/power perspective due to the rest day on MD-3	Potential for increased 'freshness' leading into MD-1 and MD
	A great approach for coaches with a deep understanding of tactical periodisation	A great approach for coaches with a deep understanding of tactical periodisation	Allows for a psychological/physical rest mid-week	Possibly allows easier physical prescription on MD-4 and MD-3
	A large contact time with players to develop physical qualities and playing style	Like a '5 Day Lead In', allows a large contact time with players to develop physical qualities and playing style	Allows a top up and overload session MD+1	Allows for a psychological/physical reset two days before the game
		Allows a top up and overload session MD+1		Allows a top up and overload session MD+1

(Continued)

	5-day lead-in	4-day lead-in	2-day lead-in	1-day lead-in
Disadvantages	More difficult to overload physical qualities due to no off/rest day in the week leading to game	More difficult to overload physical qualities due to no off/rest day in the week leading to game	Increased complexity of conditioning prescription on MD-4 due to only allowing one acquisition day vs multiple days	Possible need to combine strength and power session on MD-4 due to no MD-2 power opportunity
	Does not allow a structured recovery MD+1	Higher risk of overload through the week resulting in fatigue	Must be cognizant of residual fatigue from MD-4 when planning MD-2, particularly considerations towards max speed exposure	Potential reduced time/flow into game for tactical preparation on pitch compared to 4- and 5-day lead-ins
	Higher risk of overload through the week resulting in fatigue	Must be cautious with lower body strength doses to not bring about excessive soreness	Potential reduced time/flow into game for tactical preparation on pitch compared to 4- and 5-day lead-ins	
	Must be cautious with lower body strength doses to not bring about excessive soreness			
	No MD+1 session to top up and overload non playing group			

split into two separate groups in the transition between weekly microcycles; those who have been exposed to a high load through the match day, and those who require some form of an additional physical stimulus, due to the lack of match exposure. However, when considering a two-game per week schedule, there are more subgroups within each squad, resulting in numerous different physical statuses to be aware of. Given that players will be recovering for at least 48-hours post-match, it is highly possible that the only day which may have all players on the same training stimulus, is that on the MD-1 before the second match day (Table 10.4). At all other points throughout this microcycle, there will be players with differing physical statuses which need to be catered for on an individual basis.

Table 10.4 An example of a two games per week microcycle

Match day Code	Activity	Two games per week microcycle (congested fixture week)
MD	Session type	Match day 1
	Movement prep	Match day prep – Individual & Team
	Pitch focus	Match
	Strength & conditioning – on field	Top up conditioning <45–60 min
	Strength & conditioning - gym	Selected matches – gym for players <45–60 min
MD+1	Session type	Recovery
	Movement prep	Structured recovery modalities + Training group
	Pitch focus	Top up conditioning <45–60 min players
	Strength & conditioning – on field	
	Strength & conditioning - gym	Total body gym <45–60 min + optional UB gym for starters
MD+2/-1	Session type	Pre-match
	Movement prep	MD-1 Prehab (stretching, mobility, reactions, CNS priming)
	Pitch focus	Pre-match + priming
	Strength & conditioning – on field	Reaction games + acceleration
	Strength & conditioning - gym	Individual prep
MD	Session type	Match day 2
	Movement prep	Match day prep – individual & team
	Pitch focus	Match
	Strength & conditioning – on field	Top up conditioning <45–60 min
	Strength & conditioning - gym	Selected matches – gym for players <45–60 min

(Continued)

Match day Code	Activity	Two games per week microcycle (congested fixture week)
MD+1	Session type	OFF/recovery
	Movement prep	Rest day
	Pitch focus	
	Strength & conditioning – on field	
	Strength & conditioning - gym	
MD+2/-2	Session type	Recovery/build up
	Movement prep	Regeneration prehab (stretching, mobility, isometrics/core)
	Pitch focus	Build up
	Strength & conditioning – on field	Hurdle mobility, coordination + movement quality
	Strength & conditioning - gym	Optional upper body gym + core or extended recovery (yoga)
MD-1	Session type	Pre-match
	Movement prep	MD-1 Prehab (stretching, mobility, reactions, CNS priming)
	Pitch focus	Pre-match + priming
	Strength & conditioning – on field	Reaction games + acceleration
		Individual prep

With this type of schedule, acquisition days are essentially re-labelled as the 'match day' and the microcycle in principle becomes a 'High/Low' approach whereby players are either stimulated via match-play, or are recovering between. Consequently, the only possibility to load players from a training stimulus is when players are out of the match day squad or have inadequate match exposure (substitutes). As a result, the post-match (and proceeding day; MD+1) conditioning sessions become crucial. Within these limited opportunities, physical prescription becomes highly individualized. From a strength perspective, a micro dosing approach is preferable to maintain any injury prevention strategies put in place during previous microcycles (see *Chapter 4*). For example, post-match or MD+1 may be appropriate day to expose the non-playing group to a very small dose of posterior chain, adductor and unilateral strength work. Whereas, on-field stimulus prescriptions, such as large quantities of high-speed running (without causing any unwanted fatigue leading into the upcoming fixture), are limited to match day. It is imperative that when approaching away games, practitioners plan to recognize what each player requires the most. As a result, a sound load monitoring system put in place to track individual variations allow practitioners to truly identify what, when, and how physical work needs to be prescribed (see *Chapter 6*).

Factors to consider

There are several factors that can affect the periodisation model, such as weather, altitude, competition schedule, the, coach and travel. The following questions should be asked by practitioners working in elite soccer:

- How are training sessions planned during congested fixtures?
- What does the coaching staff want to train/develop?
- What is the influence of desired drills on the fitness status of players?
- How does the periodisation approach adapt to non-modifiables (such as weather and altitude)?

Environmental

Each environment has different weather conditions to consider when planning micro-, meso-, or macro-cycles. This external factor is potentially the most unpredictable of them all, and results in the human body responding differently to the demands placed upon it.

Hot conditions

The human thermoregulatory system is challenged in hot conditions, resulting in potentially impaired performance and increased chances for heat-related illness [18]. Thus, resulting in greater energy costs for comparative exercises, during hot circumstances [19]. Often, the external load may result equally (i.e. same physical output); however, internal load (response) is much greater during hot conditions compared to more comfortable climates. Dehydration is a main factor that can influence cognitive and physical performance [20–22]. A controllable factor that practitioners can adjust in order to acclimate to hot conditions is the training times. Altering training times during different parts of the season to avoid hot conditions can potentially expose players to better conditions for sessions requiring greater physical outputs. Furthermore, preventing players from training in the peak hot periods could potentially allow increased performance and minimize fatigue and other heat-related illnesses. However, there are many benefits associated with exposure to hot conditions.

A variety of benefits, including decrease in heart rate (during exercise) and plasma volume, can be obtained within a week of training regularly in hot conditions [23]. However, full adaptation for heat often occurs within a 10-day period [18]. With significant positive aerobic adaptations associated with short-term exposure to training in hot conditions, it is suggested that practitioners carefully periodize training times to optimize the acclimatization benefits [24]. It is suggested that players don't necessarily need to be exposed to hot conditions long-term, to obtain the physiological benefits of heat-acclimatisation. Therefore, the suggestion for practitioners is to investigate times of the year to appropriately train in the heat. The pre-season period could potentially be an optimal period to expose players to consecutive days of hot conditions, allowing for an adaptation period before the season commences [24, 25].

Cold conditions

There are various extreme conditions that teams may be exposed to during the season which can potentially alter a team's periodisation. Unlike hot conditions, athletes being regularly exposed to training and/or competing in cold weather have more negative outcomes as opposed to performance enhancements [26–29]. Therefore, playing in cold conditions may require a more extensive warm-up prior to training/matches to ensure optimal muscle temperature, as muscle temperature and neuromuscular function are linearly related [30]. Experienced cold weather athletes will usually wear breathable undergarments that are 'sweat wicking' and have a high rate of drying [31]. If garments become wet and do not dry, the athlete potentially runs the risk of cooling faster. Therefore, for teams that are occasionally exposed to cold weather environments, it is recommended to wear appropriate undergarments to assist in maintaining muscle temperature throughout activity [31].

Altitude

Balancing the acute and chronic physiological responses to altitude is essential for achieving the greatest benefit to performance [32]. To rationalize and interpret the physiological basis for altitude exposure, it is important to understand that as altitude rises, both the barometric pressure (P_b) and partial pressure of oxygen (PiO_2) decrease which leads to a reduction in the availability of oxygen that can be delivered to skeletal muscle, despite the concentration of oxygen remaining constant (20.9%) inducing hypoxic conditions [32], therefore creating inherently harder physical conditions for players during games/training. Research suggests that that there may be two windows of opportunity of optimal performance once an athlete descends from altitude, the first, within the first five to seven days upon return, with the second being three to six weeks post-altitude [33]. Furthermore, it was suggested that the acute period post-altitude training is the best time to achieve supercompensation [34]. Unfortunately, teams may be exposed to altitude for only one game which means there is not enough time to adapt to the environment and performance may be compromised due to the increased physical stress players will experience. In the lead up to such conditions, teams may choose to deload to increase the likelihood of physical readiness. Alternatively, if teams decide to perform training at altitude for an extended period of time (e.g. pre-season), it is important to understand that the equivalent load at sea level performed at altitude will be much harder physically and periodisation of training should account for this increased physical stress.

Coach

The head coach or collective coaching staff will have significant influence on periodisation for a professional soccer team. A plan may be in place for a given training session or week, however, if the coach decides to change something, then ultimately that is his/her decision to do so. This can potentially be for better or worse, but it reemphasizes the ability to be adaptable as a practitioner (see Chapters 1 and 11). Fluidity in periodisation is essential to best prepare the team for match day as sticking to the original plan when things have changed on a particular day may not be suitable. Even in the most unified of relationships between performance staff and coaching staff, changes can occur daily that were not planned for, but from a psychological or technical/tactical perspective, the coach may have made a call to increase or decrease volume/intensity. In these instances, keeping an eye on the bigger picture and where the team is at on a weekly/daily basis will assist in the future periodisation process.

Travel

Frequent travel is a common occurrence in professional soccer teams and will vary team to team depending on competition schedules and league structure. In some teams, it may be required to travel across multiple time zones (e.g. MLS in the United States). This consistent travel can have an emotional and physical cost to athletes, so it is highly recommended to have strategies in place to mitigate any negative effects [35]. Such strategies can include arriving in the environment a day or two prior to match-day, training in the host city, and hydration and nutrition interventions. Practitioners should also attempt to maintain as much of a normal preparation for match-day as you would a home game, instructing players to bring their own pillow from home to sleep on, and exposure to natural light at local times [36].

Practical application

Planning training for non-starting players

During the competitive season, large team-based training sessions to develop the necessary physical qualities can become inhibited, particularly during periods of high fixture density. The squad should display relatively comparable degrees of fitness following pre-season, but the landscape can swiftly change once the league commences, with noticeable fluctuations in fitness levels having been observed [37]. These decrements in fitness measures tend to occur due to minimal squad rotation, which subsequently creates three subset groups: regular starters, substitutes, and players left out of the squad. During congested match microcycles, it is quite common to identify disparities in high-speed running volumes when comparing starters and non-starters. Research conducted in the Premier League also discovered similar findings, with starters performing greater volumes of high-speed load throughout a week [38, 39]. With a fast turnover of matches, half of the squad are in a cycle of playing and recovering, restricting the non-starters to performing possessions and SSGs in reduced numbers, ranging from 1v1 to 6v6. This form of training certainly has its merits: it can enable both aerobic and anaerobic development, depending on the number of players involved and the duration of each possession block (see Chapter 5). However, small group training also has its limitations. For example, high-speed running and peak speed exposure are unlikely to occur when the size of the pitch is relative to the numbers of players involved in these small-sided practices, which is particularly detrimental for full-backs and wide attacking players.

Therefore, due to the restricted training content for non-starting players during the competitive season, practitioners should seek to incorporate additional training modalities to ensure individuals are exposed to high-speed running when match minutes are limited [40].

High-speed running modalities

Typically, there are two types of speed endurance (SE) interventions causing slightly contrasting physiological responses, but both forms are intended to develop fatigue-resistance qualities to tolerate recurrent explosive actions throughout a 90-minute match [41, 42]. The distinction between the two forms of training is subtle. Speed endurance maintenance develops the repeatability of high-intensity actions and is generally performed in small-sided game scenarios (2v2–4v4). Whereas, speed endurance production training, which is commonly conducted individually, improves short maximum efforts, and is performed at near maximum intensity over short bouts (<30's). Production training also requires longer rest periods to ensure there is sufficient recovery for the next repetition. With regard to training effect, intensity has a greater impact on enhancing physical performance than volume and frequency. Speed endurance fits the notion of being intense but low in volume, which is why it is a justified mode of training in an applied framework, working alongside the other critical aspects of soccer training throughout a microcycle, such as technical and tactical training.

Position-specific production drills can be contextualized based on time-motion analysis. Coaches can create individual position-specific profiles by discovering the most intense trends both in and out of possession, and where these specific actions take place on the pitch [43]. During the drill design process, practitioners should consider shorter explosive movements for central strikers, and longer locomotive patterns for full-backs and wide attacking players, which would correspond to key moments of match simulation. Once a collection of movements is formulated from match footage, practitioners can design specific drill content condensed into ~ 20–30 seconds of 'all out' bursts. This type of work is classified as supra-maximal training exceeding any 20–30 second high-speed peak bout of work during a match. Drills may incorporate

Table 10.5 General speed endurance guidelines

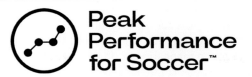

Training modality	Time	Intensity	Work: rest ratio	Sets/Reps	Training drill	Player RPE
Production	<30 seconds	90%–100%	1:>4	1–2 × 6–8	Position specific	9/10
Maintenance	1–4 minutes	70%–90%	1:3	4–5 sets	SSGs + possessions	7/10

defensive or attacking components, which would include acceleration and deceleration actions, whilst concurrently integrating technical elements, such as passing, crossing, and finishing, depending on the position (Table 10.5). Firsthand experience suggests players prefer this type of work because of game specificity. However, additional technical elements may interfere with the physical outputs when merged within a speed endurance drill, so practitioners must be cognizant of how the technical work is incorporated and should not allow it to become the limiting factor disrupting the desired physical outcome.

Practitioners should take confidence from the positive effects production training can have on elite-level soccer players. However, due to the intense nature of training prescription, caution must be taken due to the high mechanical load output. Therefore, very high-speed (sprint) running drills (>7.0 m·s^{-1}) should be progressed steadily so that players can tolerate the load without causing significantly delayed onset muscle soreness. Practitioners may also seek to utilize live GPS feedback to ensure the totalities of workload are within the prescribed optimum bandwidth range for that session and individual (see *Chapter 7*).

Planning for two games per week

With midweek fixtures, practitioners are limited to prescribing reduced volumes of sprint load (>7.0 m·s^{-1}), simply because the turnaround into the next match is imminent. In this instance, practitioners should focus on small-sided games and possessions (SE maintenance) to maintain aerobic and anaerobic conditioning, supplemented by low volume individual speed endurance production bouts, only for priority players. It is important to reduce overall physical stress on MD-2, yet expose the non-starters to some form of conditioning work. One method of choice to reduce the total high-speed distance during an individual drill is to incorporate additional technical actions and changes of direction. The player is still exposed to small doses of required metabolic load, but less invasive mechanical stress is produced.

282 Mark Read et al.

Planning for one game per week

Microcycles with one game per week allow for more creativity and offer more options to train multiple physical components. A variety of possessions and themed games (8v8–10v10) can be supplemented with speed endurance production work, with a recommendation of one or two sessions per week for priority players. Planning to perform these explosive production drills will depend on factors, such as scheduled days off, recent travel, and the physical, technical, and tactical training planned throughout the week. If 10v10 games (extensive training) are performed on a full-pitch or three-quarter-pitch dimensions, production training may well be modulated, or in some cases with certain players, not required. Each player should have individual targets for metrics deemed critical for their position to determine whether further training prescription is warranted throughout the week (*see Chapter 7*). Logistically, it is unrealistic to execute production drills with all non-starters. In this instance, a hybrid drill that combines both high-speed running with an opposed SSG practice can be implemented. This type of training drill is very efficient as technical coaches can work on specific soccer elements, such as creating 3v2 overloads, transitioning, and developing 1v1 attacking/defensive qualities, whilst also achieving a high-speed running and sprint load.

Although there is no replacement for match exposure, maintaining a sufficient level of conditioning and high-speed running load throughout the season is valuable. However, during a high-density of fixtures, practitioners are limited to implementing progressive, consistent overload to enhance physical performance. Modern-day elite soccer players with reduced match load may well be capable of physically performing in a one-off match. However, if required to play regularly in a high-density period of matches, players might be at a greater risk of injury, due to the sudden spike in high-speed load [44], particularly high-output positional groups, such as full-backs and wide attackers. To mitigate such risk, performing intense low volume production drills during less congested periods is recommended.

Practitioners and coaches involved in the design process must be aware that the perceived subjective exertion from production drills is very high. Therefore in the latter stages of the season, this type of work might be relative to other occasions within the competitive calendar. Ultimately, practitioners must communicate with the players and coaching staff to ensure the best outcome is achieved and be flexible with the weekly training plan. Production training is a justified modality to maintain and even develop physical capacity for non-starting players throughout the season if planned optimally and logically (Table 10.6).

Conclusion

Periodisation in professional soccer is a complex process that requires practitioners to factor in many variables such as environment, fixtures, training load, coach preferences, travel, and player readiness. There are a variety of ways

Periodisation 283

Table 10.6 Two microcycles for starters and non-starters (one and two matches per week)

Peak Performance for Soccer™

Microcycle with 5 day lead-in

Day		Mon	Tues	Wed	Thurs	Fri	Sat	Sun	Comments
Type		MD+2/ MD-5	MD-4	MD-3 or rest day	MD-2	MD-1	Match		With a 5 day lead-in, training can combine small rondo's, overload themes, larger-based progressions & 2× speed endurance sessions (NS).
Number of players		10–12	20–22	20–22	20–22	20–22		Rest day or full recovery at training ground	Dist >24km/h is spread across the week, but is predominantly front loaded on M-4, provided by the speed endurance intervention.
Primary conditioning objective		Post day off (moderate intensity)	Acceleration/ deceleration	Aerobic	Speed	Reactive primer			Peak speeds can be performed on M-3.
Session Duration		60'	75–90'	75'	60'	45'			M-2 is a mich lighter session due to the accumulative load from M-4/M-3. However, if M-3 reverts to a rest day, then the intensity of M-2 can increase by including 10v10 themed practices, which would also slightly increase the dist >24km/h, or include a small dose of speed endurance.
Speed Endurance (NS)			Production - PS		Production – PS Dependent on Wednesday		Non-Starters		
			1–2 sets × 6–8 reps @25–30sec		1 set × 4 @20sec		Moderate-High Speed pitch runs		Post-match running does not need to be exhaustive with a 5-day lead-in. The microcycle gives plenty of opportunity to maintain sufficient energy system training.
Hybrid Drill (NS)				2v2 attack vs defense + HSR					

(Continued)

Microcycle with 5 day lead-in

Day	Mon	Tues	Wed	Thurs	Fri	Sat	Sun	Comments
Team training drills	8v2 Rondo	4v4+3 2 groups	10v10 Possession	Light passing sequence	8v2 rondo 2 groups			
	Passing sequence	6v4 overload 2 groups	10v10 themed game	4v2+1 Rondo 3 groups	4v4+3 Possession 2 groups			
	4v4+2 Possession	4v4 SSG tournament	Peak speed >90% (2–3 reps)	Finishing drills	Unopposed tactical			
	5v5 SSG	4 players performing SE						
Total distance >7.0 m·s^{-1} (NS)		Approx. 200m	Approx. 100m	Approx. 75m		Approx. 150m		

Periodisation

Microcycle with mid-week fixture

Day	Mon	Tues	Wed	Thurs	Fri	Sat	Sun	Comments
Type	MD+2/ MD-2	MD-1	Match	MD+1/MD-2	MD-1	Match		With a mid-week fixture, training load for the non-starters is more restricted.
Number of players	10–12 (main session)	20–22		10–12	20–22			
Primary conditioning objective	Anaerobic	Reactive primer or SAQ		Acceleration	Reactive primer or SAQ			Naturally, more SSG's (<6v6's) are performed due to the starters recovery from the match.
Session duration	60'	45'		60'	45'			Training is geared towards keeping players sharp and not extensive fitness development.
Speed Endurance (NS)	Production - PS 1× set 4–6 reps@20–25sec		Non-Starters Moderate-high speed pitch runs	Production - PS 1 set × 4 @20sec		Non-Starters Moderate-high speed pitch runs	Rest day or full recovery at training ground	Speed endurance work can be conducted on <2 but intensity moderate & volume low.
Hybrid Drill (NS)				4v4 + HSR				Hybrid drills work well with smaller group training, enabling for some high speed exposure & technical work performed under fatigue.
Team training drills	8v4 Overload possession Passing sequence and acceleration 5v5 SSG	8v2 rondo 2 groups 4v4+3 Possession 2 groups Unopposed tactical		Light passing sequence 4v2+1 Rondo 3 groups Finishing drills	8v2 rondo 2 groups 4v4+3 Possession 2 groups Unopposed tactical			In this microcycle example, the game falls on M-3. Therefore, post-match work should include high-speed running blocks. Alternatively, M-2 can be utilized but with reduced volume.
Total distance >7.0m·s⁻¹ (NS)	Approx. 75–100 m		Approx. 175–200 m	Approx. 75 m		Approx. 150 m		

NS = non-starter. PS = position specific. SAQ = speed, agility, quickness. High-speed load may change depending on match involvement in which teams can periodise training, with advantages and disadvantages to each. Understanding of what can be achieved on each day with a clear collective approach from a technical/tactical, physical, psychological, and cultural perspective will assist in deciding what approach suits your club most. During congested periods in-season, practitioners must understand the implications this has on periodisation for non-starting players and what opportunities are presented to ensure appropriate levels of physical condition are maintained. Finally, it is integral that practitioners have the ability to be adaptable and fluid in the ever-changing environment that often occurs within elite soccer.

References

1 Mujika, I., et al., *An integrated, multifactorial approach to periodization for optimal performance in individual and team sports.* International Journal of Sports Physiology and Performance, 2018. **13**(5): p. 538–561.
2 Smith, D.J. and S.R. Norris, *Periodization*, in Encyclopedia of exercise medicine in health and disease, F.C. Mooren, Editor. 2012, Springer Berlin Heidelberg: Berlin, Heidelberg. p. 694–697.
3 Bompa, T.O. and G. Haff, *Periodization: Theory and Methodology of Training*. 5 ed. 2009, Champaign: Human Kinetics. 411
4 Issurin, V.B., *New horizons for the methodology and physiology of training periodization.* Sports Medicine, 2010. **40**(3): p. 189–206.
5 Kiely, J., *Periodization theory: Confronting an inconvenient truth.* Sports Medicine, 2018. **48**(4): p. 753–764.
6 Matveyev, L., Fundamentals of sports training. 1977: Progress Publishers, Fizkultura i Sport Publishers.
7 Matveev, L.P. and A.P. Zdornyj, Fundamentals of sports training. 1981: Progress.
8 Kiely, J., *Periodization paradigms in the 21st century: Evidence-led or tradition-driven?* International Journal of Sports Physiology and Performance, 2012. **7**(3): p. 242–250.
9 Kraemer, W.J., et al., *Changes in exercise performance and hormonal concentrations over a big ten soccer season in starters and nonstarters.* Journal of Strength and Conditioning Research, 2004. **18**(1): p. 121–128.
10 Cormack, S.J., et al., *Neuromuscular and endocrine responses of elite players during an Australian rules football season.* International Journal of Sports Physiology & Performance, 2008. **3**(4): p. 439–453.
11 Gamble, P., *Periodization of training for team sports athletes.* Strength and Conditioning Journal, 2006. **28**(5): p. 56.
12 Anderson, L., et al., *Energy intake and expenditure of professional soccer players of the English Premier League: Evidence of carbohydrate periodization.* International Journal of Sport Nutrition and Exercise Metabolism, 2017. **27**(3): p. 228–238.
13 Nédélec, M., et al., *Recovery in soccer.* Sports Medicine, 2013. **43**(1): p. 9–22.
14 Hornsby, W.G., et al., *Addressing the confusion within periodization research.* Journal of Functional Morphology and Kinesiology, 2020. **5**(3): p. 68.
15 Afonso, J., et al., *A systematic review of research on Tactical Periodization: Absence of empirical data, burden of proof, and benefit of doubt.* Human Movement, 2020. **21**(4): p. 37–43.
16 Morgans, R., et al., *Principles and practices of training for soccer.* Journal of Sport and Health Science, 2014. **3**(4): p. 251–257.
17 Owen, A.L., et al., *A contemporary multi-modal mechanical approach to training monitoring in elite professional soccer.* Science and Medicine in Football, 2017. **1**(3): p. 216–221.

18 Wendt, D., L.J.C. van Loon, and W.D. Marken Lichtenbelt, *Thermoregulation during exercise in the heat.* Sports Medicine, 2007. **37**(8): p. 669–682.
19 Nybo, L., P. Rasmussen, and M.N. Sawka, *Performance in the heat-physiological factors of importance for hyperthermia-induced fatigue.* Comprehensive Physiology, 2014. **4**(2): p. 657–689.
20 Judelson, D.A., et al., *Effect of hydration state on strength, power, and resistance exercise performance.* Medicine and Science in Sports and Exercise, 2007. **39**(10): p. 1817–1824.
21 Creighton, B.C., et al., *Effect of dehydration on muscle strength, power, and performance in intermittent high-intensity sports,* in Meyer, F., Szygula, Z., & Wilk, B.(Eds.), Fluid balance, hydration, and athletic performance, 2016: Boca Raton: CRC Press, p. 133–153.
22 Maughan, R. and S. Shirreffs, *Dehydration and rehydration in competative sport.* Scandinavian Journal of Medicine & Science in Sports, 2010. **20**: p. 40–47.
23 Périard, J., S. Racinais, and M.N. Sawka, *Adaptations and mechanisms of human heat acclimation: Applications for competitive athletes and sports.* Scandinavian Journal of Medicine & Science in Sports, 2015. **25**: p. 20–38.
24 Chalmers, S., et al., *Short-term heat acclimation training improves physical performance: A systematic review, and exploration of physiological adaptations and application for team sports.* Sports Medicine, 2014. **44**(7): p. 971–988.
25 Heathcote, S.L., et al., *Passive heating: Reviewing practical heat acclimation strategies for endurance athletes.* Frontiers in Physiology, 2018. **9**: p. 1851.
26 Butcher, J.D., *Exercise-induced asthma in the competitive cold weather athlete.* Current Sports Medicine Reports, 2006. **5**(6): p. 284–288.
27 Anderson, S.D. and P. Kippelen, *Assessment and prevention of exercise-induced bronchoconstriction.* British Journal of Sports Medicine, 2012. **46**(6): p. 391–396.
28 Castellani, J.W. and M.J. Tipton, *Cold stress effects on exposure tolerance and exercise performance.* Comprehensive Physiology, 2015. **6**(1): p. 443–469.
29 Castellani, J.W. and A.J. Young, *Health and performance challenges during sports training and competition in cold weather.* British Journal of Sports Medicine, 2012. **46**(11): p. 788–791.
30 Racinais, S. and J. Oksa, *Temperature and neuromuscular function.* Scandinavian Journal of Medicine & Science in Sports, 2010. **20**: p. 1–18.
31 Gatterer, H., et al., *Practicing sport in cold environments: Practical recommendations to improve sport performance and reduce negative health outcomes.* International Journal of Environmental Research and Public Health, 2021. **18**(18): p. 9700.
32 Sinex, J.A. and R.F. Chapman, *Hypoxic training methods for improving endurance exercise performance.* Journal of Sport and Health Science, 2015. **4**(4): p. 325–332.
33 Chapman, R.F., et al., *Timing of return from altitude training for optimal sea level performance.* Journal of Applied Physiology, 2014. **116**(7): p. 837–843.
34 Saunders, P.U., et al., *Special environments: Altitude and heat.* International Journal of Sport Nutrition and Exercise Metabolism, 2019. **29**(2): p. 210–219.
35 Lee, A. and J.C. Galvez, *Jet lag in athletes.* Sports Health, 2012. **4**(3): p. 211–216.
36 Leatherwood, W.E. and J.L. Dragoo, *Effect of airline travel on performance: A review of the literature.* British Journal of Sports Medicine, 2013. **47**(9): p. 561–567.
37 Mohr, M. and P. Krustrup, *Yo-Yo intermittent recovery test performances within an entire football league during a full season.* Journal of Sports Sciences, 2014. **32**(4): p. 315–327.
38 Anderson, L., et al., *Quantification of training load during one-, two-and three-game week schedules in professional soccer players from the English Premier League: Implications for carbohydrate periodisation.* Journal of Sports Sciences, 2016. **34**(13): p. 1250–1259.

39 Anderson, L., et al., *Quantification of seasonal-long physical load in soccer players with different starting status from the English Premier League: Implications for maintaining squad physical fitness.* International Journal of Sports Physiology and Performance, 2016. **11**(8): p. 1038–1046.
40 Walker, G.J. and R. Hawkins, *Structuring a program in elite professional soccer.* Strength & Conditioning Journal, 2018. **40**(3): p. 72–82.
41 Mohr, M., et al., *Effect of two different intense training regimens on skeletal muscle ion transport proteins and fatigue development.* American Journal of Physiology-Regulatory, Integrative and Comparative Physiology, 2007. **292**(4): p. R1594–R1602.
42 Mohr, M. and F.M. Iaia, *Physiological basis of fatigue resistance training in competitive football.* Sports Science Exchange, 2014. **27**(126): p. 1–9.
43 Riboli, A., et al., *Effect of formation, ball in play and ball possession on peak demands in elite soccer.* Biology of Sport, 2021. **38**(2): p. 195.
44 Gabbett, T.J., *The training-injury prevention paradox: Should athletes be training smarter and harder?* British Journal of Sports Medicine, 2016. **50**(5): p. 273–280.

11 Coach and staff integration

Jarred Marsh, David Cosgrave, Scott Guyett, Paul Caffrey and Philippa McGregor

Overview of teams within a team

A soccer team is a collection of various inter-linked departments, from a technical team, support or 'backroom' staff to management personnel and the players themselves. While the number of persons involved within this structure can vary from club to club, it is a certainty that there will always be a number of linked departments within the team itself. Understanding the team members, their specific roles and responsibilities and ensuring delegation of important tasks are crucial to ensuring the team's success (Figure 11.1).

The organogram of modern-day professional soccer clubs can be extremely detailed. Leadership positions such as a director of football/soccer generally oversee the recruitment and management of the technical team (consisting of the head coach, assistant coaches, goalkeeping coach, and fitness coach) (see *Chapter 1*). The technical team can be supported by additional 'backroom staff' departments such as the performance and medical departments. These departments can be made up of a number of individuals who have diverse roles and responsibilities within the team structure. It is therefore key to align these roles to ensure team success throughout the season. However, this is somewhat of a complex task as each individual member of the team may be influenced by personal ideas, perceptions, beliefs, experiences, and attitudes. Thus, in turn, may have a knock-on effect on the team's overall behaviour. For example, in many African countries there is still a strong association with traditional medicine and

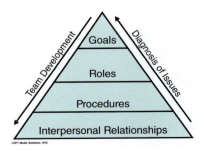

Figure 11.1 GRPI model (Adapted from Beckhard [1]).

DOI: 10.4324/9781003200420-11

ancestral beliefs. These cultural practises can have a psychological impact on a number of team aspects, such as training and match performance. Pre-match rituals may be deemed essential by the practicing player, and it is important to understand the individuals within the team and how to manage their varied personalities and beliefs in order to avoid confusion and maximise their performance.

In the same manner, the technical team and staff are all made up individuals with the same varied backgrounds. However, before their positions within the team, they are people first and foremost and understanding the person before the position is a key factor in finding a harmonious balance within the team. In many European clubs, when there is a change of management, a new manager will arrive with his/her own staff. While this can lead to faster integration and transference of the manager's philosophy into the team, it is not always allowed by the club management. In the case of a new manager entering into a fresh team environment with one (or even none) known attached staff members, it is vital to integrate into the environment to create harmony. Language barriers, cultural differences, and experiences can all play a role in the thought process and philosophy of an individual. For this reason, it is important for each member to be invested in getting to know the other individuals of the team. Developing a framework or structure within the team is the essential first step.

When establishing structures within a team, deciding upon the team's definition is the initial step towards team success. This refers to the leadership structures within the team (top-down approach vs. bottom-up). With this definition in mind, the individual members of the team are able to collectively agree upon their purpose or goals. Having common goal enables the team to then delegate responsibilities to the respective team members, in line with their agreed upon purpose. Once each individual member has been given their respective responsibilities, therefore, guidelines must be set to ensure the team members can operate freely within their specific roles. Through this structured approach, a new manager can create a framework within the team to accommodate all staff. With a shared common goal, the team will be able to have a shared consciousness and align their tasks towards a goal of the team.

Vision and mission

Each inter-linked department can operate within itself and focus on their own responsibilities and tasks. In a corporate setting, this approach might be productive. However, in a team sport setting (e.g. an elite soccer environment), each department needs to work in unison with the rest to achieve a common goal. This also applies to the individuals within the department.

Building a new team is difficult. Old habits die hard, old dogs can't learn new tricks. The phoenix doesn't always rise from the flames. Mixing new and old isn't always easy. Adding new cultures, languages, norms, beliefs, and behaviours into the cauldron of high-performance pressure could be enough to make the environment unbearable. Understanding the different stages of team formation is helpful. A new team just like a plant needs time and safety to let its roots form. Those roots can be seen as the identity that will nourish the team over time so care must be taken to allow them to grow and embed into the soil.

Psychological safety is not the seed of a fearless organisation but the soil that allows culture to grow

A new team is collective of individuals that are strangers that must find safety, norms, beliefs, and values that mirror each other. Expectations for behaviours and outcomes must be agreed at the outset. Cultural awareness and diversity training must be supported by language and communication training before any significant team effectiveness, cohesion or growth can occur. You can't just switch on teamwork. It takes time for a new team to 'gel' and work to its full potential. What's more, team members go through stages as they move from strangers to co-workers.

By developing a vision (where the department or team is going), and a mission statement (how they are going to get there), the individuals of the team can have a tangible direction to travel in. The age-old metaphor of a high-performance team being likened to a rowing boat is a great example. While the individual members of the team have individual roles to play in regard to the locomotion of the boat, they all have one clear vision – to move in a singular direction and get to the finish line. To accomplish this, they all need to focus on their mission: to execute their roles in synergistic manner and pull in the same direction. By defining a clear vision and mission, we can focus our individual and collective energy in moving the team in one direction (Figure 11.2). Be it securing promotion, moving through the group stages of an international competition, or simply surviving relegation, our success in the high-performance environment relies on us pulling together in the same direction.

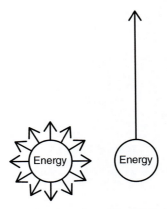

Figure 11.2 Essentialism: The disciplined pursuit of less (Adapted from Greg McKeown [2]).

Team of teams

The industrial age saw the rise of the reductionist management theory, a management style that is still used widely in many team-sport structures today. This style of management refers to breaking down systems or groups into their individual parts and assessing their output in isolation. Through this process, it is possible to assess effectiveness of the isolated departments and their linear interactions within the team. This, in turn, results in the assessment of the departments' effectiveness on the team's output. In order to achieve this structure, the decision-making members of the team must be placed at the highest point of a hierarchy or pyramid (e.g. manager), followed by mid-structure team members (e.g. assistant coaches), while the lowest members of the team are places at the bottom of the structure (e.g. support staff). Each level is responsible for engaging and instructing the level immediately beneath them.

Unfortunately, this system was designed to assess individual departments in static isolation and determining their contribution and value to the team as a whole. It is rigid in nature and not able to adapt to a complex, changing environment. In the world of elite soccer, the teams need to be agile and operate in a fluid, often chaotic environment with a shared consciousness (Figure 11.3). A recent manuscript identifying a bottom-up management solution to team operations illustrates the importance of each individual member understanding

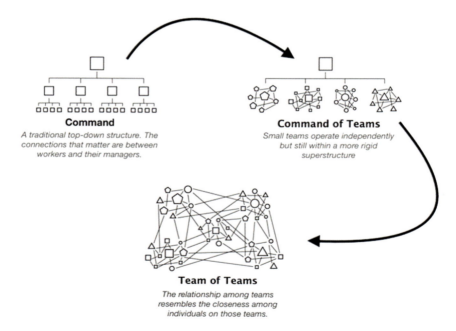

Figure 11.3 Team of teams: New rules of engagement in a complex world (Adapted from McChrystal [3]).

the various roles and requirements of the team's operation [3]. In theory, it's important for a performance analyst to understand the head coach's desired game model in order to structure and present relevant data on training and match performance. Likewise, the head coach needs to understand the detailed rehabilitation process of the medical department when a player is released back to full training after injury. In this manner, the team can operate with a shared consciousness and the micro processes within the team are synchronised towards one common goal.

To develop this shared consciousness, soccer organisations need to create trust and share a common goal (winning the domestic league, a cup final, avoiding relegation etc.). Through establishing a shared consciousness within our team structures, we are able to develop a linked 'network of networks' with individual members being able to make empowered decisions without seeking approval. Thus, the individual members can execute ideas and only need to report to management when required. In this approach, management can review the process over time and only adjust the team's direction if need be. However, it goes without saying that *it is vital to establish a shared consciousness prior to empowering the team members to make executive decisions*. Without this shared common purpose in mind, decisions may be made that are counter-productive or not aligned to the team's central goals.

Task delegation

Once a structured network is established with the team environment, delegation of performance procedures to the responsible team members is the next logical step. Delegation can be defined as getting work done through others by giving them authority and control of the work [4]. With a common goal in mind, the team staff can plan how best to approach the coming season or fixtures. Key tasks need to be delegated to ensure the goals and objectives of the team are met. This can be an important step as the tasks need to be carefully assigned to the right team members to ensure accountability, quality of delivery, and compliance.

However, it was not always easy to delegate numerous tasks to a room full of supporting staff. Managers were often reluctant to delegate tasks as the team structure was historically a 'one man show' given the lack of support staff. Teams in the 1900s did not have a plethora of soccer specialists and it was only in the early 2000s that soccer clubs saw the opportunity to enhance their team's performance through technology. It is widely known that Sam Allardyce pioneered the use of sport science, analysis, and statistics in his time as manager of Bolton Wanderers between 1999 and 2007 [5]. By empowering of his support staff, Sam Allardyce was able to delegate key performance tasks that created motivation, growth, and development for his supporting staff.

In theory, by assigning a task or responsibility to an individual team member, the group inherently recognises the competency of that team member. This is an important aspect within the elite soccer environment as trust within the technical team and support staff is paramount to success. Delegation can also be seen as an enabling tool that promotes feedback-seeking behaviour. When a task is delegated from a high position of power within an organisation (e.g. Manager), the team member is more likely to seek feedback [6]. By delegating key tasks within the team, we indirectly give power and authority to team members to actively explore and complete tasks that have been assigned to them. However, aligning the task to the central team goals is key.

Divide and conquer

When planning a complex programme, such as a preseason training camp or planning for an upcoming match during a congested period, it may be more logical to divide the process amongst a number of individuals. Therefore, the group (technical team, department, management etc.), may be able to undertake several key tasks in a short period of time. The inclusion of a group-style approach may also provide more insightful ideas. By breaking down the large, complex task of planning and preparation into smaller, more manageable processes, we may be able to lower inherent risk and increase the predictability of the process as a whole. During their successful 2019 Rugby World Cup campaign, the management team of the Springboks empowered the group of players not in the match day squad (known as the 'Bomb Squad'), to perform key analysis sessions on the upcoming matches. They were tasked to analyse the opposition players, their strength and weak areas, and even the personality traits of the appointed referees. The 'Bomb Squad' would then provide detailed feedback to management and players and highlight potential areas for the Springboks to take advantage of. As a result, the management staff showed trust in these players and empowered them. By dividing the total workload amongst the team members, the Springboks were able to create greater roles and responsibilities amongst the team members.

In the same manner, the tactical analysis for an upcoming league fixture may be conducted and presented by team members in an elite soccer environment. Defenders may be able to present key tactical attacking points to the strikers, while Goalkeepers may present key defensive points to the Defenders etc. Therefore, we could empower players to take ownership in the preparation process. Utilising the strengths of our individual members will enhance the overall team performance.

However, as with all positives, there are also negative points to the 'divide and conquer' principle. Often this style of leadership can be used to create disharmony amongst a team. Should the planning process be managed by and centred around one insecure leader, these insecurities can be used to dilute the power of the individual contributing departments involved in the planning process. Should the influence of these departments threaten the insecure leader in any way, the leader may work to create division and not cohesion within the team. It is therefore important to reinforce the elements of trust and communication within the team to ensure positive cohesion and alignment are maintained, although this may be affected by the leadership style of the manager or coach.

Conflict in the elite soccer environment

Interdependent individuals or teammates exist in two states. They cooperate or they compete. When a teammate pursues the latter, their motivation to achieve their goal will usually result in a negative outcome for the other individuals of the team [7]. Cohesive teams aim to share identities and visions and understand their context allowing them to mitigate conflict [8]. Team cohesion is the buffer to aid conflict management: cohesion is the foundations that allow leaders to directly address conflicts resulting in an atmosphere that allows them to mediate effectively [9]. Understanding where the source of conflict resonates is the first step to avoiding the negative association of conflict an environment [10]. Furthermore, investigating the 'what', 'how', 'who', and 'where' can help dissect and resolve conflict from becoming an unwanted affect.

Dealing with conflict

When seeking to understand how a conflict can be resolved within a group, it is essential to map out the motivations and power structures amongst the personnel involved [11]. The formal status of the members in the group, their afforded power, their motivation to cooperate internally, and concern for the wellbeing of the other party involved all affect the outcome. Poor cooperation between parties leads to avoidance of conflict and a gradual withdrawal from team affairs. This can also be a calculated strategy to buy time or to hope the issue resolves itself. This watch and wait tactic may hinder the conflict protagonist whilst the other party prepares their response. When an individual uses force or exerts their power to dominate the other party, it is evident that the dysfunctional team is not psychologically safe. This low concern for the other party can result in microaggressions and bullying that can undermine whole team trust if left unchecked. Leadership that uses this tactic may believe that this tactic is appropriate for certain contexts, but the reputational risk of a team casualty may not be worth the demonstration of power.

When individuals are unsure of their status and show low care for self, it is common for conflict to be avoided or prevented by accommodating another's point of view. This may be common in hierarchical, low trust or newly formed teams but also a sign of a highly respectful society. When avoiding conflict this way, teams create harmony and build trust thereby making a safe space to bring up critical issues later. Psychologically safe teams and teams that are considered a high-performance outfit will always seek to dig into an issue and find the win:win situation. By facing uncomfortable truths head on, individuals and teams that openly confront issues that face time can learn, develop trust, respect, and confidence in each other's values.

Finally, when there is no panacea and the best route to conflict resolution is not easy to navigate, mature teams will find a way to meet in the middle and seek compromise so the show can go on. Temporary solutions that benefit both parties and maintain relationships will allow both parties to feel like they mediated to their satisfaction and ensure core mission can continue.

Avoiding conflict

Teams that refuse to engage with the results of conflict, or the factors that precede it, spiral into a dysfunctional decline that affect performance [12, 13]. By removing the desire to deal with conflict head on, the team is missing a valuable opportunity to learn about itself and grow the individual members. As team members withdraw from each other tell-tale signs of quiet meetings, back-channel politics, slack discipline and loose policy enforcement become standard. Small issues may escalate into full blown team derailment resulting in large-scale restructuring of leaderships, teams, and whole organisations (Figure 11.4).

Conflict escalation

Conflict can be seen as self-reinforcing feedback loop that spirals out of control as individuals battle for supremacy or survival. Initial events that may involve a difference of opinion, perception or attitude can morph into insults, blaming and abstract unresolvable issues. As emotions run high, perception and bias may impede successful mediation leading to a compounding of negative behaviours that prevent regulation of the participants neuroendocrine response. Once conflict has embedded within a team, it is common for emotional contagion to spread to other members. Alliances and threats to the group outcomes create anxiety that negatively affect the performance of the team. Skilled third-party mediation is required to align involved individuals with the values and goals of the group thereby securing long term individual, relational, and organisation goals (Figure 11.5).

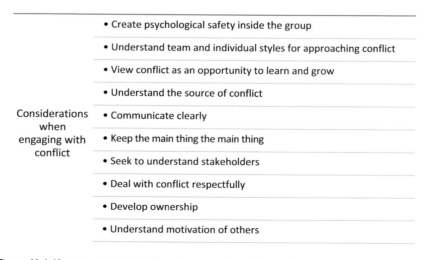

Figure 11.4 Key points to consider when engaging with conflict.

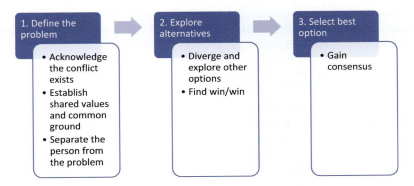

Figure 11.5 Steps for managing conflict.

Leadership styles in elite soccer

Professional soccer in England has a history of autocratic behaviours, where the coach or manager can control players either through fear and punishment or the threat of taking something away from them that they value [14]. However, in the past 20 years, leadership behaviours of soccer coaches and managers have changed, and they have begun to implement practices that empower the players, coaching, and support staff. Examples of empowerment include allowing assistant coaches to organise and oversee training sessions, allowing players a say in certain tactical strategies, or even allowing support staff such as physiotherapists/athletic trainers to give their opinion on player availability. By agreeing to these, managers are displaying a transformational style of leadership. But the question remains, *what is the best way to lead an elite soccer team?* Furthermore, what is the best way to lead a group of extremely wealthy, financially independent professional footballers?

Leadership styles are described as relatively stable patterns of behaviour displayed by leaders [15]. Furthermore, personal leadership style and strategy can vary from coach to coach. These may be influenced by upbringing, experience, their current environment, and their belief system. The leadership style of the manager or coach can have a decisive impact on the performance and retention of players in a team [16, 17]. Therefore, in order to be successful, coaching leadership styles require the team leader to have a large 'toolbox' which consists of signature strengths, self-management, and a 'give' culture [18].

Sufficient research has been conducted within the field of leadership strategies in sport [19]. A number of key leadership styles have been determined [20]. For the purposes of this chapter, we will discuss the following four:

1 Transactional Leadership
2 Transformational Leadership
3 Authoritarian Leadership
4 Democratic Leadership

Before discussing how leadership styles are applied in the elite soccer environment, it is first important to provide an overview of leadership concepts. The first concept to discuss is transactional leadership, which along with transformational leadership and laissez-faire falls within the full-range leadership model [21].

Transactional leadership

Transactional leaders are those who set objectives and promote compliance through reward and punishment. Exhibiting transactional leadership means that followers agree with, accept, or comply with the leader in exchange for praise, rewards or the avoidance of disciplinary action. The transactional leadership approach inhibits creativity and can adversely affect job satisfaction [22].

With reference to elite soccer specifically, transactional leadership refers to a manager's ability to motivate the staff and players through offering rewards for achieving set goals (think financial, status, trophies etc.). These leaders tend to be more reactive in nature and are goal focused. They tend to stay within the organisation's existing culture rather than try to change it for the better. In contrast, transformational leadership applies to managers who align their followers towards a common vision. These leaders are generally charismatic and motivate their subordinated through enthusiasm for the task at hand. They are seen as trendsetters, not afraid to change the status quo in the organisation to affect positive change and create new innovative ways of overcoming problems.

Transformational leadership

Transformational leadership is a follower-centred approach that requires the leaders to move their followers to support a future-oriented vision that goes well beyond their immediate self-interest. Transformational leaders raise the level of importance of goal setting and encourage subordinates to transcend self-interest to motivate people beyond their expectations [23]. They consider their relationship with followers a high priority and offer individualised consideration in meeting their requirements for empowerment, personal growth, and achievement (Figure 11.6).

Studies on transformational leadership have primarily involved a business, industry, or military setting, with very few being conducted in elite sport. The

Skill Set of Transformational Leaders	Behaviours Towards Followers
Creativity	Leaders to concern creativity & innovation among the followers
Visionary	Leaders provide their followers with a clear vision and mission
Team orientated	Leaders increasing awareness about teamwork
Teaching	Influence people in the process of change to teach, direct and correct them
Attention to followers	Leaders pay special attention to each individual followers needs
Motivator	Motivate followers to perform beyond the expectation
Recognition	Followers are praised by leaders

Figure 11.6 Skill set of transformational leaders (Adapted from Bass [24]).

limited studies that have been performed in the sport setting have primarily focused on collegiate athletes and the relationships between the athlete and coach or the athlete's perception of the coach's behaviour [25, 26]. Much of this literature is unanimous in the findings that a transformational style of leadership has a positive effect on the athlete's satisfaction and can increase the athlete's commitment to the overall objective. Although the sports industry provides an ideal environment to study leadership, research suggests there is no one-size-fits-all approach [27]. Leaders are not necessarily more effective because they have a gold standard set of behaviours. Instead, leaders who can apply various leadership styles in different ways for different purposes are more likely to achieve expertise [28].

Authoritarian leadership

Authoritarian leadership refers to a sole-leader within an organisation. This leadership style revolves around the Manager making all the decisions and telling his staff and players what to do. Transferring information (game model, style of play, tactical setup, etc.) is one directional. The authoritarian leader is generally task-driven but can also make decisions based on their emotional state.

Democratic leadership

In contrast to an authoritarian leadership style, democratic leadership is applied to managers who are also task-driven but allows their staff and players to interact and contribute towards the decision-making process. Teaching and learning is a two-way street with these managers and they operate with empathy, support, and robust personal relationships with staff and players alike.

Other leadership styles

Laissez-faire leaders demonstrate limited participation in organisational matters and are reluctant to offer advice and solutions to critical issues [29]. They place little importance on the completion of duties and productivity. This lack of involvement is a fundamental characteristic of laissez-faire leadership, and this style often leads to frustration and demotivation from their workers. Laissez-faire behavioural traits show little care for followers' actions and the impact they have on organisational outcomes. Therefore, for the above-mentioned reason, is has been suggested that the laissez-faire approach should not be considered as a leadership style [30].

Whilst these leadership styles have some common trends, they can vary in their approach to managing the individuals within the team. Managers, coaches, and practitioners need to develop their own leadership strategy by using these leadership styles to enhance their team and staff's performance. Understanding the variances within these styles will ultimately determine how well they can motivate their staff and players towards the club's vision and mission.

Leadership and coaching

While coaching most notably requires the teaching of sport-specific skills, coach leadership also entails the ability of the coach to establish and maintain positive interpersonal relationships. Specifically, all practitioners and coaches working directly with players, require more than just technical and tactical knowledge. Coach leadership in the elite soccer environment involves understanding the direction of the team and providing the resources and support to help it get there. Establishing a clear vision has been shown to inspire individuals towards performances targets that lead to positive athlete outcomes such as the perception of leadership effectiveness and athlete satisfaction [31, 32]. However, as previously mentioned, due to the insecure nature of soccer management, it is unlikely that managers, performance directors and other leadership roles, will be given significant time to implement their vision. It is important, therefore, that the leaders in soccer have the necessary communication skills to ensure they can get athletes to 'buy in' to the vision as soon as possible. Leaders in elite soccer must also develop role awareness, express expectations of excellence and promote collective input from their players.

Effective communication and feedback are also viewed as key determinants of effective leadership behaviours of coaches and practitioners. Without the ability to communicate, coaches, practitioners and other leaders will not be able to articulate their vision of the organisation or explain the roles and responsibilities of the athletes. However, the ability of the manager to effectively communicate is not limited to just the players. It has been highlighted that due to the evolving structures within professional soccer clubs, a manager's ability to demonstrate effective management off the pitch is becoming increasingly important [33]. Furthermore, it has been suggested that managers should adopt a dynamic, flexible leadership approach that interacts with not just the playing staff but also board members, stakeholders and supporters [34].

Additionally, suggestion has been made that athletes and coaches/practitioners working at an elite level should be encouraged to develop close and supportive relationships between them to protect themselves during the challenging periods of the season [35]. Loss of form, injury, and deselection will mean difficult decisions for the manager, and they may have to rely on the strength of the coach–athlete relationship to see them through the challenging periods of the season.

The role of the performance director

As mentioned in Chapter 1, the performance director is often the spokesperson for the performance and medical departments. Therefore, a large amount of stress is often associated with this position. Although there are numerous routes into becoming a performance director, it seems leadership qualities are the main qualification. However, a lot of other attributes are considered essential when succeeding as a performance director in the elite soccer environment. Specifically, a successful performance director exhibits not only appropriate leadership styles but also communication skills, the ability to adapt, and emotional intelligence.

Creating a high-performance culture

An integral leadership dimension highlighted is the importance of creating a high-performance culture with a particular focus on getting players and staff to buy-in to what they described as 'good habits'. Promoting a professional approach to training, lifestyle, and nutrition are examples of leadership behaviours aimed at inspiring, developing, and supporting players to reach their full potential.

The timing of when a performance director chooses to outline their expectations and standards is equally important. The first week in leading a new performance department is a key window of opportunity to set out standards and outline expectations. Failing to clarify expectations from the start of one's tenure creates a very difficult task to implement them at a later date.

A high-performance environment involves one where there is an emphasis on individual player development. A player-centred approach is a key leadership responsibility performance department, but something that probably is not prioritised enough. Practitioners who place priority on player development are able to build relationships, provide personalised feedback and develop trust between players and staff.

Role modelling

Often undervalued, there should be a high emphasis on the roles and responsibilities of the support staff when it comes to setting examples to the players. All agreed that coaching, medical, performance, and other support staff play an equally important role when it comes to leading from the front and must also adhere to the high standards set out by the manager/upper management. Team organisation, players knowing their on-pitch roles and responsibilities, game preparation, and off-pitch behaviours are often the responsibility of the support staff and are equally important when attempting to create a high-performance culture.

Adaptability and emotional intelligence

Like many high-performing environments, elite soccer poses high degrees of uncertainty. That is, at times it presents unpredictable circumstances, new/emerging information, rapid changes in people or plans and reactive responses, all of which can be overwhelming and challenging for those operating within such environments [36]. In order respond to the ever-changing landscape of such high performing environments, being adaptable has been strongly advocated as the key to thriving and gaining multiple performance advantages. Adaptation is an ongoing process that reflects our capacities to act and react effectively to stimuli we perceive as significant to ourselves and others [37]. In order to adapt, one needs to be able to step into different ways of thinking and different ways of doing according to their situation. A level of tolerance needs to be displayed to think and do things differently to how we might instinctively/ naturally choose to. There may be times we need to act fast, take our time and gather more information, support or involve others. Refining or reinventing our responses to the present situation, we find ourselves in helps to enhance our effectiveness and ultimately our performances [36]. Conversely, the opposite to this would be fixing ourselves to a preferred way of doing things, or our natural preferences, regardless of the contextual demands. Being adaptable involves recognising when our natural preferences and biases may not result in us achieving a goal, with such insight presenting a choice for us to be able to tap into different behaviours and mindsets that would be more helpful to us in any given moment. Being adaptable allow us to respond effectively to new dynamics, cultures, people, social groups, and physical environments within our organisations. Possessing characteristics such as being agile, flexible, and versatile facilitates our adaptability bringing benefits to our own performances and others we work with.

It is also useful to recognise that our adaptation can be both slow and fast processes [38]. Fast adaptation processes target aspects that require immediate responses, including when we have to regulate our emotions [39]. Slow adaptation processes involve ongoing adaptation to long-term demands, for example, developing our technical and personal competencies [40]. Thinking about adaptability as a dual temporal approach (fast and slow) in pursuit of our goals, where we strive to use personal thoughts and emotional resources to achieve an adaptation state, positions it as a function of the difference between how we perceive the environment/task (e.g. challenging and threatening) and, in turn, how we perceive our ability/capacity (i.e. self- efficacy) to interact and cope with such demands. From a performance standpoint, the important thing to note about adaptability is that it is something we can learn, develop, and grow.

> It is not the most intellectual of the species that survives; it is not the strongest that survives; but the species that survives is the one that is able to **adapt to and to adjust best to the changing environment in which it finds itself.**
> – Leon C Megginson [41]

In some situations, being adaptable to one's environment could be the most important factor that determines how successful one will be, and perhaps how long his/her tenure will last within an organisation. Adapting to any new cultural environment can be very challenging. In elite soccer organisations today, there are two main models employed in establishing a culture:

- Coach-driven model
- Club/Organisation-driven model

Coach-driven model

When implementing a coach-driven model, the culture and system of play are directed by the head coach. In this situation, the head coach is responsible for guiding the team's approach based on their personal philosophy. Oftentimes, they are also afforded the opportunity to bring multiple members of his/her staff as part of the deal. With this approach, coaches are detail-oriented and appointed based on their philosophy being aligned with the direction of the club. Ideally, the coach needs to receive support from management and achieve commendable levels of success. If a practitioner finds themselves being incorporated into a new coach's culture, they must be prepared to adapt to the new style. For instance, a sport scientist who spent most of their time analysing data for the previous coach could be expected to spend more time on the field as a fitness coach for the new coach. In this case, the sport scientist needs to be flexible and adaptable to the needs of the new head coach while providing quality care for the players for the overall success of the team. Without consistent support from management, coaches who made progress in the early years of their tenure may fail to sustain progress, resulting in the end of the coach's tenure at that club. An increase in coaching turnover may be more prevalent with a coach-driven model when organisations fail to realise the continued need to constantly adapt and build on prior improvements.

It is also essential for the performance team to recognise that they may have to adapt to various coaching models during their time at a club. Regardless of the model, the role of any practitioner is to understand the physical demands of the style of play and implement a programme to help players achieve the desired physical profiles. For all practitioners, there will be that first job and that first time you get promoted or get a job with a professional sports team where the stakes can be higher. Having experience as a licensed coach in the sport you are working in will make it easier to adapt and present the information to the coaches. Specifically, greater adherence is achieved with coaches who may not understand or agree with how much influence training data has on training sessions. Also, as professional sports technology continues to advance, whether it is GPS, HRV, AMS etc., teams will need to adjust and evolve along with these enhancements. Therefore, the 'buy in' is essential for all to ultimately succeed in an environment that is becoming increasingly more competitive. The data available to clubs increases daily, so as a sport scientist or member of a performance team, it is important to differentiate between noise and reliable information, and equally important to find the best way to present the data to the coaching staff. Ultimately, building relationships is an important factor in being successful and data can help practitioners build relationships with coaches and players, if presented effectively.

One component that has remained consistent for performance staff members over the years is the number of hours required to do the job well. Normally, the performance staff is first in and last out, analysing every piece of data possible that can help make a difference to the team's performance. Most coaches will notice and respect the amount of time and effort that the various practitioners devote to their jobs. As a result, they are often more receptive to conversations regarding adjusting training loads or incorporating specific drills. Although many coaches understand the importance of sport science and strength and conditioning, some remain reluctant to alter the training methods they are familiar with, which is why it is vital to help them adapt for the organisation to continue to develop in the best way possible. Another situation that requires practitioners to adapt is when an agreed upon methodology is discarded by coaches because results are not favourable. Being able to adapt to the current environment while remaining supportive can help the team eventually transition back to the methodology all involved agreed upon was right for the team in question.

A major drawback of this system is that once the coach departs, his entire staff usually goes with him, leaving the club back to square one once again. In addition, the average tenure for a head coach/manager is two to three years, which can make it difficult to truly change a club's culture. As a result, performance coaches, sport scientists, strength and conditioning coaches and medical staff may find themselves having to adapt to a variety of different coaches/cultures during their time at a club.

However, it is becoming more evident in organisations today that head coaches will not always be able to bring an entire staff with them to a new club. As a result, coaches will need to possess more of the softer skills to create the type of culture they want with staff members that worked with previous coaches.

Club-driven model

A different approach is to have a *club*-driven model/culture where the values and methodology are set by the club's management personnel. In the club model, standard operating procedures and expectations are made clear and followed by everyone involved; the coach is hired based on the assumption that their philosophies are in line with the existing culture of that team.

The best example of a successful team model is the New Zealand All Blacks Rugby team. As the most successful sports team in history, New Zealand's All Blacks Rugby team epitomises the team model approach. Their credence of 'No Dickheads' keeps the team from being seduced by highly talented divas that will not fit in with their non-negotiable principle of 'Whanau' which translates to 'our family, our friends, our tribe' [42]. The All Blacks team culture is unique and based strongly on New Zealand's heritage. Every individual connected to the team understands they are responsible for passing on the legacy to those who will come after them.

It is a powerful message for all coaches and practitioners that whenever you depart a team or organisation, the positive impact made should be truly evident. Strong cultures that exist such as the All Blacks are the result of all parties involved adapting behaviours to ensure the success of the team.

Regardless of whether an organisation follows either one of the two models outlined, one thing is for sure – a culture exists in all teams/companies/organisations. Whatever culture exists will have a major impact on whether the organisation is consistently successful or not. In addition, an individual's ability to adapt to that culture will determine how effectively they can influence outcomes.

Emotional intelligence

Emotional intelligence, or EQ, has previously been identified at the ability to perceive, monitor, employ, and manage emotions within oneself and in others

[43]. A similar definition for EQ was listed as the capacity to be aware of, control, and express one's emotions, and to handle interpersonal relationships judiciously and empathetically [44].

Some of the most important qualities an individual can possess in an organisation is the ability to be flexible, resilient, and humble. Improving adaptability has also been regarded as a critical emotional intelligence competency [45]. Adapting quickly to change often presents performance advantages both personally and professionally. Building momentum and psychological energy for oneself and others, making intentional choices, not just to embrace change but also to positively propel it forward are strategies that help build our adaptability and emotional intelligence capacities.

As emotional intelligence is increased, an individual's experience of work, life, and relationships are shifted [46]. A key emotional intelligence capability is being able to understand the link between our interpretation of an event and our responses to it, enabling us to choose an alternative way to feel. Achieving this facilitates higher levels of motivation and our ability to overcome setbacks and perform at our best.

EQ has been noted to be more important than intelligence quotient or IQ [47, 48]. Specifically, it has been suggested that IQ contributes 20 per cent towards life success and that the remaining 80 per cent of life success may be attributable to emotional intelligence [49]. Therefore, improving one's EQ is vital for performance as it can make individuals more productive and help build more effective relationships with the coaching staff and other co-workers in the workplace. Coleman lists the following five key elements for developing greater EQ [48, 50, 51]:

1. Self-awareness
2. Self-regulation
3. Motivation
4. Empathy
5. Social skills

Players as stakeholders

A stakeholder is someone who interacts with an organisation in the cocreation of value or experience. In this case, a soccer player interacts with the staff, players, and officials of a soccer organisation to create the soccer product that is sold in the experience economy. Players are considered internal stakeholders whilst fans would be considered external stakeholders. Players and staff would be presumed to share similar objectives with the organisation and would therefore be considered high interest stakeholders. The extent to their power within an organisation can be measured by how involved they are in decisions within the group and by how their needs are met by the leadership group. As the players are vital to the survival of the business, they should be considered primary stakeholders with high power and high interest.

The power of influence that each player has as a distinct stakeholder in the high-performance culture being created must be considered. In return, they will consider the urgency of the practitioner's request dependent on the legitimacy of the relationship shared. This symbiotic relationship must be built slowly and with care. When analysing players as stakeholders, one must consider their level of interest and assigned informal or formal power within the group, team, and club. Careful consideration of their needs and the style of communication should be considered. Communication can be formal or informal, frequent or need to know and be personal, face to face or through message. The engagement strategy can be ad hoc or structured with a frequency dependent on the urgency or significance of the relationship. The commitment level of the player should be noted as being committed compliant or resistant.

For a club culture to be embedded more efficiently, it is advisable to understand the different groups, positions, needs and demands of the various groups within it. To do this, the leadership personnel should strategically map these groups according to how they behave in different environments. The club-leadership should then plan accordingly on how they will manage each group once the stakeholder identification has taken place.

Generally, within an elite soccer club, certain groups of players will feel their needs are being met by the leadership. Whilst others may not be happy with current circumstances (Table 11.1).

Leadership must meet the needs, desires, objectives, and demands of the stakeholders and provide the economic resources to fuse internal and external motivation that will enhance their commitment to the goals of the organisation.

By managing stakeholder relations, the club is aiming to maximum return on their investment by gaining discretionary effort and, at worst, compliance from its employees. By removing any resistance or conflict via skilled stakeholder management, the leadership is pre-empting any derailment that might prevent the various groups from reaching their aligned objectives.

Table 11.1 Grouping of soccer players, categorised by their current satisfaction with environment

Being met	Not happy
Leadership group	End of contract
Starting 11	Loan player
Long term rehabber	Squad player
Youth player	Bomb squad

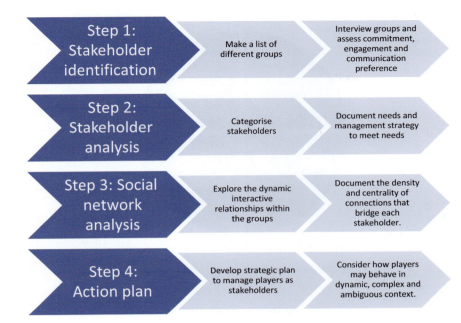

Figure 11.7 Mapping the stakeholders within an elite soccer environment.

Given the intergroup relations of a soccer club, it is wise to identify the power dynamics within each group and use tactics of influence accordingly. Understanding the legitimacy of the demands placed upon the group and the urgency of the request will allow skilled leadership to create a committed group of stakeholders that have an aligned vision of success for the club (Figure 11.7).

Understanding power and interest

The High-Power High Interest group within a playing group includes the leadership group, captains and starting 11 (Figure 11.8). This group is considered the key stakeholders and should be managed closely with personalised briefings and be kept up to date with pressing issues that affect the group. The High-Power Low Interest group should be kept satisfied to maintain their commitment to team objectives. Using existing meetings and briefings to include them in discussions will meet their needs and demands and prevent any resistance developing that could derail the group. Understanding the position of the Low-Power Low Interest group and being alert to any information that comes from them is a secure way to monitor their involvement in team affairs. Assigning a named person to monitor this group is important for team morale. It is essential the Low-Power High Interest group is kept informed of what is happening as this group is engaged and committed to the success of the group, team, and

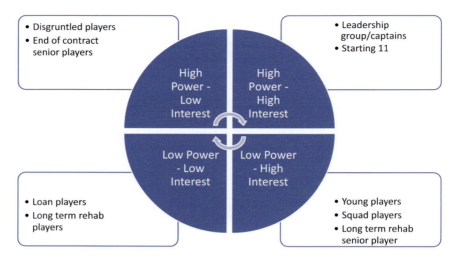

Figure 11.8 Categorising the power/interest relationships with players in elite soccer.

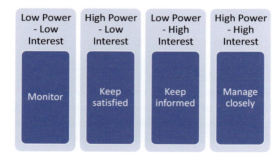

Figure 11.9 Actions to be taken as a practitioner/leader in relation to the power/interest relationship.

club and will develop more influence as the structure around the team develops (Figure 11.9). They should be given low risk tasks that allow their leadership potential to grow.

The science of influence

Understanding the science of influence is the key to building powerful committed relationships with players. Influence sits centrally in two renowned theories exploring power [52–54]. Both explore how various strengths in social settings effect followers, positively and negatively, and have become important in how individuals approach their roles as a colleague, teammates, followers, mentors, leader and importantly when leading their own context.

Influence tactics

Hard tactics include requests, legitimisation, and building coalition. Softer tactics that are more focused on getting what the other want. These tactics include rational persuasion, socialising, exchange, personal appeal, consultation, and inspirational appeals (Figure 11.10). Hard tactics are usually used by leaders who have been assigned a formal power of legitimate authority within a team. They are direct, commanding, consensus orientated, rule-based, and often hierarchical. Soft tactics on the other hand are more focused on the follower than the leader and are a source of motivation that aids task acceptance. They can be logical or emotional and focus on the strength of the relationship between the two parties. A transactional approach to aid reciprocity or consultation to reach an acceptable solution is both soft tactics that seek a give and take win–win for all stakeholders. Fusing all soft tactics with shared values and perspectives will aid the influence of inspirational appeals

Applying the appropriate influence approach

COMMITTED

When an individual stakeholder is enthusiastic about their role, and aligned on values and purpose, they are willing to go above and beyond the remit of their role in the club. This internal motivation will power the individual to carry out most requests even when met by resistance, setbacks or persistent challenges. Stakeholders who believe their counterparty to be inspirational will create a powerful relationship built on trust.

COMPLIANT

Hard leadership approaches – requesting, coalition or legitimating – have been found to create action but little enthusiasm amongst a group. This apathy results in little effort and the possibility of reduced task effort when met with resistance or setbacks. Hard influence approaches are suitable when tasks are straightforward and time of the essence.

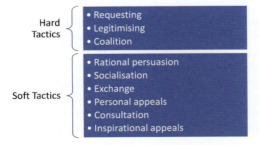

Figure 11.10 Identifying the varieties of hard tactics and soft tactics.

RESISTANT

When a group is resistant to the medium, urgency, style of the message or influence of the messenger, they will try to avoid action and refuse to accept the task, instruction, or message and will seek to derail the instruction.

To avoid this deadlock, leaders should choose inspirational appeal, consultation, personal appeals, and exchange as their tactics.

UNDERSTANDING CONTEXT

The leadership should always consider the situational context before choosing the influence tactic. For quick action on simple tasks, hard influence can be more efficient. Some examples are as follows.

- Routine tasks
- Standard procedures
- Unambiguous directives
- Urgency
- Where the leader has legitimate authority and relevant knowledge

In more dynamic situations, when there is level of complexity and ambiguity, it is important to be purposeful with time, and choose the correct set of softer tactics that will tap into the inner motivations of the stakeholder you wish to influence. Soft approaches are heard to scale, are time consuming, and involve targeted one to ones to gain commitment. For example;

- Organisation wide decisions
- Complex tasks
- Consensus seeking agreements
- Empowerment of low power stakeholder groups
- Gaining commitment to change
- Emotionally charged events
- Developing in-group leaders

Diversity in action

Diversity is more than buzz words on wall or a hiring quota in a strategic document. Teams require diversity of opinion, experience, and people. Recently, there has been a push for intersectionality where race, class, and genders intersect and are afforded equal opportunity. Diversity of opinion requires that everyone within the team has a voice. It is closely related to psychological safety (members of the team should feel safe, have a voice, and be given space to lead) and ensures all levels of the team can participate in the high-performance culture and feel their contribution is valid. A confident and curious leadership team should also make space for individuals who have a diversity of lived experience. These experienced individuals bring a personal knowledge about the world gained through direct, first-hand involvement in everyday events rather than through traditional academic pathways.

To prevent groupthink and aid creativity and innovation, it is essential that there is cognitive diversity amongst the group. As well as helping teams solve problems more quickly and effectively, cognitive diversity also prevents an echo chamber from forming in team discussions. When hiring the team, leadership should project their thoughts to five years in the future to judge what the team will look like if they hire by selecting a 'culture fit' or 'culture add' candidate. A culture-fit strategy favours candidates who match the company's DNA and would fit in well with the team whilst a culture ad model looks for people who value an organisation's standards and culture, but also brings something different that positively contributes and affects change and innovation. When making the right cultural additions, one can create a stronger organisation and shine a light on the blind spots in your high-performance model. Choosing the diverse hire over the safe hire will drive new ideas, creative ways of seeing process and new era of solving problems. Diversity of thought drives innovation.

Diversity in a high-performance team

A high-performance team that is built without diversity runs the risk of myopic group think. Sameness is when the homogeneity of a group leads to conformity and consistency and the individuals resemble each other, share values and are in balance. This can have positives as the power is held centrally amongst the group and dissipated allowing quicker decision-making and less consensus-seeking. Furthermore, this state can also have a positive effect on group dynamics and improve group cohesion. The ability to recognise that everyone is pulling in the same direction may give a competitive advantage and reduce the complications of managing a diverse group.

Diversity training allows a culture of awareness of otherness to develop. This breeds respect and patience and promotes curiosity. Slowing down the speed of decision-making also allows incubation of creativity and innovation and removes common heuristic mistakes and jumping to conclusion. The advantages of diversity are manifold. However, an elite soccer organisation needs to be prepared and patient for the move away from sameness. Cultural differences inside a team and seriously affect cohesion, dynamics, morale, and effectiveness. To enhance the positive effects of diversity, an elite soccer organisation must resource team leaders to engage all staff in diversity training, cultural awareness, and communication development. Leadership must be able to conduct a gap analysis on its supportive measures for managing a diverse team. Being able to diagnose the root cause of issues within a dysfunctional forming team will allow all new team members to feel safe and commit to the challenges of this environment.

Whilst diversity in the workplace should inspire individual thought, teamwork, creativity, and innovation, there can be serious obstacles to working together. Diverse teams find it hard to share information due to ineffective communication. This can lead to confusion, low morale, division, conflict, and decreased efficacy. Something as simple as communication is often overlooked by leadership when adding diversity to the group.

Barriers to communication in a high-performance team

There are several barriers to communication, such as the following:

Direct versus indirect communication

Understanding the cultural interpretation of giving and receiving messages is essential to a diverse team. A simple head nod may be regarding as an acknowledgement or an affirmation. Without seeking clarity that instructions are understood, it is possible for confusion to ensue. Silence may be regarded as respect in some cultures but obstinance in others.

TIP: communication experts verbal-nonverbal

Trouble with accents and fluency

A multicultural high-performance team built up of coaches, players, and staff from a variety of backgrounds creates a melting pot of languages and dialects. Group cohesion is difficult when language forms a barrier to understanding the message on-off the pitch-court. This can lead to frustration, conflict, confusion, and apathy. The team may become less engaged, motivated, independent and the negative affect on performance, culture, and collaboration is easily measured by results. Individuals can feel unnoticed, unappreciated and experts can disengage from the group as they find it difficult to get their message across.

TIP: Language lessons, interpreters, support

Different attitudes toward hierarchy and authority

Understanding the role of the group leader as a representative and advocate is essential in diverse teams. Certain team members will have come from a culture that recognises the hierarchy of mature matriarchal status whilst others have been born into a flat distributive collective. Interpreting the needs and demands of the team will give all groups the autonomy to voice their feelings in the way that feels normal to them.

TIP: Investigate cultural awareness of hierarchy, autonomy, and authority in team members.

Conflicting norms for decision-making

Cultural norms on how information is shared, with whom and what level of consensus is required, will be different amongst all diverse staff members. The level of detail required, and amount of discussion allowed will slow down decision-making but increase inclusiveness and therefore autonomy-agency-engagement

[55]. Taking a first principles approach to how the decision will be made is completely different approach to choosing the best outcome. The different ways of approaching a problem require basic agreement before hand to iron out miscommunication.

TIP: *Create a model-process on how complex and common problems are approached*

Successful approaches to handling the stresses of the diverse team

Adaptation

This requires the leadership to acknowledge the cultural gaps openly and build structures and programmes that allow the team to work around them

Structural intervention

Teams rely on process and relational congruence. Sometimes interpersonal conflict can develop that limits the cohesion of the group. Different techniques include changing the shape or makeup of the team.

Managerial intervention

Strong guidance is required when building a diverse team. Group tasks may be secondary to individual task motivation; therefore, creating an aligned vision is important.

Exit

Sometime removing a team member when other options have failed is required. Prior to that, it is important to seek understanding, mediate any conflict and create other opportunities in the organisation that may remove the obstacles to success.

Leadership must be agile and empathic to understand the needs of its team and the context of any disputes that are derailing the group. Complications that can be met head on with openness, cultural sensitivity and curiosity will give confidence to the group. Having set ground rules, norms and process guidelines for discovery of issues will remove the fear of personal conflict and move towards a collaborative approach to solving problems that are holding back the group.

Practical application of soft skills

Practitioner/coach

Although potentially problematic, a coach wants to do rondos for twenty minutes before the warm-up starts and then gives you ten minutes for a warm-up prior to 11v11 or he/she decides to talk to the team for ten minutes in cold weather following a sprint preparation warm-up etc.; it is still the practitioner's role, difficult as it may be at times, to remain upbeat and enthusiastic in front of the players and staff. Potentially troublesome situations should not be ignored by any means, but emotions should be managed and thoughts should be organised to present a case for why the previously mentioned scenarios may not be in the player's best interest. A stress response by a practitioner, whether it be verbal or purely evident in body language, could be viewed by players that the staff is not unified. If negative situations continue unchecked, something that appears as a small leak to begin with, could over time contribute to a massive problem. Any problematic occurrence should be used as an opportunity to have a private conversation with the coach to work on a solution and decide how to move forward. During conversation, explain in further detail why, possibly, the practices could be planned together in advance with flexibility to address both the technical/tactical needs and the physical performance goals to enhance players' performance. These challenging situations should be seen as an opportunity to adapt to the environment and an opportunity to improve as a practitioner. Another area where it is important to be able to adapt is when dealing with elite athletes.

Practitioner/player

The practitioner–athlete relationship is at the heart of coaching. Coaching is a process and practice within which engagement, interaction and communication between coaches and athletes occur continuously and simultaneously. The combined interactions between practitioners/coaches and players helps define the effectiveness of coaching processes and practices and ultimately the success of the coaching. The coach–athlete relationship is embedded in the dynamic and complex coaching process, providing the means through which both needs of the coaches' and athletes 'needs are expressed and fulfilled [56]. Effective coach–athlete relationships are holistic, placing emphasis on positive growth and development as well as athlete/coach and as a person [57]. Achieving effective relationships requires things like having a degree of empathic understanding; being honest and supportive; displaying levels of acceptance; being responsive, friendly, cooperative, caring, and respective, as well as displaying and offering genuine positive regard [56].

In today's environment, teams are far more diverse than they have ever been. Players and staff come from many different countries, and as a result, hold various values and beliefs. If the club has an established successful culture, the chances of scouting and signing players that fit that model are increased. As a result, the transition for new players should be easier. However, as previously mentioned, not all organisations have established a good culture and many of them operate in a dysfunctional manner. Various practitioners can be the cultural architects for the club. First and foremost, the athlete must understand that he/she is genuinely cared about. In addition, the practitioner's approach must be both professional and consistent every day. As a result, at the very least the athletes will respect the practitioners. Quite often performance coaches do their best work with the players who buy into their programmes. However, frustration can set in when players are not as enthusiastic about the same programmes.

In addition, much like the head coach needs to spend more time talking to the players who are not playing as much to get the most out of them, when needed, performance coaches must find ways to motivate the most reluctant athletes. The performance departments that adapt their programmes to help the less enthusiastic participants are the ones who bring the most value to the players and their clubs. Teams with quality practitioners that can easily adapt usually have a high percentage of their players available on match day over the course of the season. To be the most effective, it is necessary to understand the different methods and cultures that the players have come from, to help them transition to the current programme in the best way possible. It is always important to try to develop relationships and build thrust with the athletes. Performance coaches who cannot foster this environment may in fact add stress to the players, which can contribute to mental fatigue, and possibly, a decrease in performance. For example, practitioners can find themselves in the awkward position of causing tension with coaches and players by dissuading players from performing extra work post training. The concern is due to a potential overload for the player. The player, on the other hand, feels the work is necessary to keep themselves sharp for the upcoming game and the coach will want to facilitate the players wishes.

Managing training loads is obviously an important role for performance coaches/sport scientists but it is equally, if not more, important to work with the athlete to understand what they feel is necessary for them to be mentally and physically ready to perform. The ability to step out of a comfort zone, whether it is communicating with coaches or analysing and adjusting your programme to suit individual players' needs, will ultimately lead to increased productivity and development as a practitioner. These situations are an opportunity to discuss with the player and coach as to how to, collectively, design an appropriate functional training programme to help the player reach their full potential. In Dr Susan David's book, *Emotional Agility*, she discusses the importance of being able to 'move on':

> **Moving On:** Small deliberate tweaks to your mindset, motivation, and habits – in ways that are infused with your values, can make a powerful difference in your life. The idea is to find the balance between challenge and competence, so that you are neither complacent nor overwhelmed. You are excited, enthusiastic, invigorated.
>
> [58]

This principle is applicable in sports, as coaches, players and staff constantly must 'move on' – a game is played, analysed, positives highlighted and mistakes identified that require additional focus. Plans quickly shift to the next opponent in a cyclical process that takes place daily. In clubs with an effective culture, ideally this happens as a group effort with all parties involved. However, in some situations, the process still occurs in silos where most of the discussions are held by technical staff with little or no input from members of other departments, such as the sports science and medical team, who play an integral role in the team's overall performance. It is important to manage any frustrating emotions, and once again, adapt to find ways to help the team.

Practicality of soft skills in elite soccer

Many times, the methods of training executed by the head coach may be different, in terms of how to condition a team, than a performance practitioners' methods. In these situations, it is extremely important to be patient and an active listener (IE exhibit EQ and adaptability). A coach who was brought to a club to implement his model using a performance staff that he inherited may find it difficult at first to trust the expertise of the existing staff at the club. Gaining the coach's trust is key to being an effective member of the team. The time it takes to gain this trust could determine the overall success of the club.

Professional sport is a highly stressful environment and the position that is under the most stress is the head coach/manager. Practitioners need to be aware of this situation and understand that their role is supposed to help reduce the stress for a coach in terms of the amount of energy he/she needs to focus on strength and conditioning/physical performance/sports science/rehab/nutrition, etc. Practitioners may need to adapt their methodology to better serve the team. Practitioners need to learn strategies to be effective in their role in this environment while managing different personalities and sometimes different agendas. It is important to remember: if we looked at the ten best soccer teams from around the world and the ten best performance coaches, no two teams or coaches would use the same exact approach. Some coaches incorporate conditioning through tactical periodisation, made popular by Vitor Frade in Portugal and applied in multiple team sports [59]. The use of small-sided games is another popular conditioning method, while others may like to incorporate more pure running drills to achieve similar levels of fitness [60, 61]. Players also need to maximise their strength and power development. Certain coaches devote more time to strength and power work in the gym, lifting heavier weights to improve performance, whereas others use field-based sessions using lighter weights with circuits and small sided games to achieve their goals.

Regardless of the methodology of the coach, it is the job of the practitioner to find a way to enhance the programme for the players within the current framework. Establishing a cohesive working relationship can be a difficult situation and may require a great deal of patience and finesse. There is no 'best way'. A difference of opinion regarding training methods can cause some friction among coaching and performance staff. However, the coach's job is the most difficult, as he/she must deal with management, staff, players, media, sponsorship, etc. Also, he/she may be in a situation where when he/she looks out on the field, he/she does not see players that reflect the system of play that he wants his teams to play. The coach and management may also be working through an adaptation period as management tries to facilitate the coach by providing the players, he believes he needs to be successful.

Frustrations can lead to contentious and aggravating interactions with upper management about acquiring or selling players. These disappointing situations can arise in teams that have not truly established a cohesive culture. As a result, a team may operate in a roller coaster existence from year to year, as new players are brought in to fill in gaps but are not necessarily the ones the coach may want. A coach may feel pressured to make a deal because it is just a matter of who is available that can make the team better than they were the year before. During these transitional periods, the performance staff must be prepared for various changes or alterations to previous plans that are, at times, a result of a coach's frustration at the teams' results and how helpless he/she may feel when it comes to changing player personnel.

A good practitioner will be able to work with players, coaching staff and management to diffuse some of the anxiety in the environment and be a liaison to all parties involved. Younger practitioners can find these situations more challenging as the art of 'reading the room' comes with experience and is difficult to teach in a university setting. However, finessing a difficult conversation can lead to a positive outcome and an opportunity to build a trusting relationship with the parties involved [35].

The big picture

Take advantage of any opportunity given to express your thoughts to try to help educate members of the staff as to why certain methods may or may not be beneficial to the team. Understanding and observing the environment is a key tactic in deciding how to influence the process. Many excellent practitioners have tried to emphasise a particular methodology without first really understanding the Head coach's approach. As mentioned earlier, a coach's tenure at a club can be brief, so it is imperative that the performance staff works quickly to understand the coaches' methods quickly and begins working collectively as soon as possible. A practitioner who is placed in their first performance director role and inherits a staff that operates with an established system can encounter some difficult obstacles to overcome. If the approach is too authoritarian, some of the staff can end up making the transition very difficult and damage performance as a by-product of personality clashes. The total quality management (TQM) business course taught in many universities across the world could be a helpful resource [62]. Sports is a big business and understanding the principles of TQM could help practitioners as they enter new environments or the current environment changes. In a TQM effort, all members of an organisation participate in improving processes, products, services and the culture in which they work [63].

The more individuals understand how important their personal approach is and how they can adapt to their environment, the better the culture of that organisation will be. Ideally, everyone wants to work in a cohesive, collaborative, and trustworthy environment. All involved must put their egos and insecurities aside to work side by side pursuing a common goal. Having all the scientific knowledge may not guarantee success. Being self-aware and possessing the ability to adapt to various environments and personnel will enhance the possibility of having a greater impact on how efficiently one performs their role.

Conclusion

When in a leadership position in an elite soccer organisation, such as a performance director, a lot of intangible skills are required to be successful. The main objective of a leader in a high-performance environment is to create harmony across all personnel in order to achieve the organisation's vision and mission. Various skills such as leadership, conflict resolution, adaptability and emotional intelligence are required to not only get the best from the players, but the staff too. For support staff to be efficient in an elite soccer environment, the performance director can be relied on to bridge the gaps between performance, medical, and technical staffs. Understanding and applying the power of influence, via appropriate tactics, can aid in the process. Creating a healthy, diverse environment allows for best practice within an elite soccer organisation, resulting in high-performance. Whilst acknowledging the barriers and limitations with certain facets, such as communication, leadership, and decision-making, performance directors can build a high-performance environment in an elite soccer organisation with high levels of intangible skills.

References

1 Beckhard, R., *Optimizing team-building efforts.* Journal of Contemporary Business, 1972. **1**(3): p. 23–32.
2 McKeown, G., Essentialism: The disciplined pursuit of less. 2020: Currency.
3 McChrystal, G.S., et al., Team of teams: New rules of engagement for a complex world. 2015: Penguin.
4 Stonehouse, D., *The art and science of delegation.* British Journal of Healthcare Assistants, 2015. **9**(3): p. 150–153.
5 Gilmore, S. and C. Gilson, *Finding form: Elite sports and the business of change.* Journal of Organizational Change Management, 2007. **20**(3): p. 409–428.
6 Zhang, X., et al., *Leaders' behaviors matter: The role of delegation in promoting employees' feedback-seeking behavior.* Frontiers in Psychology, 2017. **8**: p. 920.
7 Deutsch, M., *A theory of co-operation and competition.* Human Relations, 1949. **2**(2): p. 129–152.
8 Hinds, P.J. and M. Mortensen, *Understanding conflict in geographically distributed teams: The moderating effects of shared identity, shared context, and spontaneous communication.* Organization Science, 2005. **16**(3): p. 290–307.
9 Tekleab, A.G., N.R. Quigley, and P.E. Tesluk, *A longitudinal study of team conflict, conflict management, cohesion, and team effectiveness.* Group & Organization Management, 2009. **34**(2): p. 170–205.
10 De Wit, F.R., L.L. Greer, and K.A. Jehn, *The paradox of intragroup conflict: A meta-analysis.* Journal of Applied Psychology, 2012. **97**(2): p. 360.
11 Thomas, K.W., *Conflict and conflict management: Reflections and update.* Journal of Organizational Behavior, 1992. **13**(3): p. 265–274.

12 Tjosvold, D., K.S. Law, and H. Sun, *Effectiveness of Chinese teams: The role of conflict types and conflict management approaches.* Management and Organization Review, 2006. **2**(2): p. 231–252.
13 Tjosvold, D., *The conflict-positive organization: It depends upon us.* Journal of Organizational Behavior: The International Journal of Industrial, Occupational and Organizational Psychology and Behavior, 2008. **29**(1): p. 19–28.
14 Ginnett, R.C. and G.J. Curphy, Leadership: Enhancing the lessons of experience. 1999: McGraw-Hill Education.
15 Eagly, A.H., M.C. Johannesen-Schmidt, and M.L. Van Engen, *Transformational, transactional, and laissez-faire leadership styles: A meta-analysis comparing women and men.* Psychological Bulletin, 2003. **129**(4): p. 569.
16 Ertureten, A., Z. Cemalcilar, and Z. Aycan, *The relationship of downward mobbing with leadership style and organizational attitudes.* Journal of Business Ethics, 2013. **116**(1): p. 205–216.
17 Soebbing, B.P., P. Wicker, and D. Weimar, *The impact of leadership changes on expectations of organizational performance.* Journal of Sport Management, 2015. **29**(5): p. 485–497.
18 Berg, M.E. and J.T. Karlsen, *A study of coaching leadership style practice in projects.* Management Research Review, 2016. **39**(9): p. 1122–1142.
19 Peachey, J.W., et al., *Forty years of leadership research in sport management: A review, synthesis, and conceptual framework.* Journal of Sport Management, 2015. **29**(5): p. 570–587.
20 Kim, H.-D. and A.B. Cruz, *The influence of coaches' leadership styles on athletes' satisfaction and team cohesion: A meta-analytic approach.* International Journal of Sports Science & Coaching, 2016. **11**(6): p. 900–909.
21 Avolio, B.J. and B.M. Bass, *Individual consideration viewed at multiple levels of analysis: A multi-level framework for examining the diffusion of transformational leadership.* The Leadership Quarterly, 1995. **6**(2): p. 199–218.
22 Bass, B.M., Leadership and performance beyond expectations. 1985: Collier Macmillan.
23 Yukl, G., *An evaluation of conceptual weaknesses in transformational and charismatic leadership theories.* The Leadership Quarterly, 1999. **10**(2): p. 285–305.
24 Bass, B.M., *Two decades of research and development in transformational leadership.* European Journal of Work and Organizational Psychology, 1999. **8**(1): p. 9–32.
25 Kent, A. and P. Chelladurai, *Perceived transformational leadership, organizational commitment, and citizenship behavior: A case study in intercollegiate athletics.* Journal of Sport Management, 2001. **15**(2): p. 135–159.
26 Horn, T., *Intrinsic motivation: Relationships with collegiate athletes' gender, scholarship status, and perceptions of their coaches' behavior.* Journal of Sport & Exercise Psychology, 2000. **22**(1–4): p. 63–84.
27 Weese, W.J., *A leadership discussion with Dr. Bernard Bass.* Journal of Sport Management, 1994. **8**(3): p. 179–189.
28 Cruickshank, A. and D. Collins, *Authors' reply to Mills and Boardley: 'Advancing leadership in sport: Time to take off the blinkers?'.* Sports Medicine, 2017. **47**(3): p. 571–574.
29 McColl-Kennedy, J.R. and R.D. Anderson, *Subordinate–manager gender combination and perceived leadership style influence on emotions, self-esteem and organizational commitment.* Journal of Business Research, 2005. **58**(2): p. 115–125.
30 Nawaz, Z. and I. Khan, *Leadership theories and styles: A literature review.* Leadership, 2016. **16**(1): p. 1–7.
31 Groves, K.S., *Leader emotional expressivity, visionary leadership, and organizational change.* Leadership & Organization Development Journal, 2006. 27(7): p. 566–583.
32 Fletcher, D. and R. Arnold, *A qualitative study of performance leadership and management in elite sport.* Journal of Applied Sport Psychology, 2011. **23**(2): p. 223–242.

33 Morrow, S. and B. Howieson, *The new business of football: A study of current and aspirant football club managers.* Journal of Sport Management, 2014. **28**(5): p. 515–528.
34 Molan, C., J. Matthews, and R. Arnold, *Leadership off the pitch: The role of the manager in semi-professional football.* European Sport Management Quarterly, 2016. **16**(3): p. 274–291.
35 Davis, L. and S. Jowett, *Coach–athlete attachment and the quality of the coach–athlete relationship: Implications for athlete's well-being.* Journal of Sports Sciences, 2014. **32**(15): p. 1454–1464.
36 Reeves, M. and M. Deimler, *Adaptability: The new competitive advantage* in M. Deimler, R. Lesser, D. Rhodes and J. Sinha (Eds.), Own the Future: 50 Ways to Win from the Boston Consulting Group, Hoboken, NJ: Wiley, 2013. p. 19–26.
37 Webb, T.L., et al., *Effective regulation of affect: An action control perspective on emotion regulation.* European Review of Social Psychology, 2012. **23**(1): p. 143–186.
38 Tenenbaum, G., et al., *Adaptation: A two-perception probabilistic conceptual framework.* Journal of Clinical Sport Psychology, 2015. **9**(1): p. 1–23.
39 Stanley, D.M., et al., *Emotion regulation strategies used in the hour before running.* International Journal of Sport and Exercise Psychology, 2012. **10**(3): p. 159–171.
40 Stambulova, N. *Talent development in sport: Career transitions perspective.* in 2006 International Society of Sport Psychology Managing council Meeting and International Forum of the Psychology of Olympic Excellence, Taipei, Taiwan, October 13–15, 2006. 2006. Society of Sport and Exercise Psychology of Taiwan (SSEPT).
41 Megginson, L.C., *Lessons from Europe for American business.* The Southwestern Social Science Quarterly, 1963. **44**(1): p. 3–13.
42 Kerr, J., Legacy. 2013: Hachette UK.
43 Salovey, P. and J.D. Mayer, *Emotional intelligence.* Imagination, Cognition and Personality, 1990. **9**(3): p. 185–211.
44 Anjum, A. and P. Swathi, *A study on the impact of emotional intelligence on quality of life among secondary school teachers.* International Journal of Psychology and Counseling, 2017. **7**(1): p. 1–13.
45 Cartwright, S. and C. Pappas, *Emotional intelligence, its measurement and implications for the workplace.* International Journal of Management Reviews, 2008. **10**(2): p. 149–171.
46 Birwatkar, V.P., *Emotional intelligence: The invisible phenomenon in sports.* European Journal of Sports and Exercise Science, 2014. **3**(19): p. 31–31.
47 Cherniss, C., et al., Bringing emotional intelligence to the workplace. 1998: Consortium for Research on Emotional Intelligence in Organizations, Rutgers University.
48 Goleman, D., Working with emotional intelligence. 1998: Bantam Books.
49 Goleman, D., Emotional intelligence: Why it can matter more than IQ. London: Bloomsbury. Katyal, S., and Awasthi, E.(2005). Gender differences in emotional intelligence among adolescents of Chandigarh. Journal of Human Ecology, 1995. **17**(2): p. 153–155.
50 Goleman, D., *Leadership that gets results.* Harvard Business Review, 2000. **78**(2): p. 4–17.
51 Goleman, D., Emotional intelligence. 2006: Bantam.
52 Lunenburg, F. C. *Power and leadership: An influence process.* International journal of management, business, and administration, 2012. **15**(1): p. 1–9. 53. French Jr, J. and B. Raven, The bases of social power In D. Cartwright, (Ed.), Studies in Social Power, Ann Arbor, MI: Institute for Social Research, 1959: p. 150–167.
54 Latané, B., *The psychology of social impact.* American Psychologist, 1981. **36**(4): p. 343.
55 Halperin, I., et al., *Autonomy: A missing ingredient of a successful program?* Strength & Conditioning Journal, 2018. **40**(4): p. 18–25.
56 Jowett, S. and I.M. Cockerill, *Olympic medallists' perspective of the althlete–coach relationship.* Psychology of Sport and Exercise, 2003. **4**(4): p. 313–331.

57 Jowett, S. and G.A. Meek, *The coach-athlete relationship in married couples: An exploratory content analysis*. The Sport Psychologist, 2000. **14**(2): p. 157–175.
58 David, S., Emotional agility: Get unstuck, embrace change, and thrive in work and life. 2016: Penguin.
59 de Lima Greboggy, D. and W.R. Silva, *The tactical periodization under the justification of the neurosciences: Habituacion and restructuring of the decision making/A PERIODIZACAO TATICA SOB A JUSTIFICATIVA DAS NEUROCIENCIAS: HABITUACAO E REESTRUTURACAO DAS TOMADAS DE DECISAO*. Revista Brasileira de Futsal e Futebol, 2018. **10**(38): p. 382–390.
60 Bangsbo, J., Aerobic and anaerobic training in soccer: [special emphasis on traning of youth players]. 2007: University of Copenhagen, Inst. of Exercise and Sport Sciences.
61 Verheijen, R., Conditioning for soccer. 1998: Reedswain Inc.
62 Talha, M., *Total quality management (TQM): An overview*. The Bottom Line, 2004. **17**(1): p. 15–19.
63 Baird, K., K.J. Hu, and R. Reeve, *The relationships between organizational culture, total quality management practices and operational performance*. International Journal of Operations & Production Management, 2011. **31**(7): p. 789–814.

Index

Note: **Bold** page numbers refer to tables and *italic* page numbers refer to figures.

absolute thresholds 170–172, **172**
academy environments, staff turnover 16–17
acceleration 38–39
acceleration-based thresholds 172, **172**
accents, in communication 312
ACL injuries see anterior cruciate ligament (ACL) injuries
active recovery 212, 264
Acute:Chronic Workload ratio (ACWR) model 154–156, *155*
acute inflammatory phase: rehabilitation process 236, 236–237; staff integration/continuum 248, *249*
adaptability 301–302; club-driven model 304; coach-driven model 302–304; emotional intelligence 304–305; fast adaptation processes 302; handling stresses of team 313; slow adaptation processes 302
adductor:abductor strength ratios 86
aerobic capacity 111–112
aerobic interval training 132
agility 112, 115, 203
altitude, periodisation 278
Anaerobic Speed Reserve (ASR) 171
anaerobic threshold 111, 112
anterior cruciate ligament (ACL) injuries 223, 230
arbitrary metrics, wearable technology 173
athletes: communication between multidisciplinary team and 204; injury (see injured athlete); performance baselines of 57; see also individual entries
athlete self-reported measures (ASRMs) 147–148, **149**

athlete workload injury cycle *152*, 153
athletic development: modern-day athlete 24–25; 9–12s (foundation phase) 25–27, **26**, **27**; 13–16s (youth development phase) 27–28, *29*; U17+ (perform) 28; U17s (earn the right) 28
authoritarian leadership 299
authority, attitudes toward 312
autonomic nervous system (ANS) 151, 152
availability 84–87; conditioning to maximise 108–109
average acceleration (AvgAcc) 120, 122, 169, 173

balance of friendliness 11
ball-in-play (BiP) time 150
ballistic training 91
Balyi, I. 22
Banister, E.W. 154
Beep tests 57, 70
beta-alanine 201, 202
BFR see blood flow restriction (BFR)
biceps femoris long head (BFLH) 227
bio-banding 49
biological age 46–49, *47*
biological maturation 46–49, *47*, *48*
block periodisation 28
blood flow restriction (BFR) 252
body surface area and body mass (BSA:BM) ratio 209
bodyweight (BW) 34, 37, 39, 194–198, 200, 203
Bomb Squad 294
Buchheit, Martin 75

caffeine 202–203
calf injuries 230; mechanisms of 234

Index

carbohydrates 194–195; game/match day 197–199, *198*; during match-play 199; post-match recovery 199–200; pre-match day *196*, 196–197
certifications 3, 3–4, *4*
Champion Data player ranking system 110
change of direction 40–41
Change of Direction Deficit (CODD) 68
change of direction (COD) qualities 26, **26**
chief executive officer (CEO) 1
chronological age 22, 46–49, *47*, 85
club-appointed role 12
club-driven model 304
CMJ *see* counter movement jump (CMJ)
coach: periodisation 279; soft skills 313–314; stress for 316
coach-appointed role 13
coach–athlete relationship 314
coach-driven model 302–304
coaching staff 58, 59; communication between performance team, leadership, and 85; contemporary issues within 5–6; leadership styles and 300
CODD *see* Change of Direction Deficit (CODD)
cohort/group testing 66–67, *68*, 69–71, *70*
cohort-related benchmarks, tests with 70, *70*
cold conditions, periodisation 278
cold water immersion (CWI) 208; external characteristics 209, **210**, 211; internal characteristics 209; protocol characteristics **208**, 208–209
cold water, recovery modalities 207–208
collagen, injured athlete 206–207
common injuries 223; hamstring muscle injuries 223, 224, *224*, 227; head injuries 231, **232**; knee injuries 230–231; lateral ankle ligament injuries 231; match injuries 223, *225*; muscle injuries 223, 224, 227–230; training injuries 223, *226*
communication: barriers in high-performance team 312–313; between coaching staff, leadership, and high-performance team 85; direct vs. indirect 312; between multidisciplinary team and athletes 204; optimising of 9; power of 15; surviving, industry 19
competitive nature 25
compression garment, recovery modalities 213
conditioning 42, *42*, 135; aerobic capacity 111–112; agility 112; with ball 119, *119*; barriers to 123–126, *124*; drill design 116–123; environment 126; finding sweet-spot 126; head coach's philosophy 125; hybrid approach 113–114, *115*; importance of 108; integrated approach 114, *115*; isolated approach 113, *115*; knowing how hard to train 125; knowing your cohort of players 123–125; to maximise availability 108–109; to optimise performance 109–110, *110*; practical application 127–134; running only prescriptions 117–119, *119*; speed 112; training approaches to 112–114, *115*; type of 110–111, *111*; use of SSG for 119–121, *120*, *121*; warm-up 115–116; without ball 118–119
conflict 295; avoiding 296, *296*; dealing with 295; escalation 296, *297*
congested periods, conditioning during 133–134, **134**
constraints *120*, 120–121, *121*
contemporary issues: within coaching-orientated staff 5–6; current issues with professional soccer players 6–7; limitations with nutritional advice 6; within medical/physio staff 6
content of gym sessions 94, 97
continuous professional development (CPD) 50
contrast water therapy (CWT) 208, 211
controlled sport-specific: rehabilitation process 238, *239*, **240**, 240–241; staff integration/continuum 250, *250*
counter movement jump (CMJ) 87, 145, 146
CPD *see* continuous professional development (CPD)
creatine 201; injured athlete 206–207
CWT *see* contrast water therapy (CWT)

daily obstacles and limitations 8–9; importance of empowerment 10; optimising communication 9; priorities and delegation 10; relationships, balance of friendliness and respect 11
David, Susan: *Emotional Agility* 315
decision-making 96, 148, 149, 248, 311; conflicting norms for 312–313
delegation 10; of task 289, 293–294
democratic leadership 299
development: biological maturation and physical development 46–49, *47, 48*; education 49–51; limitations and challenges 46–52; mobility and stability 32, 32–33; movement competency 33, 33–34, *35*; phases of

21–24; psychological wellbeing and performance mindset 51–52; qualities for 30–32; specialisation model *vs.* late specialisation models of 22, **23**; strength 34
differential-RPE (dRPE) 147
digital natives 25
direct communication 312
diversity 310–311; in high-performance team 311–312
'divide and conquer' principle 294
DLS *see* Dynamic Stress Load (DLS)
drill design 116; common errors with 122, **122**, *123*; peak match intensity and 116–117, *117*; running only conditioning prescriptions 117–119, *119*; use of SSG for conditioning 119–121, *120*, *121*
drills 114; position-specific production drills 280; Y-drill, ways to progress 41, *41*
drop jump (DJ) 145
DSI *see* Dynamic Strength Index (DSI)
Dynamic Strength Index (DSI) 89
Dynamic Stress Load (DLS) 173

eccentric exercises 93–94, 236
eccentric hamstring strength 86
Eccentric Utilization Ratio (EUR) 146
education 49–51
effective coach–athlete relationships 314
effective communication 300
Elite Player Performance Plan (EPPP) framework 21
elite soccer: conflict in 295–297; leadership styles in 297–300; practical application of wearable technology 175–181; practicality in 316–317; recovery in 190–193; self-report measurement 148
elite soccer, coach role in: contemporary issues 5–7; professional soccer structure 1–5
Emotional Agility (David) 315
emotional intelligence (EQ) 304–305
empowerment 10, 297, 298
energy, injured athlete 205
energy system development guide 42, *42*
English Premier League 64, 65, 130, 171, 193
environment: conditioning 126; creation of 46
environmental factors, periodisation 277; altitude 278; coach 279; cold conditions 278; hot conditions 277–278; travel 279
EPPP framework *see* Elite Player Performance Plan (EPPP) framework
EQ *see* emotional intelligence (EQ)

EUR *see* Eccentric Utilization Ratio (EUR)
exercise selection: common exercises used 92–94, **93**; injury prevention exercises 94
exercising HR (HRex) 151, 152
exit, handling stresses of team 313
extensive session, periodisation 261
extensive training days 44
external motivation 306
external training load **142**, 142–143, 166; monitoring of 182
extrinsic motivation 12

fast adaptation processes 302
fat 193, 196, 197, 209
fatigue 143–144, 152, 189, 192
feedback 13, 19, 27, 116, 176, 178, 179, 181, 294, 296, 300
fibre type profiling 85
Fight of Flight Response 190
first team, staff turnover 16
fitness-fatigue continuum 260
fitness, testing for 77–78
5-day 'lead-in' methods 265, **266–269**
5-Day Training Model 43
fixture congestion 94, 96, **97**
fluency, in communication 312
FootEval 77
FOR *see* functional overreaching (FOR)
force plate testing 145–146
force-velocity curve *90*, 90–91; power prescription 91, **92**
foundation phase (9–12s) 25–27, **26**, **27**
4-day 'lead-in' methods 265, 270, 271, *271*
frustrations 299, 312, 315, 317
functional overreaching (FOR) 189, 190

game/match day (MD) nutrition 197–199, *198*
general macronutrient requirements 194; carbohydrates 194–195; fat 196; protein 195, *195*
generation Z 25, 27
global positioning system (GPS) 10, 114, 144, 145, 238, 261; wearable technology 165, 168–169
glucose transporters type 4 (GLUT4) 206
glycogen 197–200
goalkeeper reports, wearable technology 176–178
GPS *see* global positioning system (GPS)
graded exercise testing (GXT) 168
grey zone 130
group cohesion 312

group-style approach 294
gym-based progressions 34, *35*
gym sessions: content of 94, 97; scheduling for seven-day microcycle 94, **95**
gym strength-programme 7

hamstring muscle: risk to 64–65; strength exercises 87
hamstring strain injuries (HSIs) 85, 224, 227, 251; mechanisms of 231–233, **233**, *233*; muscle injuries 224, 227; strength testing 243, *243*
hard leadership approaches 309
hard tactics 309, *309*
head coach: game-model of 123; periodisation 279; philosophy 125
head injuries 231, **232**
heart rate (HR) 146–147, 165, 261; hot conditions, periodisation 277; measures 174–175, **175**; monitoring, wearable technology 167–168; responses 151–152
heart rate recovery (HRR) 151, 152
heart rate thresholds/zones 174, **175**
heart rate variability (HRV) 151, 152, 175
hierarchy, attitudes toward 312
higher purpose, practitioners 11–12
high-intensity interval training (HIIT) 77
'High-Low' loading model 130, 263
high-performance culture 301, 305, 310
high-performance professional soccer 14–15
high-performance team 291; approaches to handle stresses of 313; barriers to communication in 312–313; communication between coaching staff, leadership, and 85; diversity in 311–312
High-Power High Interest group 307, *308*
High-Power Low Interest group 307, *308*
high-speed running (HSR) 166, 244, 265, 270, 272, 276, 280; ACC/DEC *177, 178*; modalities of 280–281, **281**; sprint *177, 178*
hip and groin injuries 229; mechanisms of 234
hip thrusts 93
Hoff test 77
hot conditions, periodisation 277–278
HSIs *see* hamstring strain injuries (HSIs)
HSR *see* high-speed running (HSR)
human physiology: investigation of 57; systematic testing of 57
human thermoregulatory system 277
hybrid conditioning approach 113–114, *115*
hybrid (intensive/extensive) training days 45
hyper personalisation 25

IGT *see* Integrative Governor Theory (IGT)
implicit vs. explicit learning 26, **27**
indirect communication 312
individual testing 68, *68,* 72–73, *73,* **74**
influence tactics 309, *309*
injured athlete 204–205; creatine, omega-3, and collagen 206–207; energy 205; immobilization/atrophy stage 204; protein 205–206; rehabilitation phase 204–205
injuries 83–84; incidence of 227; rates of 86, 89
injury delay period 153, *154*
injury mechanisms 231; calf 234; hamstrings 231–233, **233**, *233*; hip and groin 234; rectus femoris 234
injury prevention: and availability 84–87; exercises 94; programmes 84
injury risk *152,* 152–153, 166, 167; ACWR model 154–156, *155*; training load and 153–154, *154*; training stress balance 154
injury risk tests 57–58, 60, 69, *69,* 71; cohort considerations *70*; individual considerations 73, *73*; positional considerations *71*
InStat Index 110
integrated conditioning approach 114, *115*
integrated training approach 110, *110*
integration, value of 5
Integrative Governor Theory (IGT) 144
intelligence quotient (IQ) 305
intensity: level of 120–121; peak match 116–117, *117*
intensive session, periodisation 261
intensive training days 44
interest, understanding of 307–308, *308*
internal motivation 306, 309
internal training load **142**, 142–143; consequence of 166, *166*
International Olympic Committee 204
international role *13,* 13–14
Interval Shuttle Run Test (ISRT) 70
intramuscular tendon injuries 227–229, *228*
intrinsic motivation 12, 52
IQ *see* intelligence quotient (IQ)
isolated training approach 113, *115*
isometric testing 88, 244
ISRT *see* Interval Shuttle Run Test (ISRT)

joints, mobility vs. stability of 32, 32

key performance indicators (KPIs) 12, 14, 85; application of testing in RTP 244; decision-based RTP model 241, 241; testing in RTP setting 242, 242–243, 243; training and match data as 244, 245, 246, 247
knee injuries 230–231
Krogh, August 57

laissez-faire leadership 299
landing training 38
large-sided games (LSGs) 128
lateral ankle ligament injuries 231
leadership 306; communication between coaching staff, performance team and 85; gap analysis 311; in high-performance environment 318; hiring team 311; understanding context 310
leadership structures, team 290
leadership styles 297–298; authoritarian leadership 299; and coaching 300; democratic leadership 299; laissez-faire leadership 299; transactional leadership 298; transformational leadership 298, 298–299
'lead-in' methods 264; 1-day 272, **273–274**; 2-day 271–272; 4-day 265, 270, 271, 271; 5-day 265, **266–269**; match day (-1) (reactive/preparation session) 270; match day (-2) (moderate area session with speed) 270; match day (-3) (large area session) 270; match day (-4) (tight area session) 270
licensed massage therapist (LMT) 211
ligament injuries 230
linear-based sports 167
LMT see licensed massage therapist (LMT)
load management 86, 139, 144, 148, 151, 154, 156, 244
locomotor demand 144, 146, 151
longitudinal reports, wearable technology 178, 178–179
long-term athletic development (LTAD): initial goal 31; pathway of 21–23; pyramid of 30, 30
Low-Power High Interest group 307, 308
Low-Power Low Interest group 307, 308

LSGs see large-sided games (LSGs)
LTAD pathway see long-term athletic development (LTAD) pathway

magnetic resonance imaging (MRI) 227–228
managerial intervention, handling stresses of team 313
manual massage therapy 211–212
massage therapy 211–212
match day (MD): match nutrition 197–199, 198; 'top up' conditioning 130–131, 131, **132**
match day-1 (MD-1) 194, 196, 197, 272, 275
match day-2 (MD-2) 179, 272, 281; re-group for 133; warm-up on 133
match day-3 (MD-3) 94, 96; two-day split (total body) 97–98; two-day split (upper and lower body) 98
match day-4 (MD-4) 94, 96; two-day split (total body) 97; two-day split (upper and lower body) 98
Match Day +1 (MD+1) 194, 212, 272, 276
Match Day +2 (MD+2): second-day recovery ('re-entry') days 45; testing 242–243
match-minute exposure 85
match nutrition: game/match day (MD) 197–199, 198; during match-play 199; post-match recovery 199–200; pre-match day (MD -1) 196, 196–197
match-play workloads, field-based progressions 244, 245
maturity offset 48, 48
Matveev, L.P. 259
maximal fitness tests 59
maximal oxygen uptake (VO_{2MAX}) 111
maximal strength 59, 66, 88, 90, 91
maximum aerobic speed (MAS) 10, 42, 70–71, 77, 171
Maximum Multistage 20m Shuttle Run Test (MMSRT) 70
maximum velocity (V_{max}) 10, 31, 39–40, 59, 73, 87, 114, 171, 244
MDT see multi-disciplinary team (MDT)
medial collateral ligament (MCL) injuries 230–231
medical assessments, advancement in 58
medical staff 85; contemporary issues within 6
Mendez-Villanueva, Alberto 75
metabolic conditioning 237

328 Index

metabolic power (P$_{MET}$), wearable technology 173–174
metric integration 110
micro-cycle period 108
microcycles: lead-in 264–274; models 262–264; multiple games per week 272, 275–276, **275–276**; perfect training plan 262, **263**; prelude 264; for starters and non-starters 282, **283–285**
microdosing 40
Midweek Recovery 44
mission, of teams 290–291
MMSRT see Maximum Multistage 20m Shuttle Run Test (MMSRT)
mobility 32, 32–33; and stability 32, 32–33
modern-day athlete 24–25
modern-day professional soccer clubs, organogram of 289
modifiable factors, injuries 84, 109
Modified 505 (M505) test 68
monitoring 139–140; approach to problem 140, 140; assessing fatigue 143–144; of external training load 182; injury risk (see injury risk); subjective-objective/ internal-external 141–143, **142**; testing 57–58; training processes 141; understanding physical demands of soccer 144–145
monitoring strategies: heart rate responses 151–152; physical performance analysis 149–151; rate of perceived exertion 146–147; self-report measures of wellbeing 147–149, **149**; use of force plate testing 145–146
monotony 44, 45, 238
most demanding passages of play (MDPP) 242, 245
motivation 12, 51, 75, 146, 295, 309; external 306; extrinsic 12; internal 306, 309; intrinsic 12, 52
movement competency 33, 33–34, 35
movement experience 30, 31, 33
movement selection 34; acceleration 38–39; change of direction 40–41; conditioning 42, 42; maximum velocity 39–40; patterns and examples 34, **36**; periodisation options 36–37; plyometrics 37–38, 38; power 37; prescription options 36–37; ways to progress Y-drill 41, 41
multi-disciplinary team (MDT) 5, 8, 13, 14, 124, 246; communication between athletes and 204

multiple games per week 272, 275–276, **275–276**
muscle imbalances 84
muscle injuries 223–224; calf injuries 230; common ligament injuries 230; hamstring injuries 224, 227; hip and groin injuries 229; incidence of injury 227; intramuscular tendon 227–229, 228; quadricep injuries 229–230
muscle protein synthesis 205
muscle strength 84, 86

needs analysis 64–65; categories and rationale 65–69
nervous system and role in recovery 190
New Zealand All Blacks Rugby team 304
NFOR see non-functional overreaching (NFOR)
nitrates 203–204
nitric oxide (NO) 203
non acquisition days 133
non-functional overreaching (NFOR) 189, 190
non-linear sprint training 39–40
non-modifiable risk factors 84, 85
non-starting players, planning training for 279–280; high-speed running modalities 280–281, **281**; planning for one game per week 282, **283–285**; planning for two games per week 281
NordBord 71, 244
Nordic hamstring exercise 93, 94
nutrition 189, 193–194, 213; general macronutrient requirements 194–196; match nutrition 196–200; periodisation 261–262; and recovery 191–192
nutritional advice, limitations with 6

'off the ball' exercises 132
Olympic lifting exercises 93
omega-3 fatty acids, injured athlete 206–207
1-day 'lead-in' methods 272, **273–274**
1-RM back squat test 88
one-size-fits-all approach 126, 127
on-field conditioning 43
order of session 45
overloading 153, 190
overreaching 127, 190
overtraining syndrome (OTS) 189, 190

pain free vs. pain threshold rehabilitation 251
'paralysis by analysis' 87

parasympathetic alterations 190
passive recovery 264
PBM see Psychobiological Model of Fatigue (PBM)
peak height velocity (PHV) 22, 23, *48*, 48–49; stages of 24, *24*
peak match intensity 116–117, *117*, 150
peak oxygen uptake (VO$_{2peak}$) 171
peak speed exposure 280
percussion massager 212
performance: barriers to 123–126; measurement of 109
performance-based process 235
performance-based tests 67, *69*; cohort considerations 70; individual considerations 73, *73*; positional considerations *71*
performance department 3, 101; modelling 7–8; practitioners in 8
performance director, role of 300; high-performance culture creation 301; role modelling 301
performance mindset 51–52
performance practitioners 17, 19, 21; holy grail for 126; running only conditioning prescriptions 117–119, *119*
performance staff 59, 60, 113, 303; problems within 6
performance tests 57–58; approach 60–61, *61*; parameters 61–63, *62*; test exercise selection 63–64
periodisation 259, 286; assessing variables 260–261; environmental factors 277–279; intensive and extensive 261; microcycles 262–276; practical application 279–282, **281**, **283–285**; recovery/nutrition 261–262; resistance training 261; visual representation of structure 259, *259*
PHV see peak height velocity (PHV)
physical demands, understanding of 144–145
physical development 46–49, *47*, *48*
physical performance analysis 149–151
physical qualities 21, 24, 30, 31, 33, 36, 42, 52, 65, 69, 83, 88, 116, 128, 270–272, 279
physiological demand 146
physiology, recovery modalities 207–208
physio staff, contemporary issues within 6
planes of motion 31, 34
platelet-rich plasma (PRP) injections 252
player-centred approach 301

PlayerLoad (PL) 173
players: availability of 108–109; durability and resilience of 85; grouping of soccer player 306, **306**; knowing your cohort of 123–125; mapping stakeholders within soccer environment 307, *307*; science of influence 308–310; soft skills 314–316; as stakeholders 305–310; sweet-spot for 126; tracking and monitoring (see monitoring); understanding power and interest 307–308, *308*
player-tracking technology 166
plyometric-based exercises 91
plyometric progression system 37, *38*
plyometrics 37–38, *38*, 93
plyometric training 37, 38, 237
positional testing 66–67, *68*, *71*, 71–72, *72*
position-specific high-speed-running protocol 110, *110*
position-specific production drills 280
post-exercise HRV 175
post-match recovery, nutrition 199–200
power 37, 261; of influence 305–306; understanding of 307–308, *308*
power-based exercises 91
power training 37, 39; content of gym sessions 97; fixture congestion 96, **97**; importance of 83–84; misconceptions of 99; scheduling 94, **95**, 96; two-day split 97–98
practical application, conditioning 127; alternatives for volume 132–133; during congested periods 133–134, **134**; grey zone 130; match day 'top up' 130–131, *131*, **132**; starting point 127–129, **129**
practical application, of soft skills: big picture 317–318; practicality in elite soccer 316–317; practitioner/coach 313–314; practitioner/player 314–316
practical application, of wearable technology 175, *175*; delivering data 176–180; displaying change 179; goalkeeper reports 176–178; longitudinal reports *178*, 178–179; primary barriers of delivery 179–180; reporting 176, *177*
practical application, periodisation 279–282, **281**, **283–285**
practitioner–athlete relationship 314
practitioners 83; fixture congestion 94, 96, **97**; higher purpose 11–12; high-performance management 148;

live tracking for 181; need to learn strategies 316; operating as solo practitioner 7–11; in performance department 8; positive effects production training 281; previous work experience 4, *4*; roles within industry 12–14; soft skills 313–316; strength-testing parameters 88–89; surviving industry 16–19; training-recovery cycle 141; unwritten laws of industry 14–15
pre-match days (MD-1) 45; nutrition *196*, 196–197
pre-match rituals 290
pre-season games-based conditioning programme 128–129, **129**
pre-season testing 58–60, 86
priorities 9, 10, 33, 113, 207, 265
production training 280, *281*, 282
professional soccer: common strength and power tests performed in 87, *88*; players, issues with 6–7; unwritten laws 14–15
professional soccer structure 1; certifications 3, 3–4, *4*; different names/roles/titles 2–3; hierarchy 1, *1*; sport staff 1–2, *2*; value of integration 5
programming 42–43; on-field conditioning 43; training models 43–44; types of training days 44–45
protein 195, *195*; injured athlete 205–206
Psychobiological Model of Fatigue (PBM) 144
psychological safety 291, *291*
psychological wellbeing 51–52

quadriceps: injuries 229–230; strength 86

rate of force development (RFD) 31, 90–92, 146
rate of perceived exertion (RPE) 128, 146–147, 261
reactive speed days 45
reactive strength index (RSI) 146
re-conditioning phase: rehabilitation process 237–238, *238*; staff integration/continuum 249, *250*
recovery 189, 190–191; active/passive 264; nervous system role in 190; nutrition and 191–192; periodisation 261–262; sleep 191; training load and *192*, 192–193
recovery modalities 207, 262; active recovery 212; cold water and physiology 207–208; compression 213; factors affecting cold water immersion methodology 208–211; massage therapy 211–212
rectus femoris, injury mechanisms 234
reductionist management theory 292
regular maximum velocity exposures 31–32
rehabilitation process: acute inflammatory phase *236*, 236–237; controlled sport-specific and RTP phase 238, *239*, **240**, 240–241; designing framework 235–241; key performance indicators (see key performance indicators (KPIs)); phases of 235; re-conditioning phase 237–238, *238*; staff integration/continuum 246, 248–250
rehydration 200
relationships 11; creating and managing 17
relative thresholds 170–171
reliability: of tracking technologies 145; wearable technology 166–169
reporting, wearable technology 176, *177*
resistance training, periodisation 261
respect 11, 36, 46, 51, 99, 198, 241, 295, 296, 303, 311, 312, 314
Rest and Digest Response 190
resting HR (RHR) 151
resting HRV 152, 175
restoration day 264
rest periods 45
return to play (RTP) 227–228, *228*, 253; blood flow restriction in 252; calf injuries 230, 234; hamstring strain injuries 231, 233; key performance indicators, rehabilitation process 241–246; pain free vs. pain threshold rehabilitation 251; phase, rehabilitation process 238, *239*, **240**, 240–241; phase, staff integration/continuum 250, *250*; platelet-rich plasma injections 252; quadricep injuries 229–230; rehabilitation process 235
RFD see rate of force development (RFD)
roles, within industry: club-appointed role 12; coach-appointed role 13; international role *13*, 13–14
rolling-duration method 116, *117*
Romanian/stiff leg deadlift 93, **93**
RPE see rate of perceived exertion (RPE)
RSI see reactive strength index (RSI)
RTP see return to play (RTP)
running: conditioning with ball 119, *119*; conditioning without ball 118–119; variables in 117

scheduling, strength and power training 94, **95**, 96
Schneider, C. 152
science of influence 308; committed 309; compliant 309; influence tactics 309, *309*; resistant 310; understanding context 310
second-day recovery ('re-entry') days (MD+2) 45
second ventilatory threshold (VT$_2$) 171
self-care 17–18, *18*
self-fulfilling prophecy 227
self-report measures, of wellbeing 147–149, **149**
semi-automated video-based tracking technologies 144, 145
sensitivity 62, 62
sensitivity-specificity quadrant 62, *62*
session-RPE (sRPE) 147
shared consciousness 292–293
single leg jumps (SLJ) 145, 146
sleep 191, 213
SLJ see single leg jumps (SLJ)
slow adaptation processes 302
smallest worthwhile change (SWC) 179
small-sided games (SSGs) 112, 128; use for conditioning 119–121, *120, 121*; warm-up for 115–116
soccer: exercise selection in 92–94; physical evolution of 65; strength and power in 83–84; understanding physical demands of 144–145
soccer-specific testing 75–76; testing for fitness 77–78; testing for speed 76; testing for strength 76
soft skills, practical application: big picture 317–318; practicality in elite soccer 316–317; practitioner/coach 313–314; practitioner/player 314–316
soft tactics 309, *309*
soft tissue injuries 152, 236, **236**
solo practitioner, operating as 7; daily obstacles and limitations 8–11; modelling performance department 7–8
specificity 62, *62*, 63
speed 112; testing for 76
speed and acceleration metrics 170; absolute thresholds 171–172, **172**; relative thresholds 170–171
speed endurance (SE) interventions 280
split stance exercises 92
sport-related concussion (SRC) 231
sport science 19; accreditation process for 4; advancement in 58; department 1

sport scientists 1–3, 76, 139, 151, 153, 156, 303, 304, 315
sport staff 1–2, *2*
sprinting 112; type injuries 231, **233**, *233*
squat jump (SJ) 145, 146
SRC see sport-related concussion (SRC)
stability 32, 32–33
staff integration/continuum: acute inflammatory phase 248, *249*; athlete-centred approach 246, *248*; controlled sport-specific and return to play phases 250, *250*; re-conditioning phase 249, *250*; return-to-play continuum 248, *249*
staff turnover 16; academy environments 16–17; first team 16
standard day in-season 8–9
strength 34, 39; assessing 87–89, *88*; importance of 83–84; injury prevention and availability 84–87; testing for 76
strength and conditioning (S&C) practices 83, 84, 87; cultural differences 99–101, *100*; limitations 98–99
strength-power modules 90–92
strength-testing parameters 88–89
strength training 261; content of gym sessions 97; fixture congestion 96, **97**; misconceptions of 99, *100*; scheduling 94, **95**, 96; two-day split 97–98
stretching type injuries 231, **233**, *233*
stretch-shortening cycle (SSC) 37, 237
structural intervention, handling stresses of team 313
subjective-objective/internal-external monitoring 141–143, **142**
super compensation 189, 235
supplements 201; beta-alanine 202; caffeine 202–203; creatine 201; nitrates 203–204
surviving, industry: attributes to survive 17–19; communication 19; continual learning and work ethic 19; creating and managing relationships 17; expectancies and working conditions 18–19; self-care 17–18, *18*; staff turnover 16–17
SWC see smallest worthwhile change (SWC)
switch off 264, **273**

Tactical Periodisation approach 262–263, 265
tailored nutrition strategy 192
task delegation 293–294
TBD see trap bar deadlift (TBD)
team cohesion 10, 295

teams: divide and conquer 294; GRPI model 289, *289*; psychological safety 291, *291*; task delegation 293–294; team of teams 292, 292–293; vision and mission 290–291
technical mastery 40
technical team 289, 290
testing 57; categories with associated influential attributes 66, *66*; cohort 66–67, *68*, 69–71, *70*; for fitness 77–78; individual 68, *68*, 72–73, *73*, **74**; for injury risk 71; performance, monitoring, and injury risk 57–58; performance tests 60–64; positional 66–67, *68*, *71*, 71–72, *72*; pre-season 58–60, 86; for speed 76; for strength 76; types of *69*, 69–74
testing battery 62–63; in elite soccer 72, **74**
tests with-related benchmarks, tests with 72, *72*
30-15 Intermittent Fitness test (30-15$_{IFT}$) 57, 77
time of day 45
total quality management (TQM) 317
TQM see total quality management (TQM)
tracking technologies: injury risk (see injury risk); validity and reliability of 145
training age 46–47, *47*, 49
training days, types of 44–45
training impulse (TRIMP) 168, 174
training load (TL) 153–154, *154*, 165, 168, 315; and recovery *192*, 192–193
training load–recovery relationship 193
training models 43–45
training processes, monitoring of 141
training-recovery cycle 141
training stress balance (TSB) model 154
transactional leadership 298
transformational leadership *298*, 298–299
trap bar deadlift (TBD) 92
travel, periodisation 279
2-day 'lead-in' methods 271–272
two-day split programmes: total body 97–98; upper and lower body 98
2-Game Week 43–44

U17+ (perform) 28
U17s (earn the right) 28
unwritten laws, practitioners 14–15

validity: of tracking technologies 145; wearable technology 166–169
Velocity-Based Training 25
vision, of teams 290–291
Vitamin C 207

warm-up 115; elements of 115–116; on MD-2 133
wearable technology 165–166, *166*; arbitrary metrics 173; average acceleration 173; global positioning system 168–169; heart rate measures 174–175, **175**; heart rate monitoring 167–168; metabolic power 173–174; methodological considerations 181–182; practical application of 175–181; speed and acceleration metrics 170–172; utilising live data 181; validity and reliability 166–169
wellbeing, self-report measures of 147–149, **149**
work economy 111
World Anti-Doping Agency (WADA) 6

Y-drill, ways to progress 41, *41*
young player: components of power training 37; enrolled in (online) educational programmes 50; exposed to higher training loads 191; holistic development of 46; physical development of 46; soccer performance for 30; technical mastery 40; working through exercise progressions 36
youth development phase (13–16s) 27–28, *29*
youth development programme (YDP) 38
Yo-Yo intermittent tests 57, 58, 70, 77

Zdornyj, A.P. 259